Health Services Management

Readings & Commentary

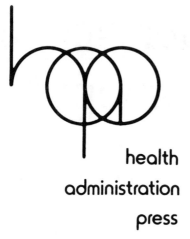

health

administration

press

Health Services Management

Readings & Commentary

Fourth Edition

Edited by
Anthony R. Kovner
Duncan Neuhauser

Health Administration Press
Ann Arbor, Michigan 1990

95 94 93 92 91   5 4 3 2

The editors are grateful to the authors and publishers for their contributions to this book. Because of the variety of sources, references were not changed to a consistent style, but follow the citation style of the book or journal in which they first appeared.

Library of Congress Cataloging-in-Publication Data

Health services management : readings and commentary/edited by
    Anthony R. Kovner, Duncan Neuhauser. — 4th ed.
    p. cm.
    Includes bibliographical references.
    ISBN 0-910701-54-7
    1. Health facilities — Administration. 2. Health
services administration. 3. Hospitals — Administration.
I. Kovner, Anthony R. II. Neuhauser, Duncan.
RA971.H43 1990 362.1′068 — dc20   89-26945 CIP

Health Administration Press
A division of the Foundation of the
  American College of Healthcare Executives
1021 East Huron Street
Ann Arbor, Michigan 48104-9990
(313) 764-1380

Dedicated
to

Anna and Sarah   Ann and Steven

Contents

Preface xi

Introduction xiii

I THE ROLE OF THE MANAGER

Commentary 3

1 The Work of Effective CEOs in Four Large Health
   Organizations
   Anthony R. Kovner 14

2 Industry Distinctiveness: Implications for Strategic
   Management in Health Care Organizations
   Roice D. Luke and James W. Begun 35

3 American College of Healthcare Executives Code of Ethics
   Introduction by *Duncan Neuhauser* 56

4 Viewing the Health Care Manager
   Anthony R. Kovner 71

5 The Proper Way to Live: Remarks on the Teaching of
   Hospital Administration
   John R. Griffith 80

II CONTROL

Commentary 93

6 Controlling Hospital Organizations
   John R. Griffith 102

7 Improving the Effectiveness of Hospital Governing Boards
   Anthony R. Kovner 121

8   Simplified Manual Systems for Clinical Management: The
    Internal Management Report
    *Richard Owens, Patricia Fairchild, Annette Pierce, and
    Ronald Goldberg* 132

9   Control Aspects of Financial Variance Analysis
    Steven A. Finkler 149

10 The Medical Management Analysis System: A Professional
    Liability Warning Mechanism
    Joyce W. Craddick 167

11 The Quality of Medical Care and the 14 Points of
    Edwards Deming
    Duncan Neuhauser 180

           III   ORGANIZATIONAL DESIGN

Commentary 189

12 Foundations of the Hospital Organization
    John R. Griffith 196

13 Vertical Integration and Diversification of Acute Care
    Hospitals: Conceptual Definitions
    Jan P. Clement 224

14 Decentralized Management in a Teaching Hospital
    *Robert M. Heyssel, J. Richard Gainter, Irvin W. Kues,
    Ann A. Jones, and Steven H. Lipstein* 236

15 Technical and Structural Support Systems and Nurse
    Utilization: Systems Model
    Ramesh K. Shukla 246

           IV   PROFESSIONAL INTEGRATION

Commentary 263

16 Justice as a Prelude to Teamwork in Medical Centers
    André L. Delbecq and Sandra L. Gill 270

17 Physician Leadership in Hospital Strategic Decision Making
    Anthony R. Kovner and Martin J. Chin 282

18 Work Satisfaction among Hospital Nurses
    Clifford J. Mottaz 298

19 The Medical Staff of the Future
    Stephen M. Shortell 316

V ADAPTATION

Commentary 347

20 Implementing Change within the Academic Medical Center
    Cecil G. Sheps 359

21 Strategy Making in Health Care Organizations:
    A Framework and Agenda for Research
    *Stephen M. Shortell, Ellen M. Morrison, and
    Shelley Robbins* 369

22 Adapting to the Age of Competition: A Paradigm Shift for
    Voluntary Hospitals
    Tasker K. Robinette 397

23 The Rural Wisconsin Hospital Cooperative: An Evolving
    Systems Model Based on Traditional Community Values
    Tim Size 407

VI ACCOUNTABILITY

Commentary 425

24 The Patient as Partner: A Competitive Strategy in Health
    Care Marketing
    Scott MacStravic 432

25 The Politics behind the Building of a High-Tech, High-Cost
    Medical Center
    Bruce Murphy and John Pawasarat 442

26 Improving the Quality of Work Life in Hospitals:
    A Case Study
    Martin D. Hanlon and Deborah L. Gladstein 464

27 The Dilemma between Competition and Community Service
    Bruce C. Vladeck 480

Annotated Bibliography 491

Index 503

About the Editors 513

Preface

The fourth edition of *Health Services Management: Readings and Commentary* reflects its established reputation and its usefulness in the classroom. In addition, although the organization of the book remains the same, the new material in this edition responds to the continuing and exciting developments in health services management.

Introduction

Anthony R. Kovner
Duncan Neuhauser

In 1978, it was a challenge to find enough good articles to fill the first edition of this book. Since then, however, there has been explosive growth in the health care management literature. We now have authoritative work on a range of topics, reflecting both the growth of the profession and the establishment of health services management as a field of study. Indeed, the field and its accompanying literature have expanded to the point where health services management can be studied from a variety of approaches, including management specialty areas, related social sciences, health care systems and organizations, health professions, and topics and issues. Each approach offers a different perspective, and each one has a substantial body of associated literature. The challenge today is not one of finding *enough* material, but of finding an approach to the literature that allows access to the most useful and relevant information for health care managers.

This book addresses that challenge by using organization theory as its structure to link the specific area of health care with the larger literature on management. The levels of organization diagrammed in Figure 1 provide a framework for our discussion of management in health care. The central focus here is on the role of health services managers—how they try to modify and maintain an organization within contextual limits. The organizations described in the studies that follow provide direct patient care services. These include hospitals, nursing homes, ambulatory care facilities, and health maintenance organizations, among others. We have tried to choose articles related to various types of health organizations.

LEVELS AND ISSUES

There are many different ways of conceptualizing an organization such as a hospital, group practice, or nursing home. One can use an

FIGURE 1

Manager, Organization, and Environment

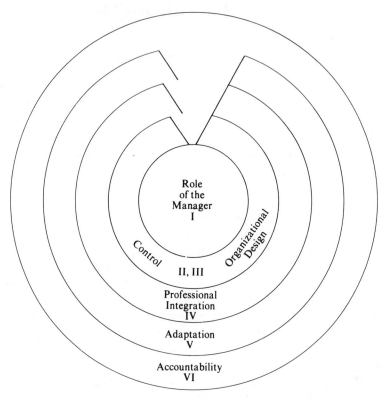

Section of Book	Key Issues	Organizational Space	Some Relevant Academic Disciplines and Schools
I	The role of the manager	The manager	Psychology, decision sciences, ethics, social psychology, organizational behavior
II, III	Control, organizational design	Management, internal organization	Management science, microeconomics, accounting, industrial quality control
IV	Professional integration	Internal organization	Sociology, organization theory, cultural anthropology
V	Adaptation	Organization, environment	Economics, finance, political science
VI	Accountability	Environment, organization	Philosophy, law, history

organization chart, draw sociometric diagrams, indicate the flow of production based on inputs, process, and outputs, write its history, describe its key policies, and so forth. Each of these is appropriate, depending on the questions being asked. We use a different conceptualization.

Here the organization is viewed as a set of concentric rings (Figure 1). At the center is the senior manager and his or her role—the immediate context. At one remove, in the second ring, the manager undertakes to design the structure of his or her organization, to specify procedures, to use resources, and to provide a feedback mechanism to evaluate performance. The third ring (Professional Integration) represents the interaction between management and professional members of the organization, including physicians. The fourth ring (Adaptation) is concerned with how the organization can and must respond to fit its present and future environment. The fifth ring (Accountability) is concerned with how the environment imposes requirements for responsiveness on the organization.[1]

This diagram makes the manager the sun and provides a heliocentric view of the organization. Another diagrammatic perspective might be used if this were a book for patients, doctors, or trustees. We use this conceptualization because our book is written for those who are or who wish to be health services managers. This is not to deny the usefulness of other ways of viewing the organization.

The outline of this book follows the form of Figure 1, starting from the center and moving outward. The sections, described below, focus on key problems and issues at each level in the organization.

Section I, The Role of the Manager, is concerned with the immediate context within which managers work, how they spend their time, the importance of judgment, the kinds of problems by which they are challenged, and the opportunities and constraints they face in implementing change and sustaining the organization.

In large organizations, managers cannot work face-to-face with all employees. Rather, they must specify their activities indirectly, relying on other managers, formal rules, hierarchy, budgets, information systems, and impersonal techniques for control and evaluation. Sections II and III cover Control and Organizational Design. To varying degrees, managers will be successful in structuring and monitoring the organization to achieve their view of organizational purpose.

Similarly, organization members will respond to these efforts in varying degrees with independent actions, resistance, or cooperation. A critical problem is the degree to which professionals, especially physicians, are integrated into the organization. This is addressed in Section IV, Professional Integration.

Management must adapt both to changes in the organization's internal structure and function and to the organization's specific environment, as discussed in Section V, Adaptation. Management must be accountable to the community or publics served, as is indicated in the readings in Section VI, Accountability. These last two sections are concerned with the health services organization's interface with suppliers of needed resources such as manpower, funding, legitimacy, and information.

At the center of the circle, managers are able to influence what happens. Moving toward the periphery, their influence steadily declines and is replaced by other forces. This is shown schematically in Figure 2, where managers' influence flows in diminishing strength from left to right. The influence of others (government, patients, professionals, employees, comanagers, and so on) flows with diminishing strength from right to left. The slope and height of the diagonal line, reflecting the balance of these forces, should be viewed as varying through time and depending on the manager, the organization, and the environment.

Figure 3 presents, in an oversimplified way, examples of issues and problems at various levels of the organization that are within or outside the manager's sphere of influence. A more accurate representation would indicate that each of these issues and problems is more or less influenced by the manager at varying times and to varying degrees in certain types of organizations facing certain types of environments.

Managers have most control over the structure and function of their own office (role of the manager). They can, to a considerable extent, decide how to spend their time, what problems to take on in what order,

FIGURE 2

The Flow of Influence Within a Health Services Organization

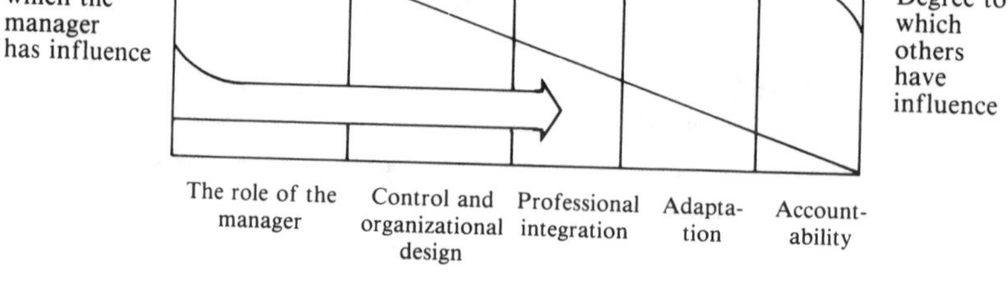

FIGURE 3

Examples of Issues and Problems Associated with Different Levels of the Organization

Degree to which manager can influence activities

I The role of the manager	Leadership style How the manager spends his or her time What the manager does Whom the manager talks to The management team Who they are What they do	Manager's personality and previous experience Limits of the manager's capacity Authority of office Actions of trustees
II,III Control, organizational design	Structure of organization Procedures Resources Information systems Incentive systems Scope of services provided	Resource limits Technological imperatives Information overload Delays, distortions
IV Professional integration	Labor relations Morale Skill mix of staff Personnel policies Level of conflict	Values of staff Historical organizational structure Professional organizations, unions Informal groups
V Adaptation	Community perception Funding Supply of manpower	Social history Competition Government regulations
VI General environment	Health behavior	Socioeconomics Prevalence of illness Value systems

Degree to which
the manager cannot influence activities

who should be on the management team and what they should do, and so forth. However, managers' experience, work background, physical capacity, and personality are to some degree fixed and beyond their ability to change. They also exert some control over the authority of their office and the actions of their comanagers and trustees.

At the next level, managers can impose structure and specify control and information systems, but only within the limits of resource availability and technological imperatives. Information and control systems cannot be complete, exhaustive, or immediate in their effects; they are not error-free and are often costly in money and managerial time.

Managers' design and control efforts will be met with varying degrees of acceptance by workers, professionals, and patients, all of whom sometimes act independently of and are at odds with managers. There is often little managers can do to change the attitudes of doctors, union officials, and patients.

At the environmental level, managers have some modest influence on legislation, regulation, third-party financing, community values, and other organizations' actions. However, much of the specific behavior of groups and organizations in the environment of the organization and most of the general environment is beyond their control or influence.

PERFORMANCE REQUIREMENTS AND ORGANIZATIONAL THEORY

A second way of conceptualizing health services organizations is in terms of general performance requirements, such as goal attainment, system maintenance, adaptive capability, and values integration. The performance of a society, an organization within society, and sub-components of an organization can be judged by these four requirements.[2] The usefulness of this perspective lies in its emphasis upon each of various aspects of the manager's job in organizational terms. System maintenance and values integration have been neglected in the health services management literature, but they are as important for managers as goal attainment and adaptive capability. In organizational terms, system maintenance and values integration represent resource investment, while goal attainment and adaptive capability often involve costly expenditures of funding, managerial time and energy, and organizational legitimacy.

Goal attainment deals with the ability of the organization to achieve its goals as defined by its governing body, often with substantial advice from its top management team. These goals are usually some combination of growth, a high-quality product, profit, and improving the health of a defined population. Goal attainment is sometimes called *effectiveness, outcome, achievement,* or *efficiency.* The extent to which stated goals are attained is a reflection of the accountability of an organization to its governing body. The extent to which the organization's goals are appropriate is a measure of the accountability of the governing body to the interest groups that sustain it.

System maintenance concerns organizational performance in self-renewal. Are the organization's members and suppliers stable over time, or are these relationships in the process of disintegrating? System maintenance includes the degree to which revenues match expenses, new staff match departing staff, obsolescing plant and deteriorating equipment are replaced, and incentive systems are appropriate to the level of effort required. It includes the maintenance of rules, procedures, and information systems. Alternative terms for system maintenance are *integration, structure, stability*, and *homeostasis.*

Adaptive capability involves organizational performance in changing to meet and cope with new conditions. Organizations must be innovative (proactive) and responsive (reactive). One indicator of adaptive capability is the presence or absence of specialized units that are primarily concerned with this function, such as long-range planning groups. Change is necessary for the organization to continue to survive and achieve its goals. Other terms specifying adaptive capability include *change orientation* and *organizational responsiveness.*

Values integration deals with organizational performance relative to congruence of the values of organizational members with the organization's goals and of organizational values with larger societal values — for example, the extent to which management and health services professionals are committed to the ideals of high-quality care, team effort, compassion, and continuing education. To the extent that the values of personnel are consistent with organizational goals, there may be less misuse of organizational resources. To the extent that organizational goals are consistent with societal goals, the organization may find it has higher prestige and access to more resources.[3]

Recently, the concept of "corporate culture" has received a lot of attention. The specific cultures of different organizations have been described, particularly as they relate to goal attainment and innovation. Hospitals and medical centers often have strong cultures built on long histories, religious traditions, and notable individuals. The American Hospital Association's (AHA's) library has collected over 360 published histories of American hospitals, and their collection is far from complete. Some corporate cultures and values are shared by all members. In others, management and workers see the company very differently. This interest in corporate cultures has been fueled by the recognition that management styles differ in Japan, France, Sweden, and Germany, to name a few examples.

If shared values are important, how can leadership reshape corporate culture? How do you change a hospital where the following comment is frequently heard: "Only people who can not get a job anywhere else work here"? How do you create an environment where employees are compelled to make the following remark: "This hospital really appreciates its employees. It's a joy to practice here and I am proud to be here, particularly in this time when so few people are going into nursing and so many doctors are discouraged." Addressing this issue requires an evaluation of employee, management, and organizational expectations and performance.

The four performance requirements or variables outlined above appear in the writings of a number of organization theorists. These writers often use different terms, some of which have differences in nuance and meaning. Table 1 summarizes the concepts of some of these writers. One could spend a lot of time in scholarly comparison of subtle similarities and differences between the concepts of these writers. Such detail is not appropriate here, but some discussion may be useful in relating the subject matter of this text to organizational theory.[4]

Some writers, like Katz and Kahn, make a major distinction between effectiveness and efficiency. They equate efficiency with a narrowly defined degree of goal attainment and effectiveness with the degree to which the organization meets our four performance requirements.[5] Other writers, particularly economists, would consider the goal of long-run rate of return on invested capital as the one organizational end; the other performance requirements would be simply means to that end. The resolution of these two apparently conflicting views lies in part in the concept of long-run return. The efficiency-effectiveness writers consider efficiency as today's efficiency, profitability, or such, while the economic writers consider the whole future stream of return discounted to present value. These ideas are summarized diagrammatically in the first column of Table 1.

Ecology based on Darwinian theory of species survival would equate goal attainment with survival. To turn survival from a life-or-death dichotomy into a continuous variable of the number of species surviving is analogous to the industrial concept of share of the market. In ecology, system management is analogous to the biological concept of homeostasis. Adaptive capability might subsume both adaptation and evolution (analogous to innovation). Ecology does not appear to concern itself with species values. This appears to be distinctive to the observation of human behavior.

A widely used classification of measurement of quality of care in health services includes outcome, process, and structure. Outcome might be related to goal attainment, while process and structure might be

TABLE 1

A Comparison of Some Performance Requirements with Selected General Theories of Organization

Performance Requirements	Efficiency, Effectiveness	Quality of Care	Ecological	Parsons*	Caplow**	Becker and Gordon†	Lawrence and Lorsch‡	Etzioni§	Schein‖	Other
Degree of goal attainment	Efficiency, ends, effectiveness	Outcome	Survival or share of the market	Goal attainment	Achievement	Owner's goals	Performance	—	—	Output, productivity, profit, rate of return
System maintenance	Effectivness, means	Structure and process	Homeostasis	Integration	Stability and integration	Specification of procedures and resources	Differentiation and integration	—	—	Support, control; Responsiveness to environment, development, growth, adjustment
Adaptive capability	Adaptation, innovation	—	Evolution	Adaption	—	—	—	—	Leadership, change	
Values integration		—	—	Latency	Voluntarism	Goal congruence	Employee orientation	Coercive, utilitarian, normative	Culture	Loyalty, commitment, member values

*Nicos Mouzelis, *Organization and Bureaucracy* (Chicago: Aldine, 1971), chapter 7.
**Theodore Caplow, *Principles of Organization* (New York: Harcourt, Brace & World, 1964).
†Selwyn Becker and Gerald Gordon, "An Entrepreneurial Theory of Formal Organization," *Administrative Science Quarterly* 11 (1966): 315–44.
‡Paul Lawrence and Jay Lorsch, *Organizations and Environment* (Cambridge: Harvard University Press, 1972).
§Amitai Etzioni, *A Comparative Analysis of Complex Organizations* (New York: Free Press, 1961).
‖Edgar Schein, *Organizational Culture and Leadership* (San Francisco: Jossey-Bass, 1985).

viewed as measures of system maintenance. This schema does not include the measurement of quality of care associated with adaptive capability. (This might measure the speed at which a hospital undertakes new treatment techniques and, conversely, how quickly it discards outmoded technology.) Nor does the schema consider a quality-of-care measure associated with values. (Such a measure would include characteristics such as professional commitment to the value of excellence of patient care.)

Talcott Parsons' AGIL schema can be matched to the four performance requirements used here. Parsons' terms — goal attainment, integration, adaptation, and latency — are analogous to our goal attainment, system maintenance, adaptive capability, and values integration.

Another typology is Theodore Caplow's SIVA schema: stability, integration, voluntarism, and achievement. Achievement is similar to goal attainment. Stability and integration might be viewed as part of system maintenance, while voluntarism is similar to values integration.

Becker and Gordon's entrepreneurial theory of formal organization has some parallels. They assume legal ownership of a formal organization and an owner's goal. System maintenance might subsume their concepts of specification of procedures that increase information to the owner (visibility of consequences) and procedures that regulate behavior (specification of resources). The issue of values is subsumed in their concept of goal congruence. They go on to predict relationships between these variables and organizational innovation.

Lawrence and Lorsch's conceptualization of organizations is somewhat similar. For them, performance is analogous to goal attainment. Their differentiation and integration are the two key components of system maintenance. They propose that one reason for differentiation is the need for employees to maintain different orientations (similar to values).

Amitai Etzioni has two different works of particular relevance here. In his article "Two Approaches to Organizational Analysis," he argues for the rejection of goal attainment as a useful model for organizational analysis, preferring a systems model. (His goal model parallels the idea of efficiency, while his systems model parallels the idea of effectiveness.) Also relevant is his book *A Comparative Analysis of Complex Organizations*, in which he develops a typology based on three types of organizations: coercive, utilitarian, and normative. In coercive organizations, such as jails, members (inmates) are hostile to organizational goals. In utilitarian organizations, such as businesses, the workers are mostly indifferent to corporate goals. In normative organizations, such as religious groups, members are deeply committed to organizational goals.

Thus, Etzioni's theory is based on member values and is similar to the concept of goal congruence developed by Becker and Gordon.

Schein describes the creation of corporate cultures through leadership. He sees culture (values) as both stable (systems maintenance) and changeable (adaptation). One role of leadership is to shape a culture consistent with goal attainment.

Bolman and Deal present another typology for understanding organization.[6] They see four major theoretical perspectives that apply to understanding organization: rational-structural, human resource, political, and cultural-symbolic. The authors call for a systems theory that integrates these theoretical perspectives. Because these four theories attempt to explain organization, they cut across both levels and performance requirements and could be added as a third dimension to the two-dimensional diagram in Figure 4.

In addition to the terminology of these theorists, a number of other terms are used to describe the four performance requirements: output, profitability, and rate of return are measures of degree of goal attainment; support and control are measures of system maintenance; development, responsiveness to the environment, growth, and adjustment are measures of adaptive capability; and loyalty and commitment are measures of values integration.

Thus the four performance requirements can be used to relate a number of different organization theories and to connect the readings that follow with the larger organizational behavior literature.

The readings in this book are organized along two dimensions: issues

FIGURE 4

Levels and Issues, and Performance Requirements

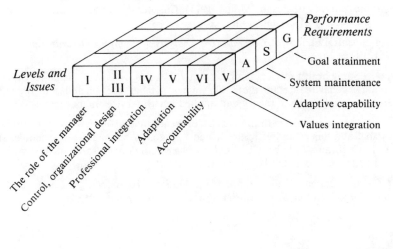

and levels, and performance requirements. The four performance requirements can be related to each of the five issues and levels specified earlier, as shown in Figure 4.

Note that the different performance requirements have varying relevance to different issues and organizational levels. These relationships will be considered in the section commentaries.

USEFULNESS OF THE CONSTRUCTS

We believe there is value in organizing materials around levels and issues of the organization because this is the context in which managers function. Managers typically are responsible for work activities at a given level of the organization and spend most of their time identifying and responding to issues and problems.

We believe there is also value in organizing materials by performance requirements because this can help health services managers and managers-to-be in applying the valuable insights of organizational theory and in understanding theory itself. We make this statement with the full recognition that most organization theorists have not yet been concerned in a meaningful way with the practical applications and significance of theory. We hope that this book may contribute to such a movement.

NOTES

1. The idea for Figure 1 comes from Robert Sutermeister, who put the production workers at the center of his circle. See Robert A. Sutermeister, *People and Productivity*, 2d ed. (New York: McGraw-Hill, 1969).

2. The best description of this can be found in Nicos Mouzelis, *Organization and Bureaucracy* (Chicago: Aldine, 1971), Chapter 7; and his critique of Talcott Parsons' theory of organization.

3. Amitai Etzioni, *A Comparative Analysis of Complex Organizations* (New York: Free Press, 1961).

4. Some health services managers may find this linkage to the larger organizational behavior literature of little interest. It has been included in order to effectively link general theory and applied health services management.

5. More common definitions of effectiveness and efficiency are effectiveness as goal attainment and efficiency as cost of goal attainment. For example, see A. L. Cochrane, *Efficiency and Effectiveness* (London: Oxford University Press and Nuffield Provincial Hospitals Trust, 1972).

6. Lee Bolman and Terrence Deal, *Modern Approaches to Understanding and Managing Organizations* (San Francisco: Jossey-Bass, 1985).

SELECTED BIBLIOGRAPHY

PERFORMANCE REQUIREMENTS

Becker, Selwyn, and Duncan Neuhauser. *Organizational Efficiency.* New York: Elsevier, North Holland, 1975.

Caplow, Theodore. *Principles of Organization.* New York: Harcourt, Brace & World, 1964.

Etzioni, Amitai. *A Comparative Analysis of Complex Organizations.* New York: Free Press, 1961.

____. "Two Approaches to Organizational Analysis: A Critique and a Suggestion." *Administrative Science Quarterly* 5 (September 1960): 257–78.

Jaques, Elliott. *A General Theory of Bureaucracy.* New York: Halsted Press, 1976.

Katz, Daniel, and Robert Kahn. *The Social Psychology of Organizations.* New York: Wiley, 1966.

Kimberly, John, and Robert H. Miles. *The Organizational Life Cycle.* San Francisco: Jossey-Bass, 1980.

Lawrence, Paul, and Jay Lorsch. *Organization and Environment.* Cambridge, MA: Graduate School of Business Administration, Harvard University, 1972.

Mohr, Lawrence B. *Explaining Organizational Behavior.* San Francisco: Jossey-Bass, 1982.

Nystrom, Paul C., and William H. Starbuck. *Handbook of Organizational Design.* 2 vols. New York: Oxford University Press, 1981.

Parsons, Talcott. "Suggestions for a Sociological Approach to the Theory of Organizations." *Administrative Science Quarterly* 1 (June 1956): 63–85, 224–39.

Pfeffer, Jeffrey. *Organizations and Organization Theory.* Boston: Pitman, 1982.

Scott, W. Richard. *Organizations, Rational, Natural and Open Systems.* 2d ed. Englewood Cliffs, NJ: Prentice-Hall, 1987.

SYSTEM MAINTENANCE

Barnard, Chester. *Functions of the Executive.* Cambridge, MA: Harvard University Press, 1964.

Cohodes, Donald, and Brian Kinkead. *Hospital Capital Formation in the 1980s.* Baltimore: Johns Hopkins University Press, 1984.

Galbraith, Jay. *Designing Complex Organizations.* Reading, MA: Addison-Wesley, 1973.

Kilman, Ralph H., Louis R. Pondy, and Dennis P. Slevin. *The Management of Organization Design.* 2 vols. New York: North Holland, 1976.

Kotter, John P. *Power in Management.* New York: Amacom, 1979.

Lipset, Seymour. *Union Democracy*. New York: Doubleday, 1962.

Meyer, Marshall. *Environments and Organizations*. San Francisco: Jossey-Bass, 1978.

Mintzberg, Henry. *The Structuring of Organizations*. Englewood Cliffs, NJ: Prentice-Hall, 1979.

Parsons, Talcott. *Structure and Process in Modern Societies*. Glencoe, IL: Free Press of Glencoe, 1960.

Selznick, Philip. *Leadership in Administration*. Evanston, IL: Row Peterson, 1957.

Tannenbaum, Arnold S. *Control in Organizations*. New York: McGraw-Hill, 1968.

von Bertalanffy, Ludwig. *General System Theory*. New York: Braziller, 1968.

Zald, Mayer. *Power in Organizations*. Nashville, TN: Vanderbilt University Press, 1970.

GOAL ATTAINMENT*

Bass, Bernard M. *Stogdill's Handbook of Leadership*. New York: Free Press, 1981.

Cummings, L. L., and Donald P. Schwab. *Performance in Organizations*. Glenview, IL: Scott, Foresman, 1973.

Dubin, Robert, George C. Holmes, Floyd C. Mann, and Delbert C. Miller. *Leadership and Productivity*. San Francisco: Chandler, 1965.

Ghorpade, Jaisingh. *Assessment of Organizational Effectiveness: Issues, Analysis, Readings*. Pacific Palisades, CA: Goodyear, 1971.

Goodman, Paul S., Johannes M. Pennings, and associates, eds. *New Perspectives on Organizational Effectiveness*. San Francisco: Jossey-Bass, 1979.

Nash, Michael. *Making People Productive*. San Francisco: Jossey-Bass, 1985.

Price, James I. *Organizational Effectiveness: An Inventory of Propositions*. Homewood, IL: Irwin, 1968.

Raia, Anthony. *Managing by Objectives*. Glenview, IL: Scott Foresman, 1974.

Schulberg, Herbert, Alan Sheldon, and Frank Baker. *Program Evaluation in the Health Fields*. New York: Behavioral Publications, 1969.

Sutermeister, Robert A. *People and Productivity*. New York: McGraw-Hill, 1969.

Zammuto, Raymond F. *Assessing Organizational Effectiveness*. Albany, NY: SUNY Press, 1982.

---

*This categorization of references is an oversimplification because many of the references deal with other aspects of organizational behavior as well.

ADAPTIVE CAPABILITY

Argyris, Chris. *Management and Organizational Development*. New York: McGraw-Hill, 1971.

Bennis, Warren. *Changing Organizations*. New York: McGraw-Hill, 1966.

____. *Organizational Development*. Reading, MA: Addison-Wesley, 1969.

Burns, Tom, and G. M. Stalker. *The Management of Innovation*. London: Tavistock, 1961.

Daft, Richard, and Selwyn Becker. *Innovation in Organizations*. New York: Elsevier, 1978.

Dalton, Gene. *Organizational Change and Development*. Homewood, IL: Irwin, 1970.

Etzioni, Amitai. *Studies in Social Change*. New York: Holt, Rinehart and Winston, 1966.

Goodman, Paul S., and associates. *Change in Organizations*. San Francisco: Jossey-Bass, 1984.

Guest, Robert. *Organizational Change*. Homewood, IL: Irwin, Dorsey Press, 1962.

Hage, Jerald, and Michael Aiken. *Social Change in Complex Organizations*. New York: Random House, 1970.

Kaufman, Herbert. *The Limits of Organizational Change*. University, AL: University of Alabama Press, 1971.

Lawrence, Paul, and Davis Dyer. *Renewing American Industry*. New York: Free Press, 1983.

Lawrence, Paul, and Jay Lorsch. *Developing Organizations*. Reading, MA: Addison-Wesley, 1969.

Pennings, Johannes M., and associates, eds. *Organizational Strategy and Change*. San Francisco: Jossey-Bass, 1985.

Quest, Robert, Paul Hersey, and Kenneth Blanchard. *Organizational Change Through Effective Leadership*. Englewood Cliffs, NJ: Prentice-Hall, 1977.

Rogers, Everett M. *Diffusion of Innovations*. 3d ed. New York: Free Press, 1983.

VALUES INTEGRATION

Anderson, Odin W. *Health Care: Can There Be Equity?* New York: Wiley, 1972.

Bass, Bernard M. *Leadership and Performance beyond Expectations*. New York: The Free Press, 1985.

Bendix, Reinhard. *Work and Authority in Industry*. New York: Harper & Row, 1956.

Chandler, Alfred, Jr. *The Visible Hand*. Cambridge, MA: Harvard University Press, 1977.

Deal, Terrence E., and Allen A. Kennedy. *Corporate Cultures*. Reading, MA: Addison-Wesley, 1982.

Field, Mark. *Soviet Socialized Medicine*. New York: Free Press, 1967.

Heclo, Hugh. *A Government of Strangers: Executive Politics in Washington*. Washington, D.C.: Brookings Institution, 1977.

Kilmann, Ralph, Mary Saxton, Roy Serpa, and associates, eds. *Gaining Control of the Corporate Culture*. San Francisco: Jossey-Bass, 1985.

Lindblom, Charles E. *Politics and Markets*. New York: Basic Books, 1977.

Ouchi, William G. *Theory Z*. Reading, MA: Addison-Wesley, 1981.

Schein, Edgar. *Organizational Culture and Leadership*. San Francisco: Jossey-Bass, 1985.

Sutton, Francis X., Seymour E. Harris, Carl Kaysen, and James Tobin. *The American Business Creed*. New York: Schocken Books, 1962.

I

The Role
of the
Manager

A leader is best
When people barely know that he exists.
Not so good when people obey and
  acclaim him,
Worst when they despise him.
Fail to honor people,
They fail to honor you;
But of a good leader, who talks little,
When his work is done, his aim fulfilled,
They will say, "We did this ourselves."

—Lao Tzu

ILLUSTRATION I

New York University Medical Center Position Description

POSITION TITLE:	Vice President for Institute of Rehabilitation Medicine	OBJECT CODE: 100 GROUP: E-1, Executive
REPORTS:	Executive Vice President	JOB CODE: 0008

PRIMARY FUNCTION

The Vice President for the Institute of Rehabilitation Medicine shall be the chief administrative officer of the Institute responsible for its patient care services and programs.

DUTIES AND RESPONSIBILITIES

Administers, directs, and coordinates all activities of the hospital to carry out its objectives in provision of health care, furtherance of education and research and participation in community health programs.

Responsible for the operation of the hospital, the application and implementation of established policies and for liaison between the medical staff and the departments of the hospital.

Organizes the functions of the hospital through appropriate departmentalization and delegation of duties. Establishes formal means of accountability from those to whom duties have been assigned.

Prepares reports for and attends Steering Committee meetings regarding the total activities of the hospital as required.

Reviews and acts upon the reports of authorized inspecting agencies. Implements the control and effective utilization of the physical and financial resources of the hospital.

Participates, or is represented in community, state and national hospital associations and professional activities which define the delivery of health care services and aid in short- and long-range planning of health services and facilities.

Commentary

Anthony R. Kovner
Duncan Neuhauser

How does one compare the management of health services organizations with the management of other organizations? Large health services organizations are typically smaller than large businesses, so health services managers are more often generalists than specialists. The goals of health services organizations are often more complex than those of manufacturers of raw materials and finished products, or even of service organizations such as banks and insurance companies. For health services organizations, goals include patient care, research, teaching, and community service, whereas the goal of business organizations is primarily profit, regardless of the function or service performed. Greater complexity of goals implies increased problems in organizational integration and less possibility of hierarchical movement, at least above the level of department head. The health services manager must gain consensus for disparate organizational goals, not merely ensure that workers carry out mandated goals.

Compared to business executives, health services managers typically have less authority over the professionals who work in the organization. Specifically, they have less control over the organizational activities of physicians, who are usually not employees of the organization.

Because of their weaker organizational role, health services managers may be less willing to undertake significant change. They must worry about their own survival as well as about goal attainment. Often they are rewarded not for improving the delivery system or reducing unit costs, but for keeping the medical staff content. The dilemma is this: key internal interest groups neither particularly desire nor see the need for change, yet managers know that those who supply necessary resources are demanding change. Thus health services managers must adapt their organizations to meet the demands of those who provide resources, while placating internal groups.

The health services industry is becoming increasingly goal oriented.

Purchasers of care are demanding lower prospectively set prices, documented and demonstrable quality, and responsive services. At the same time, competition from existing or new organizations is increasing, and health services managers must be concerned with organizational adaptation to these pressures.

Financing is more complex in health services organizations than in other service organizations. Health services managers must understand and be able to manipulate sources of funds. The product of health services organizations is difficult to specify; therefore managers must have patience and perseverance in applying quantitative techniques, which are more relevant to the structure and process than to the outcomes of medical care. Change is often resisted because there is no standardized output by which it can be measured. For example, if managers wish to lower the skill level of the nursing staff or to eliminate health screening tests with low cost-benefit ratios, they require professional legitimization in the face of physician objections that this would lower the quality of care. Sometimes there is no expert consensus concerning the outcomes of many clinical procedures.

Other than financing, there is no organizational factor that is unique to health services. For example, universities often are of similar size, are nonprofit, and produce a service that is difficult to measure. Although the features of health care organizations can be found elsewhere, the combination of such features makes the field unique. If only because the health services sector of the economy is so large (over 10 percent of the gross national product), there is good reason to teach management specifically in terms of health services organizations. Such teaching is more relevant for those seeking jobs in the health services sector and is appropriate so long as it is done within the context of general management.

The role of the health care manager has changed substantially over time. Up to the 1920s the only health care organizations needing management were hospitals, and the typical hospital of those days was as complex as a small nursing home is today. The manager needed to know all the details of hospital work and instruct a largely unskilled work force.

After World War II, there were more skilled department heads—in nursing, social work, medical records, dietetics, engineering, laboratory work, and so on. The manager's role changed to one of creating an organizational climate that would allow these specialists to perform well.

Medicare and Medicaid, introduced in 1965, both reflected and fostered the growing complexity and costs of hospital care. This opened an era of environmental complexity. New organizations appeared, such as health maintenance organizations (HMOs), nursing homes, neighborhood health centers, regulatory agencies, and third parties. Health care management was no longer synonymous with hospital management, and the hospital manager had to adapt to a much more complex environment.[1]

In the 1980s, with the growth in competition and multi-institutional delivery systems, the managerial role changed once again, at an unprecedented rate. Steady-state organizational management was transformed into creative leadership of complex organizational systems.

ORGANIZATIONAL SETTINGS

In analyzing what health services managers do, it is useful to examine their work in different types of organizational settings. Typical organizations include a nonprofit community hospital, a for-profit nursing home, a public teaching hospital, and a for-profit group practice.

Within these organizations, the manager's job can be compared along three dimensions. First, how much discretion or autonomy do managers have within the organization? For example, to what extent do managers determine how they spend their own time? Do they initiate significant work programs or merely react to the initiatives of others? Second, on what tasks and with which groups and programs do managers spend most of their time and energy? Are they primarily involved in generating necessary resources and surveying the environment for changing trends in the availability of resources, or are they primarily technical specialists in financial planning or community relations? Finally, to what extent are managers directly involved in the production process? Do they hold accountable those who coordinate the organization's work processes, or are they merely concerned with maintaining harmony among organization members? The following descriptions of work in such organizations are hypotheses based on work experience, on discussions with other health services managers, and on reviewing the literature.

A NONPROFIT COMMUNITY HOSPITAL

The manager's job will vary significantly depending upon hospital size, complexity, auspices, and environment. One type of hospital is nonprofit, suburban, nonteaching, medium-sized (270 beds), and part of a small, regional, multihospital system of nine hospitals, most of them about the same size. Its technology is of medium complexity (higher than a doctor's office, lower than a university teaching hospital). Much of the hospital was constructed after World War II. It serves a middle- and high-income population. Although it faces little competition from other hospitals, it does face increasing competition from ambulatory care facilities (operated by its own attending physicians) and potential competition from HMOs.

In this hospital there are four or five managers other than department heads and medical officials. There are three levels of management: managers (other titles for managers include president, director, and administrator), associate managers, and assistant managers. The top manager's job involves planning with other hospitals in the system, marketing, development of physician-managers, and identification and control of hospital costs. Top managers have increasing discretion or autonomy in their work as a result of prospective payment and falling inpatient occupancy. The key problems the hospital faces concern retaining market share and developing an integrated care system; therefore, critical tasks involve adaptation to external pressures. Other managers in the community hospital are generalists, but they are increasingly forced to deal with technical matters such as planning, marketing, information systems, and costing and pricing. They receive assistance in those matters from functional specialists at system headquarters.

Entry-level managers in the community hospital are involved as staff on new projects, but they also supervise several departments such as housekeeping, dietary, and maintenance. They may also be involved in assuring compliance with regulations by supervising activities related to hospital accreditation and by preparing disaster plans and drills.

A FOR-PROFIT NURSING HOME

Nursing homes are more homogeneous organizations than hospitals because they are smaller and less complex. One type of nursing home is for-profit, is located in the suburbs, has 50 to 100 beds, but is not part of a chain. The available technology is relatively simple. The nursing home is a nonteaching facility with middle-income patients. Unlike the nonprofit hospital, the nursing home faces a market that is not highly competitive. The manager directs rather than facilitates activities. There is little confusion about ownership, and organizational goals are clearly defined. Physicians are organizationally weak. They do not spend much of their time with their nursing home patients, nor do they derive much of their income from their nursing home practice.

Managers in such facilities have limited discretion because resources are limited. Their critical tasks concern internal operations, on which they spend more time than on relations with external groups. Since revenue is often fixed, a key problem is controlling costs at an acceptable level of quality, not increasing the size of the market or obtaining additional capital or physicians. Managers are generalists who perform directly such technical functions as personnel and purchasing. Since there may only be a single general manager, there is not much opportunity for work specialization. The manager is more concerned with system maintenance than with change. He or she is concerned with maximizing profits consistent with organizational survival and is very concerned with production.

The entry-level manager is the only manager or the manager's chief assistant; typical tasks include dealing with patients and their families, purchasing, personnel, billing, and complying with government rules and regulations. In a chain of nursing homes, many of these specialized activities would be performed centrally.

A PUBLIC TEACHING HOSPITAL

Another type of hospital is governmental, urban, teaching, and large (750 beds). Its technology is highly complex. This particular hospital is new, replacing an older facility, and it is the only facility in its catchment area that serves a low-income population. The hospital does not have a high occupancy rate, as nearby hospitals attract middle- and upper-income patients.

In the public hospital there are 20 managers other than department heads and medical officials. There are four levels of management, and department heads may be required to have a master's degree or comparable proficiency. The top manager's job is primarily external and political, because the hospital is part of a municipal hospital system and is affiliated with a large private medical school whose university hospital is nearby. Typically there is a deputy manager who is in charge of internal operations. Key problems the hospital faces include attracting and retaining professional staff, billing, negotiating reimbursement, and fostering community and minority relations.

The entry-level manager in this hospital typically supervises one department such as central services, is an administrative assistant to an associate director, or is a staff analyst in the financial affairs or personnel department.

FOR-PROFIT GROUP PRACTICE

Another type of health services organization is a group practice that is under for-profit auspices. Professionals own the professional corporation. Located in the suburbs, the group has 15 to 20 physicians and employs about 60 nonprofessionals. Its technology is of medium complexity. The group was established recently, has no teaching affiliation, serves a middle- and upper-income population, and faces competition from other providers. The medical group sees patients primarily on a fee-for-service basis but also on a prepaid basis as part of an independent practice association (IPA).

The tasks of managers in the group practice include planning, negotiating for the group with the IPA plan, influencing decisions made by medical staff, directing nonprofessional activities, and supporting professional activities. Managers have both external and internal responsibilities; they are concerned with relations with other organizations and with routine internal administration. Managers are both generalists and specialists; for example, they may make and implement contracts with the IPA and develop or modify systems for physician reimbursement. Group practice managers may be more concerned with change than with support activities. Because a particular medical group is a new organization, the manager is largely involved in program development. Thus, he or she is more often an initiator of change than a facilitator.

As in the for-profit nursing home, the entry-level manager is often the top manager or chief assistant to the top manager. An entry-level manager in a group practice typically is involved in planning the physical facility, hiring nonprofessionals, planning patient flow and staffing patterns, and establishing a billing and information system.

Although the roles and tasks of health services managers differ in the four types of settings described, many health services managers perform similar roles and tasks across organizations. The work of managers in all fields typically consists of coordinating organizational activities, relating the organization to its environment, and integrating worker behavior so that it reflects adequate identification with and commitment to the organization's goals. Typically, the means that managers use to carry out these functions include meetings, phone calls, memos, and tours or visits. There are many excellent general management texts that cover these typical roles and activities.[2]

THE READINGS

In "The Work of Effective CEOs in Four Large Health Organizations," Kovner describes how four managers cope with episodes of management activity. Building on observations and interviews, Kovner describes how the managers choose episodes and how they decide how much time to devote to each situation.

Luke and Begun explain the distinctive elements of health management, including the market for health care, which is unique in that health care can be a needed service for all persons, irrespective of ability to pay;

the powerful role of clinicians in institutional management; and the cultural commitment to the value of equal access.

The American College of Healthcare Executives has propounded, revised, and updated a code of ethics for health managers for the last 50 years. That statement has been included here as an example of the standards that have guided and influenced health services managers over the years.

In "Viewing the Health Care Manager," Kovner describes the activities, skills, and personal characteristics of the health care manager. Griffith's article, on the other hand, is directed toward teachers of hospital administration rather than toward managers. This article is included because it emphasizes the importance of values as opposed to techniques. Griffith describes the obligations of faculty as leaders, researchers, and teachers. A similar assessment is needed of the obligations of health services managers—to their communities, to their employees, and to themselves.

It is difficult to generalize about the successful manager because requirements vary in different settings, and contrasting styles of management may be equally effective, even in similar settings. Managers say that the support of superiors and subordinates, integrity, persistence, assertiveness, and speaking skills have a strong effect on their performance, and that class ranking and need for power have no significant effect. We suspect that knowledge of the job also has a lot to do with success.

Despite the difficulty of isolating managerial contributions to organizational goals and the failure to make such goals operative, managers find their performance is increasingly being questioned and evaluated by trustees, physicians, regulators, staff, patients, and consumers. Performance requirements are each addressed, directly or indirectly, in the following chapters.

Performance Requirements

The five chapters in this section are discussed below in terms of the four performance requirements. In addition, Table I.1 summarizes the authors' statements.

GOAL ATTAINMENT

Kovner's study of four CEOs focuses on effectiveness and results. These outcomes are not easy to measure because managerial "episodes" are components of longer campaigns. Griffith suggests that successful goal attainment by the hospital is related to community satisfaction with the process

TABLE I.1

Perspectives on Performance Requirements
and the Role of the Manager

Readings	Goal Attainment	System Maintenance	Adaptive Capability	Values Integration
Kovner "Work of CEOs"	Effectiveness results	Stability & viability	Where to focus effort	
Griffith	Hospitals serve communities			Values central to hospital management
Luke & Begun	Success	Structure	Strategic adaptation	Community culture
ACHE		Obligations to clients	Changing ethics	The ethics of health management
Kovner "Viewing . . ."	Motivating	Resource allocation	Scanning the environment	Managerial beliefs and style

of health care. Community satisfaction may be more difficult to achieve than physician and trustee satisfaction.

Luke and Begun propose that successful health care organizations will be focused on the local market, decentralized, and tied to community cultures. In "Viewing the Health Care Manager," Kovner suggests that the manager's ability to motivate others is critical to success.

SYSTEM MAINTENANCE

The manager's role in maintaining the organization has various components. For example, according to Kovner, the effective manager must be concerned with organizational viability and stability. Luke and Begun state that, in order to achieve this stability, health care organizations need to have structures that are diversified and decentralized. The American College of Healthcare Executives Code of Ethics describes the manager's obligations to clients and patients. Fulfilling these obligations contributes to system maintenance by encouraging patients to return to the same centers for services. Kovner includes resource allocation as a managerial activity.

ADAPTIVE CAPABILITY

Kovner's CEOs differ in where they choose to focus their efforts, reflecting varying degrees of and attitudes toward adaptive capability. Luke and Begun see strategic adaptation to local market conditions as vital and argue that the approaches needed for strategic planning are different in health care than in other fields. The evolution of the ACHE Code of Ethics reflects adaptive changes in health care delivery. Kovner also points out that scanning the environment to stay informed of changes in the health care community is an important activity of the health manager.

VALUES INTEGRATION

Griffith suggests that values determine the kinds of hospitals we have, that the spirit of altruism that exists in hospitals is an important contribution to communities, and that hospitals are entitled to funds "on the same basis as the local art museum or local whiskey dealer—namely, that the expenditure will be the proper way to live." Reasonable people might not agree on whether or not consensus exists among Americans about these matters or on how consensus is reached.

Luke and Begun say that the successful health care organization should be tied to its community's culture. The ACHE Code of Ethics reflects underlying values such as honesty and integrity, which are integral to the values of the organization. In addition, the manager's style and beliefs can reflect personal values and can be perceived as such by organization members (Kovner).

ADDITIONAL TOPICS OF INTEREST

Additional topics of interest include what managers do in health planning agencies, management consulting firms, and insurance organizations, and how managerial roles in freestanding organizations compare with those in multi-unit organizations. These and other related issues, such as the politics of managing in health organizations and the manager's participation in ethical considerations, are compelling topics for research.

The literature on managerial style in health services organizations is sparse. Little has been written concerning fit between managerial skills, attitudes, and persona and the particular characteristics of health services organizations. No research has adequately evaluated various ways of organizing top management teams, such as determining desired numbers and levels of managers for health services organizations of varying sizes and complexity. It is also difficult to find good articles on managerial incentives and compensation in health services organizations. However, the selected bibliography below provides some useful sources on management-related topics. Readers should also refer to the annotated bibliography at the end of the book.

NOTES

1.   Duncan Neuhauser, *Coming of Age—The 50 Year History of the American College of Hospital Administrators and the Profession It Serves 1933-1983* (Chicago: Pluribus Press, 1983).

2.   See, for example, Leslie W. Rue and Lloyd L. Byars, *Management: Theory and Application*, 4th ed. (Homewood, IL: Irwin, 1986).

SELECTED BIBLIOGRAPHY

Bellin, Lowell E. "The Health Administrator as Status Seeker." *Journal of Medical Education* 48 (October 1973): 869-904.

Bellin, Lowell E., and Lewis E. Weeks, eds. *The Challenge of Administering Health Services: Career Pathways*. Washington, DC: AUPHA Press, 1981.

Brown, Lawrence D. "The Political Economy of Management." In *Politics and Health Care Organization*, 75-128. Washington, DC: Brookings Institution, 1983.

Brown, Ray. *Judgment in Administration*. New York: McGraw-Hill, 1966.

Feldman, Saul. "The Middle Management Muddle." *Administration in Mental Health* 8 (Fall 1980): 3-11.

Goldsmith, Seth. *Health Care Management: A Contemporary Perspective*. Rockville, MD: Aspen, 1981.

Hardy, Clyde T., Jr. "Survival Through Dependency." *Medical Group Management* 32 (July-August 1985): 18-25.

Harvey, James D. "Evaluating the Performance of the Chief Executive Officer." *Hospital & Health Services Administration* 23 (Spring 1978): 5-21.

Herzlinger, Regina E. "The Failed Revolution in Health Care—The Role of Management." *Harvard Business Review* 2 (March-April 1989): 95-103.

Johnson, Richard L. "The Power Broker—Prototype of the Hospital Chief Executive?" *Health Care Management Review* 3 (Fall 1978): 67-73.

Kinzer, David M. "Turnover of Hospital Chief Executive Officers: A Hospital Association Perspective." *Hospital & Health Services Administration* 27 (May-June 1982): 11-33.

Kovner, Anthony R. "The Hospital Administrator and Organizational Effectiveness." In *Organizational Research on Health Institutions*, edited by Basil Georgopolous, 355-94. Ann Arbor, MI: Institute for Social Research, The University of Michigan, 1972.

————. *Really Trying: A Career Guide for the Health Services Manager*. Ann Arbor, MI: Health Administration Press, 1984.

Levenson, Dorothy. "Martin Cherkasky at Montefiore." *Montefiore Medicine* 6, no. 2 (1981): 43–54.

Light, Harold L., and Howard J. Brown. "The Gouverneur Health Services Program—An Historical Review." *Milbank Memorial Fund Quarterly* 45 (October 1967): 375–89.

Longest, Beaufort B., Jr. "The Contemporary Hospital Chief Executive Officer." *Health Care Management Review* 3 (Spring 1978): 43–53.

————. *Management Practices for the Health Professional*. Reston, VA: Reston, 1980.

McNerney, Walter J. "The Role of the Executive." *Hospital & Health Services Administration* 21 (Fall 1976): 9–25.

Miller, Dulcy B., and June T. Barry. *Nursing Home Organization and Operation*. Boston: CBI, 1979.

Munson, Fred C., and Howard S. Zuckerman. "The Managerial Role." In *Health Care Management*, 2d ed., edited by Stephen M. Shortell and Arnold D. Kaluzny, 38–72. New York: Wiley, 1988.

Myers, Beverlee. *A Guide to Medical Care Administration*. Washington, DC: American Public Health Association, 1965.

Neuhauser, Duncan. *The Relationship between Administration Activities and Hospital Performance*. Chicago: Center for Health Administration Studies, 1971.

Pfeffer, Jeffrey, and Gerald R. Salancik. "Organizational Context and the Characteristics and Tenure of Hospital Administrators." *Academy of Management Journal* 20, no. 1 (1977): 74–88.

Pointer, Dennis D., and Dennis W. Strum. "A Framework for Management Assessment in Health Services Organizations." *Hospital & Health Services Administration* 26 (Summer 1981): 81–95.

Shortell, Stephen M. "Managerial Models." *Hospital Progress* 58 (October 1977): 64–69.

Summers, James W. "Closing Unprofitable Services: Ethical Issues and Management Responses." *Hospital & Health Services Administration* 30 (September–October 1985): 8–28.

Torrens, Paul R. "Administrative Problems of Neighborhood Health Centers." *Medical Care* 9 (November–December 1971): 487–97.

Veninga, Robert. "Administrator Burnout—Causes and Cures." *Hospital Progress* 60 (February 1979): 45–51.

Viguers, Richard T. "The Politics of Power in a Hospital." *Modern Hospital* 96 (May 1961): 89–94.

Wentz, Walter J., and Terrence F. Moore. "Administrative Success: Key Ingredients." *Hospital & Health Services Administration* 26 (Spring 1981): 85–93.

Zuckerman, Howard S. "Redefining the Role of the CEO: Challenges and Conflicts." *Hospital & Health Services Administration* 34 (Spring 1989): 25–38.

1 | # The Work of Effective CEOs in Four Large Health Organizations

Anthony R. Kovner

Large health care organizations are changing rapidly and they face increased competition and increased risk of organizational failure. We know little about the contribution that chief executive officers (CEOs) make to the survival and effectiveness of their organizations. We do not know a great deal about what CEOs say they do, nor about how what they do is seen by those with whom they work. In a previous article, I wrote that CEOs must "assume more power and be held more accountable," for health care organizations to survive and grow in an increasingly turbulent environment. [1] Here I suggest that we take a more analytic look at what CEOs do in order to evaluate their performance better.

One way of looking at what CEOs do is in terms of "episodes" of their work. An episode of work is defined as a cluster of activities performed or participated in by a CEO on a particular subject or topic. Examples include responding to a clinical chief's request to start a satellite clinic, or asking for a profit and loss analysis of a new diagnostic center.

Much of the general management literature focuses on functions of management such as planning, coordinating, and controlling [2], or on

Reprinted from *Hospital & Health Services Administration* 32 (August 1987): 285–305, with permission, Health Administration Press.

Funding for this study was provided by The Pew Memorial Trust. The author wishes to thank the four chief executive officers who graciously welcomed him into their organizations. He is grateful to them as well as to Art Brief, Chris Kovner, John Griffith, and Steve Shortell for their comments on early drafts of this paper.

the roles managers assume, such as negotiator, figurehead or entrepreneur [3]. As a result of shadowing the CEOs, and at the same time reading about episodes of illness as units of analysis in medical care [4,5]. I have come to believe that in evaluating CEOs and other managers, more attention should be paid to analyzing the work that they do, particularly as related to organizational objectives. The activities of CEOs can be categorized by subject or topic. (For an example of activities performed during the day by a CEO, see Appendix A. For an example of an episode of work performed by a CEO during a three-day period, see Appendix B.) Although this study was not designed to analyze episodes of CEO work, episodes emerged during data analysis that I believe are worthy of further exploration.

Episodes of work can be analyzed in terms of subject matter; those involved in a variety of interactions; the type of response required by the action; the CEO's choice regarding which episodes to manage and which to delegate or ignore; the time the CEO chooses to devote to managing or participating in different episodes; and results per managed episode as determined by costs in CEO time and use of other organizational resources.

Focus on work episodes can assist in evaluating what a CEO should be doing in relation to work expectations and performance. This type of analysis can sharpen or focus CEO attention on objectives and how time is spent. It can also result in necessary changes in organizational objectives.

This article is organized into four main sections: a description of the study undertaken; perceptions within the organization of CEO effectiveness; preliminary and sample measurement of episodes of CEO work; and crosscutting themes regarding CEO effectiveness in large health care organizations.

STUDY METHODOLOGY

This exploratory study was carried out between January 1, 1986 and July 31, 1986 in four large health organizations in a large eastern city. CEO selection was based on five or more years of tenure as CEO of a large local not-for-profit health organization with gross revenues in 1984 of $85 million dollars or more and with 500 employees or more. The organizations were selected to represent a mix by size and mission. Finally, of those CEOs who met the study criteria, I chose four who, in my opinion, were effective managers.

Each CEO was interviewed twice for three hours and shadowed for five consecutive working days during one week chosen by the CEO.

Eight to nine close associates inside and outside the organization, as
selected by the CEOs, were interviewed; each interview lasted from 60 to
75 minutes. The associates were selected to represent a range of persons
with whom the CEO has worked closely. (See Appendices C1 through 3
for the CEO and associate interview questions.) Available documents
such as annual reports, articles written by or about the CEO and the
organization, and financial analyses were reviewed. During the interviews and observations, copious but not verbatim notes were taken.
Daily notes were typed to facilitate data analysis and following typing,
the author summarized data and isolated themes. What follows is an
analysis of the data filtered through the author, who teaches health
management and who has managed several health organizations.

To preserve anonymity, CEOs and organizations have been given ficti-
tious names. Short paragraphs describing each CEO and health care
organization follow.

SITE #1: WASHINGTON MEDICAL CENTER AND
CEO T. GEORGE

Washington Medical Center has over 1,000 beds, more than 5,000
employees, and gross annual revenues of over $300 million dollars. It is
part of an academic health center with over 2,000 faculty and has a
mission of excellence in teaching, research, and service. Technology and
mission are complex at Washington Medical Center and the hospital is
therefore less susceptible to being centrally managed. Because of ample
resources and a strong reputation, Washington Medical Center is
believed to face relatively low environmental turbulence in terms of
threats to operating finances or market share.

T. George is 64 years old, was educated as a physician, has worked at
the hospital for more than 30 years, and has been in his present position
for more than 15 years.

SITE #2: VAN BUREN HOSPITAL AND
CEO L. MARTIN

Van Buren Hospital has over 500 beds, more than 1,500 employees,
gross revenues of over $85 million dollars, and is the smallest of the four
observed organizations. It lacks tertiary facilities, provides a broad range
of ambulatory care services in high volume, and serves a low-income as
well as a middle-income population. Relative to the other organizations
in the sample, Van Buren Hospital is believed to be lower in organizational complexity, providing primary and secondary care only, and not
emphasizing teaching or research missions. The hospital is believed to

face a relatively stable environment because most of the residents in its two primary service areas receive hospital service at Van Buren Hospital and because most of Van Buren's services are provided to such residents.

L. Martin is over 55 years old, has a master's degree in public health, and has worked at the hospital in his present position for more than 15 years.

SITE #3: CLEVELAND HOSPITAL AND CEO T. GROVER

Cleveland Hospital has over 500 beds, more than 2,000 employees, and gross revenues of over $100 million dollars. Its primary missions are service and teaching as it is strongly affiliated with a local medical school. Cleveland Hospital is believed to be middling in organizational complexity relative to the other three organizations because it combines two hospital sites and emphasizes a teaching as well as a service mission. Its environment is believed to be more turbulent than that facing either Washington or Van Buren Hospital as it faces competition from neighboring hospitals from which it is not distinctive with regard to product mix. Also contributing to the turbulence is the dispersed nature of its patients and physicians and the hospital's problematic finances which allow little margin for error with regard to acceptable losses from operations.

T. Grover is in his mid-forties, has a master's degree in public health, and has worked at Cleveland Hospital for more than 15 years, with more than 5 years as CEO.

SITE #4: WILSON HMO AND CEO S. WOODROW

Wilson HMO is a prepaid group practice plan or group model health maintenance organization. The Wilson system has over 4,500 employees, with gross revenue over $700 million. The HMO has more than 900,000 members. The organizational complexity is believed to be high relative to the other three organizations. Unlike the hospitals, Wilson HMO combines financing health care with the responsibility for its provision. The plan interacts with nine independent medical groups, has several subsidiaries, and because of its large size has many sites and facilities distributed over a wide geographic area. The environment Wilson operates in is turbulent, because of the number of well-financed new competitors that are entering its service area.

S. Woodrow is in his mid-fifties, has a master's degree in public health, and has worked in his present position for more than five years.

Previously, he served for more than five years as CEO of another large HMO.

PERCEPTIONS OF MANAGERIAL EFFECTIVENESS

It is difficult to sum up in any meaningful way the CEO and associate responses to questions about CEO effectiveness or my observations after twenty days of shadowing the CEOs. Therefore, I will focus on the responses by CEOs to questions on CEO effectiveness, accomplishments, strategies, as well as on their current projects. Some crosscutting themes selected from the gathered data are summarized across organizations in a later section of this paper.

T. GEORGE (WASHINGTON MEDICAL CENTER)

George's response on what makes an effective CEO at Washington Hospital reveals one who practices a collegial style, communicates effectively with clinical chiefs, and most importantly recruits clinical chairmen and assists them in recruitment. George emphasized the importance of having an academic medical school background so that "no translator" is needed in frequent interactions with chiefs.

George's accomplishments as perceived by his associates include holding together the hospital and the academic factions; putting personal interests last (his institutional perspective); supporting the development of new technology; assisting in the recruitment of academic leaders; and involving the institution in long-range planning. One associate cited George's survival in the job as a key accomplishment.

George finds the primary barriers to getting things done relate to people. He says that he doesn't hand down orders but talks about problems, that consensus is easier to reach than people think it is. The opportunities at Washington Medical Center to get things done are relatively unlimited; the problem is that George doesn't take the time to assess and prioritize them. What George has learned over the years is how to assess and deal with a situation in a short time. George comments that one reason why a person should not stay in the job for twenty years is the degree of inflexibility in approach that develops over time. His tremendous advantage now is that he knows the job. Perhaps he knows it so well that he doesn't think generally, flexibly, or creatively enough about what ought to be done.

Associates see George as getting things done by touching base with people who are important in implementation and who are experienced with similar issues. He is seen as delegating a great deal, as being persistent, and by one associate as "not having much life outside of Washington Medical Center." Another associate says that it can take George a long time to make a decision, but when he decides, it has been well thought through.

Unlike those of the other CEOs, and because George is in the process of retiring next year, his responses to future agendas deal with what the hospital needs to accomplish this year. This includes gaining approval for certificate of need for a major rebuilding program, adjusting to DRG reimbursement, searching for his successor, and implementing a guest relations program.

George's associates see him trying to position Washington Medical Center for the future with regard to affiliations for managed care and for teaching, obtaining approvals and financing for major hospital renovation, coping with possible occupancy problems related to diagnosis-related group (DRG) reimbursement, keeping pace with technology, and maintaining a "good operation."

L. MARTIN (VAN BUREN HOSPITAL)

Martin responded that being a good CEO at Van Buren Hospital means using the hospital as an instrument to convert resources into appropriate use for the neighborhood. He says that he tells an honest and continuing story about what the hospital is trying to do. Almost everything that he has said the hospital was going to do has been done, with little operating capital and no endowments.

Martin's accomplishments, as viewed by associates, include the hospital's serving the community better through the establishment of a neighborhood health center, the development of a completely modern hospital, the creation of a large housing complex for the elderly, the planned nearby construction of a nursing home, and the development of a small for-profit company. One of his associates says that based on operations before Martin took over, the hospital wouldn't have survived without him. His associates say that Martin has attracted and held excellent administrators and has an acute sense of the opportunities in hospital development and management.

Martin believes that the "easiest way" (which he does not follow) to be a CEO is to be weak. In that way, no single individual can be held accountable, risk is eliminated; mistakes are "ours," not "yours." He sees insufficient funds as the primary barrier to managing effectively at Van Buren. A significant barrier for some CEOs is defending themselves against current activities so as to inhibit their ability to do the things that they ought to be doing. Martin says that the CEO needs the self-confidence that inspires people to believe that something is good if the CEO says it is. The major pitfall for a CEO at Van Buren, according to Martin, is "not knowing what you are doing." The toughest decisions are in the area of risk; converting an abandoned factory into a modern hospital, for example.

Martin says that he will leave behind the sense that the CEO is really key to hospital effectiveness in setting the style, attitudes, and spirit, signaling whether this is a risk-taking place or not, and defining institutional choices.

Martin is seen by associates as using his tremendous sense of logical reasoning to accomplish things, and as doing things quickly once a decision has been made. He is said to investigate thoroughly and to be well prepared. His associates say that they know what Martin's plans are and how he feels about their performance. They say that Martin does not use meetings or committees, and is a firm believer in responsibility tied to individuals.

Martin says that both his short-range and long-range agendas include understanding neighborhood need and adjusting to meet it. This means continued development of services for older people and ambulatory services for people in a community area not served by private physicians. He is talking about merger possibilities, acquiring a long-term care unit as a partner and improving performance for the for-profit diagnostic center. Martin says that the most difficult thing is maintaining everyone's confidence and trust in allowing the hospital to accomplish these goals. He fears setting up new relationships and redefining the hospital mission in a merger.

Martin's associates see him as creating an environment in which Van Buren Hospital can "thrive not merely survive"; developing a health care system with other hospitals in this part of the city; and doing this under the restrictions placed on the hospital by government regulators.

T. GROVER (CLEVELAND HOSPITAL)

Grover responds that the effective CEO at Cleveland Hospital must be concerned with satisfying the objectives developed with the governing board. He says that he enjoys seeing people excited about objectives, and that he is effective because of his ability to accomplish objectives. To be effective at Cleveland Hospital, Grover says that the board must understand the CEO's objectives and find them acceptable.

Grover's associates see his main accomplishments as the merger with another hospital; the rebuilding of Cleveland Hospital; developing a vision of the future understood by trustees, physicians, and managers;

building a fine administrative staff with special skills; keeping the hospital alive throughout several financial crises; and dealing successfully with the board.

In order to get things done, Grover says that he tries to foster respect through reasonableness, intelligence, and patience; and to build a collegial atmosphere around a work effort. He speaks of the commitment and compulsiveness required to do the CEO job effectively at Cleveland Hospital.

Grover's associates see him using such means as educating the board, visualizing the practical steps required to implement new ideas, supporting staff with enthusiasm, and not taking problems to others without having a solution to reach goals. They say that Grover has a knack for understanding how interested parties will view his decisions. One associate says that Grover gets things done in a hands-on way; another, that he delegates while keeping the reins tight.

Grover says that his present agenda is preparing the hospital for the long term. This involves improving financial stability and market viability of programs; developing positive relationships with community groups, managed care companies, and regulators; clarifying the hospital's relationship with the medical school; and, for the longer term, developing a local regional health system.

His associates perceive Grover as trying to keep the hospital afloat, merge with other local hospitals, and rationalize Cleveland Hospital's relationship with the medical school. In addition, he is seen as expending a tremendous amount of energy on operations, in "meeting the payroll, handling the State Health Department citations, and pulling doctors apart and so forth."

S. WOODROW (WILSON HMO)

Woodrow responds that he would like to be concerned mainly with implementation of policy and review of operations but currently he must handle operations, such as developing the programs of medical groups, meeting with consumers, and reviewing market strategies.

The main things that his associates see Woodrow as accomplishing at Wilson are taking the physicians from group practice to full health maintenance organization (HMO) status; the HMO's owning all the medical group facilities and equipment; influencing the board to move into new regions (markets, products, marketing to commercial accounts); and leading Wilson staff into adopting a corporate mentality as opposed to a government mentality. According to one associate, "Woodrow accomplished what others said couldn't be done without losing anyone we wanted to keep."

Woodrow says that to get things done at Wilson HMO he must be a good conceptualizer and yet be flexible in the face of changing circumstances. Wilson's CEO must be a practical politician with thick skin who builds the confidence of those working in the organization. Being wedded to a corporate ideology would be a major pitfall. The CEO requires management skill and flexibility, Woodrow adds, using new approaches and modifications of existing ones with political skills to win support for objectives. The CEO must be tenacious and flexible. Woodrow says that his subordinates respect him because he knows what he's doing. Woodrow says that he had to instill a degree of accountability and insecurity in others to improve managerial performance.

Woodrow's associates say that he gets things done by giving people responsibility and holding them accountable; by asking, then expecting things to get done without disruption to other people. He (like Martin) is said to be able to convey to a group a sense of authority and candor whether or not he is being candid. Woodrow is said to devise strategies to allow constituents to see changes as in their interest and to have a good sense of timing. One associate said that Woodrow forces issues, not in terms of exact timing or form, but in terms of their resolution and direction. He understands the use of power in negotiation.

Woodrow says his current agenda is to mold an organization that can effectively compete, to continue upgrading management and programs, to promote the organization's public image more aggressively, to expand existing product and service areas, and to restructure his role in all of this.

Woodrow's associates see him trying to maintain Wilson's customer base and expanding into existing and neighborhood markets, conducting educational programs for physicians related to marketing efforts, modernizing and building new facilities and developing new product lines. They see him trying to develop a sense of pride in the organization and trying, according to one associate, to assure that the organization survives the national shakedown of HMOs without "losing the organization's sense of integrity and social purpose."

USING WORK EPISODES FOR EVALUATION

Although considerable time was spent in this study recording and categorizing activities and episodes of work, the methods used are problematical in specifying adequate operational definitions. For example, in Table 1.1 below, activities #4, #5, and #6 were defined as separate,

TABLE 1.1

Episodes of Work—S. Woodrow: Wilson HMO

. . .
3. CEO performs follow up to job interview by phone.
4. CEO responds to medical group directors' request for expansion of facilities.
5. CEO informs medical director of desirability of one medical group.
6. CEO is informed of physician's perceptions of a hospital which is owned by Wilson HMO.
7. CEO responds to request to discuss performance appraisals.

although the three activities occurred during the same meeting. Activities #5 and #6 are informational only. It may be argued that activities #4, #5, and #6 should be counted as one activity rather than as three. Conversely, a very long merger meeting in which CEO Martin was participating was counted by the observer as one activity of work, even though several separate topics (I categorize them as subactivities) were dealt with during the same meeting. These included finances, medical staff, and population characteristics of utilizers at the two hospitals.

Appendix A and B illustrate the texture of episodes and activities. Appendix A lists 25 management activities for CEO George on a Monday of 12 hours at work. Twenty of the activities are brief, lasting ten minutes or less, or usually five minutes or less. These activities range from a trustee requesting the name of a physician for a friend to the chief financial officer telling the CEO that a local not-for-profit organization wishes to sell property to Washington Medical Center. Examples of longer (lasting over 30 minutes) activities are CEO participation with the dean of the medical school in separate performance reviews of two clinical chairmen and a CEO interview with a physician interested in management whose primary appointment would be in the department of medicine.

Appendix B lists eight activities on a Monday through Wednesday which constitute a partial episode of management for CEO Martin. The episode concerns Van Buren Hospital's sharing obstetrics-gynecology (OB-GYN) services with a nearby hospital. This episode began before and ended after the period of observation by the author. Merger talks having lapsed between these two hospitals, CEO Martin wishes also to end the agreement to share OB-GYN physician services and has indicated this to the other CEO. A summary of the activities in this episode in which Martin participated follows.

On Monday, Martin reviews the facts of the situation with his chief operating officer (COO), meets with the two physicians involved who were formerly co-chiefs at Van Buren Hospital to let them know what they can expect when Dr. B. returns to Van Buren and to confirm the time of his return. On Tuesday, Martin and the COO review the two physicians' reactions to Van Buren's offer and how they plan to work together in the future. Later that day the COO tells Martin that Dr. B. has called the CEO of the other hospital who will expect Martin's call. On Wednesday, the COO tells Martin that the co-chiefs want a bottom-line financial commitment before Dr. B. leaves the other hospital. Martin tells the COO to prepare a sample agreement. Later, Dr. B. drops by to discuss with Martin how the two co-chiefs will function together when he returns. Late on Wednesday, Martin calls the CEO at the other hospital concerning terminating the shared services agreement as quickly as possible.

It is suggested that one way of evaluating what CEOs do is to analyze CEO activities and episodes and compare results per episode and fit of managerial time spent across episodes with organizational objectives. Part of this analysis concerns merely counting the number of activities and episodes by CEO.

In this study the number of activities and episodes were tallied for the four CEOs and the activities per episode were calculated for a Monday through Friday period of observation, as shown in Table 1.2.

The scores are included here to indicate the variance in what CEOs do and to suggest that hypotheses can be derived and tested associating CEO activities and episodes of work with different sets of organizational circumstances. The data collected in this study suggest the following hypotheses:

1. When organizational complexity and environmental turbulence are high, the CEO will participate in a large number of episodes and in many activities per episode.

TABLE 1.2

Episodes and Activities of CEOs for Three Days of One Week

CEO	Episodes	Activities	Activities Per Episode
George	58	111	1.9
Martin	21	52	2.5
Grover	53	115	2.2
Woodrow	60	106	1.8

2. When organizational complexity and environmental turbulence are low, the CEO will participate in a small number of episodes and in a small number of activities per episode.
3. When organizational complexity is high and environmental turbulence is low, the CEO will participate in a large number of episodes and in few activities per episode.
4. When organizational complexity is low and environmental turbulence is high, the CEO will participate in few episodes and in a large number of activities per episode.

CROSSCUTTING THEMES

Some crosscutting themes suggested by the responses to the interviews regarding CEO effectiveness in large health organizations include (1) the importance of setting CEO and trustee expectations regarding CEO performance, (2) the lack of transferability of CEOs across large health care organizations, (3) the importance of visible results from CEO choice of managerial work, and (4) the impact of increasing organizational size and complexity on the executive office in large health care organizations.

SETTING EXPECTATIONS FOR CEO PERFORMANCE

Large health care organizations are difficult to manage effectively because of differing opinions on organizational objectives and the contribution of management. CEO contribution to organizational effectiveness is not specified in the study nor are the four CEOs evaluated for it.

Some implicit setting of expectations did occur for each of the four CEOs. This took place during the initial hiring process and again during the long-range planning process among managers, trustees, and medical staff at three- to five-year intervals in two of the four organizations studied.

There are good reasons why neither organizational objectives nor CEO contributions to their attainment are being set in these organizations. These reasons include a lack of pressure to set objectives and the cost in time and conflict in attempting to set them. I believe that it will be increasingly difficult, however, for large health care organizations to retain their market share or to grow in the future without stated expectations for organizational and CEO performance. Objectives are necessary in making decisions on scope of services and levels of cost and quality, and in validating the CEO's role in implementing them.

LACK OF TRANSFERABILITY ACROSS
ORGANIZATIONS

Fiedler has emphasized that leadership characteristics vary with the nature of the situation [6,7]. Managers who are effective in facing certain circumstances in one type of organization may be ineffective in another organization.

The four observed organizations vary with regard to mission, available resources, political constituencies, organizational complexity, and turbulence of environment. These differences affect the work that CEOs do as well as the roles they play and the functions they perform. In such a situation, the choices that CEOs make among episodes of work are likely to be associated with the circumstances faced by their organization. On this point, regarding Washington Medical Center, CEO George comments:

> The most important aspects of this job have to do with quality of patient care . . . and a participation in the academic side sufficient to ensure that the academic side is held up well. . . . You must work with your chiefs to develop objectives consistent with the institutional objectives but especially tailored to the needs of that department. . . . It's a mistake to think that you will direct these people in a very distinctive way.

Contrast this with CEO Martin's observations on managing Van Buren Hospital: "I also leave behind the sense that the CEO is really 'key'; he sets the style, attitude, and spirit; signals whether this is a risk-taking place or not; defines institutional choices. . . ."

It is obvious that these two examples point to the differences in the type of work that effective CEOs perform. Regarding episodes of work, a CEO facing circumstances like those at Van Buren Hospital should involve himself more thoroughly in fewer projects. A CEO who participates less intensively in more projects at Van Buren would manage less effectively there. A CEO facing circumstances like those at Washington Medical Center should manage in yet another way to be effective.

In accounting for the assumed effectiveness of the CEOs observed, I am struck by the long tenure of the CEOs involved. All four CEOs had been at least eight years in their present positions, and had held similar tenure in preceding positions. I believe that tenure is related to perceived predictability of CEO behavior, making it possible for organizational leaders to focus on the work that must be done rather than on jockeying for position and worrying excessively about job security and autonomy.

VISIBLE RESULTS AND CEO CHOICE

Health care is a service that is difficult to measure. Profits are an ambiguous index of success for large nonprofit health care organizations. The data in this study suggest that CEO effectiveness in such organizations is measured by trustees and medical staff leadership primarily in terms of the visible achievements of the organization. Construction or renovation of a building, refinancing a mortgage, obtaining a government grant, hiring a new chief of service, ranking highly in a national survey—are all visible results. Less visible are accomplishments in such areas as improving the technical quality of care and the amenities of service, encouraging the career development of managers, and decreasing the unit cost of providing services of acceptable quality both within and outside the institution. Though these less visible areas may be as important for organizational survival and growth, they will tend not to be seen as equally important factors in evaluating CEO effectiveness, and therefore CEOs are likely to devote less time to managing them—at least until specified accomplishments can be suitably measured.

Although observation of CEOs and interview responses in the study indicate that CEOs commonly engage in activities in the less visible areas referred to above, organizational objectives were not specified in these areas. Often they were not specified for the more visible areas either, other than in general terms. For example, CEO Grover cites Cleveland Hospital's mandate as being able to provide "accessible high-quality human services with public health and medical education." How does he or the board or the medical staff know, for example, what the expected or acceptable levels of achievement regarding provision of high quality care are? Or, to what extent are public health and medical education objectives being met with regard to prenatal care? Many measures of CEO effectiveness in important areas are difficult to quantify and agree upon, but the observations and data in this study suggest that CEOs, boards, and medical staffs place too little emphasis on the benefits of goal specification. However, it is recognized that goal specification has its own costs and can generate internal conflict.

Progress is being made by studying CEOs and institutions in the less visible areas. Interviewees were questioned specifically about CEO involvement in cost containment and quality assurance. The responses indicated that costs are being contained primarily through regular budgeting processes and in response to external regulatory controls. Technical quality standards are increasingly being set and implemented. This is partly in response to state regulatory initiatives, particularly in the areas of physician credentialing, delineation of privileges, and reviewing physician work as indicated in the medical record. Another area of CEO involvement in quality as indicated by the data is in the selection and termination of clinical chiefs of service.

INCREASING ORGANIZATIONAL SIZE AND COMPLEXITY AND EXECUTIVE WORK

The final crosscutting theme addresses the increasing size and complexity of the organizations studied and the implications for organizing the executive office. For example, Washington Medical Center is already a vast and complex institution with a mission of excellence in teaching, research, and service. Now it must also consider creating affiliated networks for teaching and service, along with medical staff for managed care organizations. Simultaneously, funds must be raised and approvals must be obtained for a massive facility reconstruction program. Cleveland and Van Buren Hospitals are discussing merging with each other and other neighboring hospitals, and both are diversifying more heavily into areas other than inpatient medical care. Wilson HMO is developing new products (individual practice associations and preferred provider organizations) and expanding into new regions. Both Wilson HMO and Cleveland Hospital have recently acquired other health care organizations through mergers.

In all four organizations, despite the presence of a chief operating officer, the CEO remains involved in operations at the main site. The CEO spends less time than three of the CEOs desired or thought appropriate on growth and development activities such as program development and evaluation of key operating officers. Paradoxically, associates say of three of the CEOs that they do not spend sufficient time on operations (less than was previously spent) because of heavy involvement in organizational response to external pressures such as regulation, competition, and, for hospitals, the threat of declining inpatient occupancy. Two of the CEOs say that they are hesitant to place chief operating officers in complete charge of operations either because COOs are not fully trusted or because the CEO is reluctant to yield responsibility. In all four organizations, COOs do not seem to be specifically developed to take over as CEOs. Through analysis of episodes of work CEOs and others can more easily detect when too much or too little CEO attention is being paid to certain organizational objectives, and gauge in a timely way when the case for organization restructuring becomes compelling.

Conclusion

This paper suggests that CEO effectiveness should be analyzed in terms of the work that CEOs do in relation to specific health care organization objectives. The work of CEOs can be categorized and analyzed in terms of episodes and activities. Further it is suggested that CEOs and trustees set expectations regarding CEO performance; that there may be a lack of transferability of CEOs across large health organizations; that bias exists in CEO work toward that involving visible results; and that the position of chief operating officer be further developed in terms of greater responsibilities and possible designation as the next CEO.

References

1. Kovner, A.R. Issues in the structure and process of hospital governance. *Frontiers of Health Services Management* 2(1): 4–33, August 1985.

2. Gulick, L. Notes on a theory of organization. In L. Gulick and L. Urwick (eds.). *Papers on the Science of Administration.* New York: Institute of Public Administration, 1937.

3. Mintzberg, H. *The Nature of Managerial Work.* New York: Harper & Row, 1973.

4. Strauss, A., S. Fagerbaugh, B. Suczek, and C. Wiener. *Social Organization of Work.* Chicago: The University of Chicago Press, 1985.

5. Hornbrook, M.C., A.V. Hurtado, and R.E. Johnson. Health care episodes: Definition, management, and use. *Medical Care Review* 42: 163, Fall 1985.

6. Fiedler, F.E. A Contemporary Model of Leadership Effectiveness. In Berkowitz (ed.). *Advances in Experimental Social Psychology.* New York: Academic Press, 1964.

7. Fiedler, F.E. Validation and extension of the contingency model of leadership effectiveness: A review of empirical findings. *Psychological Bulletin* 76: 128, August 1971.

Appendix A

EPISODES OF MANAGEMENT ACTIVITY FOR CEO
T. GEORGE ON A MONDAY (12 HOURS)

	Episode	*Time Spent*
1.	Trustee requests the name of a doctor for a friend. CEO refers to chief operating officer (COO).	Brief (10 minutes or less)

2.	Other CEO calls indicating that his institution will not be part of a third organization's affiliation network for managed care.	Brief
3,4.	CEO participates with the dean in separate performance reviews of two clinical chairmen.	Long (31–60 minutes each)
5.	CEO conducts job interview of a physician whose primary appointment would be in the Department of Medicine.	Long
6.	CEO calls Director of Nursing in response to a question about the number of nursing students in the hospital.	Brief
7.	CEO indicates support for a development project in response to M.D. request and communicates this to the Director of Development.	Brief
8.	CEO agrees to give blood.	Brief
9.	CEO requests publicity for laudatory article.	Brief
10.	CEO is requested to review space plans by a clinical chief in a new building. He agrees.	Brief
11.	CEO is requested to facilitate admission of a patient in response to a trustee request to a nursing home affiliated with the hospital. CEO follows up.	Intermediate (11–30 minutes)
12.	CEO is told that a study on operating room efficiency is proceeding.	Brief
13.	CEO informs CEO of another hospital of the search process for his successor.	Brief
14.	CEO is informed that M.D.'s wife is pleased with award the M.D. has received.	Brief
15.	CEO is informed that an assistant administrator is working on "Do Not Resuscitate" guidelines.	Brief
16.	CEO asks how lawyers are dealing with development of other property in the face of resistance from a historic preservation group.	Brief
17.	CEO is informed that an assistant administrator is responding to the State Health Department investigation of a complaint about emergency services.	Brief
18.	CEO is told by community relations staff about relocation plan related to sale of a property to a private developer. CEO will visit the building into which tenants will be relocated.	Intermediate
19.	CEO is told about VIP who has been admitted (the brother of a potential large donor). CEO will visit.	Brief

20.	Physician complains to CEO that a new building obstructs the view of a plaque for a previously honored physician. The CEO will follow up.	Brief
21.	CEO is told about locals who wish to sell a property. He asks for more information.	Brief
22.	CEO tells donor that room which donor paid to refurbish is ready for viewing.	Brief
23.	Lawyer requests CEO's permission to attend an educational conference. CEO grants request.	Brief
24.	CEO is informed that another VIP is a patient in the Emergency Services Area. CEO will visit.	Brief
25.	CEO is told about other available job. CEO says he is not interested.	Brief

APPENDIX B

ACTIVITIES OF ONE MANAGERIAL EPISODE FOR
L. MARTIN: A MONDAY THROUGH WEDNESDAY
PERIOD

TOPIC: SHARED OB–GYN SERVICES WITH
ANOTHER HOSPITAL

Monday

1. CEO reviews the situation with his COO. He wants to confirm that Dr. B. will return to Van Buren Hospital after the agreement for shared services is terminated. This was agreed to by both parties if merger talks failed.
2. CEO meets with the two M.D.s, codirectors of OB-GYN, and the COO. CEO summarizes his position and the co-chief involved agrees with the summary. CEO says he will attempt to satisfy the co-chief professionally and financially and to know when he can return to Van Buren Hospital. The co-chief says whenever it is agreeable to the two CEOs. CEO concludes by saying he wants to strengthen Van Buren Clinical service.
3. CEO tells CEO of second hospital (with whom he is conducting merger talks) about the other hospital's offer to hire Dr. B and that Dr. B will be returning to Van Buren Hospital.

Tuesday

4. CEO meets with COO who says that the co-chiefs are satisfied with a more costly financial package and who should be in charge of what among the two codirectors.

5. CEO meets with COO who says Dr. B. called. Dr. B told the other hospital medical director of his decision and that CEO would be calling their CEO. Dr. B will meet with their medical director on Thursday. CEO says that now this is Dr. B's decision. COO says that "I didn't want to hear what their hospital had to offer and that Van Buren Hospital would be fair."

Wednesday

6. CEO meets with COO who says the co-chiefs want bottom line commitment before Dr. B leaves the other hospital. Dr. B. wants the same money as he's earning now without taking the money from Dr. C. CEO says that for the money, Dr. B. can build a department with young obstetricians and Van Buren also gets a director of medical education. This gives the hospital some of Dr. C's time as it proceeds with merger talks with the second hospital. He asks the COO to write down the quid pro quo for all parties.
7. Dr. B. drops by and the CEO reviews merger talks with him. Dr. B. doesn't want the co-chief, Dr. C., to step down prematurely. He says that the timing has to be resolved. The CEO says that Dr. B. should concentrate on what has to be done to make the service relevant in the market place. He will continue as director of medical education . . . the CEO will ask Dr. C. to represent the clinical directors in merger talks. He will be needed for this purpose.
8. CEO calls the CEO of the hospital terminating the shared service agreement. He says that Dr. B. indicates he wants to return home to Van Buren Hospital. Does the other CEO have any thoughts on the matter? CEO explains that once someone has decided to leave, their staying will be ineffective.

APPENDIX C-1

STRUCTURED INTERVIEW QUESTIONS FOR FIRST
CEO INTERVIEW

1. When you took over as CEO, what strong wishes, thoughts, aspirations, ambitions did you have in mind?
2. When you were selected for your CEO tasks, were you given a specific charge by the Board? Did that charge differ significantly from what you yourself saw had to be done? What did you hope to be able to do beyond the expectations of the Board?
3. What did you see had to be done in and to the organization in order to achieve those goals? That is, what policies, practices, perceptions, methods, attitudes did you perceive had to be changed?
4. How did you go about changing policies, practices, perceptions, methods and attitudes?
5. Looking back on it now, how well did you succeed in making those changes? Did they produce the effects you were striving for? How do you know?
6. Describe your job. Being very effective in the job means what?
7. What were the toughest decisions you have had to make as a manager? Why?

8. If you were to point out one or more major pitfalls for persons in your job, what would they be?
9. When you want to leave your organization, what managerial changes do you want to leave behind? That is, what will indicate that you have had an enduring effect on your organization?
10. Who among your peers has done something in his or her organization that you wish you had been able to do in yours? Why can't you do it?
11. What stories do people tell about you?

Appendix C-2

STRUCTURED INTERVIEW QUESTIONS FOR
SECOND CEO INTERVIEW

1. What makes for an effective manager in your organization?
2. How are you evaluated? By whom? How do you evaluate yourself?
3. What are the barriers to managing effectively in your organization and how do you overcome them?
4. What are the opportunities for managing effectively in your organization and how do you take advantage of them?
5. To what extent are you an effective manager? How can you be more effective?
6. How did you learn to be an effective manager in this organization? What have you learned?
7. What is your agenda for the short term? For the long term?
8. How will you accomplish these? Through what networks?
9. How is your job changing?
10. How is your job performance changing?
11. How do you influence the cost of medical care in your organization? Give examples!
12. In what ways do internal and external groups affect your ability to and the ways in which you influence costs?
13. Why don't you do more to control costs in this organization?
14. How do you influence the quality of medical care in this organization? Give examples.
15. In what ways do external and internal groups affect your ability to and the ways you influence quality?
16. Why don't you do more to assure quality in this organization?
17. Are there any comments or thoughts you would like to share relevant to this study with regulators, other managers, educators, and researchers?

Appendix C-3

STRUCTURED INTERVIEW QUESTIONS FOR
INTERVIEWS WITH CEO ASSOCIATES

1. What is your background? How long and where have you worked with the manager? What are those problems or issues on which you have worked most closely with the manager?

2. What are the key things one needs to understand about this business and this organization to truly understand the context in which the general manager works?
3. What are the key things he has done, good or bad, in his job? Why did he do that? What impact did it have?
4. How do you normally interact with him? When and for how long? How does he get things done? What is he trying to do? What are the sources of his power?
5. How would you describe him as a manager? As a person?
6. How would you rate his performance? Why?
7. In what ways has he changed in the way he manages or what he manages and why?
8. What stories do people tell about him?
9. How does he influence the cost of medical care in your organization? Give examples!
10. How does he influence the quality of medical care in your organization? Give examples!

2 | Industry Distinctiveness: Implications for Strategic Management in Health Care Organizations

Roice D. Luke
James W. Begun

The significant changes now occurring in the health care industry have been widely chronicled by observers and practitioners alike. The consensus appears to be that the industry, having discovered the big-business model, is well on its way to a true private-industry approach to providing health care to the nation's ill. The predicted consequences of this development are far-reaching. One analyst recently suggested that "It's only a question of time before the major hospital companies consume . . . all of the nursing home companies. I don't foresee any of the nursing home companies standing alone in five or six years"[1]. A major securities analysis firm foresees market penetration of 30 percent of the population

Reprinted from *Journal of Health Administration Education* 5 (Summer 1987): 387–405, with permission, Association of University Programs in Health Administration.

This paper was prepared as part of a project on multi-institutional health systems education funded by the W.K. Kellogg Foundation and jointly coordinated by the Hospital Research and Educational Trust of the American Hospital Association and the Association of University Programs in Health Administration.

for health maintenance organizations (HMOs) and 40 percent of the population for preferred provider organizations (PPOs) by 1990, with a "radical transformation" of the health care system that "will take the form of a wide array of economically based delivery systems that will be truly competitive and completely deregulated"[2].

The danger with such views is that they embrace a traditional business model without fully considering the possible moderating effect of distinctive factors within the health care industry. The dramatic growth of large multihospital systems, at least until recently, has led many to assume that the horizontal strategy for system growth would dominate the industry. However, not only does horizontal expansion represent a small portion of organizational growth and restructuring within the industry, but recent shifts in strategy, even among multi-institutional systems, suggest that predictions such as those mentioned above may not prove reliable in the long term.

From the perspective of curriculum design, an even larger question must be addressed than one focusing on dominance among strategic patterns of growth. It has been traditional to assume that because of the distinctiveness of the health care industry, a unique curriculum in health administration is justified. However, as the field adopts business approaches to management, it is incumbent upon faculty to determine the degree to which the linkage between industry distinctiveness and curriculum remains.

The implications of a changing industry for the design of curricula in health administration programs must therefore be carefully considered. In many ways, developments in the field create no special difficulties for the design of curricula, as health administration programs have historically emphasized the fundamentals of management, an emphasis long formalized in accreditation requirements. Yet the enormity of change and the limited time period within which it is occurring make reassessments of and measured adjustments in curricula an absolute necessity.

In what areas are modifications in health administration curricula potentially most needed? This is a question considered by the W.K. Kellogg Foundation when it funded efforts to develop educational materials for use in training individuals who might eventually function in multi-institutional systems in the health care field. The implicit question posed by the Foundation's funding decision was, are there any areas in health administration education that may need greater emphasis or development, given the needs of present or future administrators in multi-institutional systems?

There are many possible answers to that question. It is a premise of this article, however, that the greatest need for educational development lies in the area of health care strategic management. This is because the changes in the field stem essentially from a revolution in the environment of health care, a revolution that is increasingly causing health care organizations to be strategically oriented; they are struggling to adapt in ways that even a decade ago were considered unthinkable. It follows that if revisions in curricula are needed, priority must be given to the area of strategic management. General management issues do arise out of recent developments in the field, but the factors precipitating change are primarily external to health care organizations; hence, future leaders in the field must be prepared to help their organizations adapt to an uncertain future.

It is an additional premise of this article that educational development and innovation should give priority to the content of strategy more than to the process of strategic decision making [3]. This is because the elements of health organization strategy are more likely to be linked to the distinctive features of the field than are the techniques of decision making, which themselves should be relatively generalizable across industries. This implies, of course, that the health care field is not only distinctive, but that its distinctiveness is sufficient to justify the search for strategic elements that may be unique to health care organizations.

We suggest, in fact, that before private-industry models of strategic behavior are integrated into our teaching, we should (1) assess whether or not any of the vestiges that once may have distinguished our industry from others remain, and (2) if they do, determine the significance of such distinctiveness for organizational strategy. It is thus the purpose of this article to discuss areas of industry distinctiveness and to derive implications for the strategic management of health care organizations and for teaching strategic management in health administration programs.

INDUSTRY DISTINCTIVENESS PRIOR TO THE 1980s

For the better part of this century, the health care field has been assumed to be highly distinctive and deserving of special attention (or inattention, as the case may be). Many characteristics could account for this, including the fragmented structure of the industry, the unusual behavior of hospitals (which have been conceived of as cooperatives within which physicians maximize their incomes [4] or as "conspicuous producers" of sophisticated staff, equipment, and facilities [5]), and the tendency for federal and state governments to single out the industry for special regulatory and reimbursement controls. Of all the special traits, however, there is one that not only has been important historically, but should continue to affect the evolution of the industry as it moves toward the private-industry model: the centrality of patient need in the organization and financing of health services.

Before the era of diagnosis-related groups and major multi-institutional systems, students of the field had attempted to identify those few factors that account for the health care industry's special features. A unique market structure had evolved, but it was unclear whether this was merely an aberration of history or a product of some fundamental structural distinctiveness. In the 1960s, the noted economist Kenneth Boulding produced a classic paper postulating an answer to this question. In his article on the concept of need, Boulding captured a fundamental underpinning of the subdiscipline of health economics: the pervasive role played in the economics of health care by consumers who seek care to ameliorate perceived needs and whose decisions cannot be assumed to be made either autonomously or rationally [6]. Such consumer behavior violates the assumption of consumer sovereignty and gives rise to a sociological concept known as the sick role [7,8].

We suggest that the concept of need is so central in its importance that nearly all of the truly distinguishing characteristics of the field are tied to it. Many industries have complex technologies, mixes of both the public and private sectors, or poorly defined and thus not easily marketable services. But with only a few exceptions (the field of law comes to mind) does the lack of independence and the irrationality of the consumer, as embodied in the concept of need, play such an important part in the structuring of markets, roles, and organizations as is true in the health care field.

We explore the importance of patient need by focusing on three additional characteristics that have been identified by others as being unique to the health care field, but that have their roots in the concept of need: (1) market failure, (2) the professional dominance of physicians, and (3) an overriding public concern with the value of equal access. Figure 2.1 expresses graphically the relationship between each of these characteristics and the concept of need.

MARKET FAILURE

In another classic paper in health economics written in the early 1960s, Kenneth Arrow argued persuasively that it is the uncertainty inherent in medical care problems and the concomitant demand for information by ill people that most distinguish the market for health services:

> The value of information is frequently not known in any meaningful sense to the buyer; if, indeed, he knew enough to measure the value of information, he would know the information itself. But information, in the form

FIGURE 2.1

Traditional Sources of Distinctiveness in Health Care

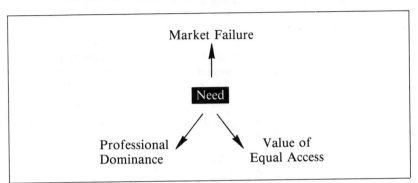

of skilled care, is precisely what is being bought from most physicians. . . .
The elusive character of information as a commodity suggests that it
departs considerably from the usual marketability assumptions about
commodities.

That risk and uncertainty are, in fact, significant elements in medical
care hardly needs argument. I will hold that virtually all the special features
of this industry, in fact, stem from the prevalence of uncertainty. [9]

Arrow contended that neither the content of information sought by
sick persons for relief of medical problems nor the value of that information could easily be determined. As a consequence, such information
could not be marketed with the same efficiency as that achieved in the
exchange of basic commodities, leading, in effect, to the failure of medical care markets (see Pauly [10] for an extension of Arrow's arguments
and Arnould and Debrock [11] for a more recent discussion of market
failure).

An additional point Arrow developed is that weaknesses in the structure of demand have contributed not only to the failure of health care
markets (relative to what might ideally be expected under the competitive
model) but to the creation of many unique social institutions organized
in response to these failures, thus contributing to still other distinctive
features in the health care industry.

Thus while Boulding and Arrow differed somewhat in the specific
dimensions they emphasized, both traced the distinctiveness of the field
to consumers and consumer difficulties in "demanding" medical care.
Arrow overlooked consumer irrationality due to illness (an essential fac-

tor underlying the concept of need), but clearly recognized the importance of uncertainty (an additional underlying factor) as a complicating factor in the structure of consumer demand.

PROFESSIONAL DOMINANCE

In another classic work, this time in the field of medical sociology, Eliot Freidson emphasized the powerful and distinctive role that physicians play in the health care field. At the heart of their influence, he argued, is their ability to claim "medical emergency" on behalf of their patients, contributing to a significant extent to a position of dominance in health care organizations, particularly in hospitals:

> The physician is able to intervene in many places in the hospital and justify his intervention on the basis of a "medical emergency"—a situation in which the well-being of a patient is said to be seriously in jeopardy and in which it is the physician alone who knows what is best done. We all are familiar with the dominant symbolic image: the interruption of orderly routine by a violent convulsion, heart failure, a hemorrhage. . . . While this no doubt happens on occasion, far more common in the hospital is the labeling of ambiguous events as emergencies by the doctor so as to gain the aid or resources he believes he needs. [12]

To a large extent the claim of medical emergency is based upon the same features Boulding and Arrow observed, namely, the uncertainty and threat inherent in the medical care problem and the complexity of the information needed to diagnose and treat that problem. As a result physicians and, to some degree, other health professionals have been able to create dual lines of authority in health care organizations [13,14] and to fragment public and private efforts to control the health care industry [15]. Professionals, of course, play important roles in other industries, too. But rarely have they gained so much autonomy in and influence over so complex a field as health care. Physicians' dominance is directly tied to their ability to use the concept of need to bolster their claim to autonomy in work.

THE VALUE OF EQUAL ACCESS

From the beginning of sophisticated, modern medicine, the public has recognized the need to assure, within limits, equal access to health services. How best to realize this value has been the subject of considerable debate. Nevertheless, there is little doubt that concern for equal access has been at the heart of many of this century's public programs [16,17].

The rationale for the concept of equal access in the health care field is primarily tied to the critical contribution health care makes to assuring that the basic rights required of a just society are preserved for all. Daniels expressed this point effectively:

> [We] can account for the special importance ascribed to health care needs by noting the connection between meeting those needs and the opportunity range open to individuals in a given society. This suggests that the principles of justice governing the distribution of health care should derive from our general principles of justice guaranteeing fair equality of opportunity (cf. John Rawls, 1971:Sect.14). Specifically, health care institutions will be among a variety of basic institutions (for example, educational ones) which are important because they insure that conditions of fair equality of opportunity obtain. [18]

Failure to provide needed treatment obviously could lead to the impairment of a person's ability to function normally in life. The concept of need, as Daniels clearly pointed out, is thus central to the argument for equality of opportunity. When combined with the essentially paternalistic dimension of need that Boulding developed, the equality of opportunity requirement gives a special public dimension to the health care field that often translates into a justification for public intervention into the financing and regulation of health services delivery.

INDUSTRY DISTINCTIVENESS BEYOND THE 1980s

In all, the health care field has developed a distinctive pattern. Health care has traditionally been conceived as outside the domain of private commodities and private markets. Industry fragmentation, the low priority given to efficiency, acceptance of the unusual relationship between physicians and health delivery organizations, and the apparent incongruity of health services delivery and the profit-making, marketing, and strategic behavior of health care organizations all have been justified by reference to the characteristics mentioned above. But now that we have entered the late 1980s, it appears that the usual assumptions about the distinctiveness of the health care field may no longer hold. Competition has taken hold, efficiency is the watchword of effective performance, and profit making and its companion concepts are becoming commonplace in the field.

Is it possible for the basic characteristics of a field to change so dramatically? To answer this, we must determine what has changed and what has not. Certainly the modus operandi of health administration has changed. It has been altered, perhaps permanently, by the incentives emanating from the health insurance industry and the federal government. Further, society has become more willing to accept entrepreneurial behavior in a historically need-based industry.

But what about the weaknesses in the market for health services, the dominance of the physician, and the concern for equality of access? It is probably true that the first of these, market failure due to an ineffective consumer, is changing, due to insurance companies' emergence as the "new consumers" of health services. Their changing role is prompted by enormous new pressures exerted by enlivened consumers of health insurance—large corporations, governments, and other insurance-purchasing organizations driven by a need to contain expenditures for health benefits.

The other two derivatives of the concept of need, however, should retain their importance in the field. The principle of equal (or at least assured) access may, in fact, emerge even more explicitly to protect those disenfranchised by the new system of delivery. The ongoing debate about the two-tiered health care system reflects continuing societal concern about how the changes in the field might affect our ability to assure that all persons receive needed health care services.

The field is less likely to be successful in assuring that the core of its business—the diagnosis and treatment of ill individuals—is properly buffered from the pressures of environmental and organizational change. We suggest that this may, by default, be accomplished through the agency of the physician. The dramatic changes already observed in the field do not appear to be altering the clinical relationship between patient and physician, although the business relationship most certainly will change as expected modifications in payment and organizational strategies take their course. The well-established autonomy of physicians in the technical or clinical zone of work also does not appear to be threatened. Reviewing physicians' "professional dominance" in light of recent changes in the health system Freidson noted, "It is true that they [physicians] are not wholly autonomous, but when one takes into account the operation of the invisible hand of the market in constraining the self-employed, putatively 'free' professional, they never were" [19]. In sum, the changes now underway should not alter significantly the legally sanctioned role of the physician ultimately to be responsible for the care of the patient. Thus physicians, drawn ever more into the world of cost containment, will retain their ability to claim medical emergency—a claim likely to be reinforced by the need to shepherd sick people through an increasingly market-driven and more bureaucratic health care delivery system.

And, of course, patient need—the root of these and possibly other distinctive features—remains a probable constraint on the restructuring of the health care industry. How then will the continuity in underlying characteristics affect patterns of change in the organization and delivery of health services? How will change affect the teaching of strategic management in health administration programs? Some indications of the new order are already visible. Others will require some speculation.

IMPLICATIONS FOR THE ORGANIZATION AND DELIVERY OF HEALTH SERVICES

Continuity in the concept of need and its derivatives should have important implications for how the health care industry restructures itself. Specifically, we will be concerned with the effect of the continuing role of the physician as agent for the patient and with the continuing requirement that all citizens be assured access to needed health services. We argue that these factors will filter or constrain the demands for cost control, corporate reorganization, and other changes affecting health care organizations. The aggregate effect of these demands is that the complexity of the environment faced by health care organizations has increased tremendously, producing a need to balance conflicting goals and address traditional sources of resistance.

As indicated in Figure 2.2, we suggest that the filtering effect is likely to be reflected in unique organizational (with emphasis on the strategic) and governmental adaptive responses to significant environmental change. In what follows, we highlight selected responses and then con-

FIGURE 2.2

Strategic Adaptation and Government Response in a
Rapidly Changing Health Care Environment

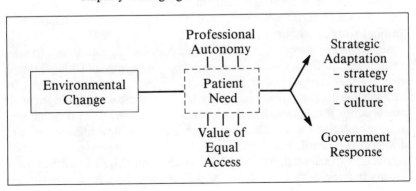

sider their implications for the teaching of strategic management in health administration programs.

STRATEGIC ADAPTATION

Responses to environmental change should occur in organizations within each of the major areas likely to be manipulated by administrators for purposes of adapting strategically: organizational strategy, structure, and culture [20,21,22]. Some specific organizational responses are discussed below.

Strategy

Major complexities involved in arranging integrated systems of delivery will force health care organizations to give priority to strategic issues at the local level. While much attention is being given to horizontal consolidation and the megafirm, another rapidly emerging form of organization is garnering increasing notice. At the grassroots of the changing health care system are a large number of complex systems that are being organized at the local or community level in response to complex patterns of community need and demand. These include many small multi-institutional systems, many actively developing hospitals (independents or members of systems), HMOs, and other permutations and combinations of systems, all of which are driven by factors imbedded in system integration at the local level [23]. Some of the factors affecting organization and delivery at the local level are physician organization, insurance competition, and history and tradition.

Physician organization. Despite the powerful forces leading to consolidation within the health care industry, the extent to which these will lead to consolidation of physicians beyond the local level is unclear. For many reasons, some of which have already been discussed, it is reasonable to assume that physicians will become organized, but predominantly around local referral networks, informal colleague relationships, and hospital staff appointments.

Insurance competition. Insurance organizations will consolidate to take advantage of obvious economies in larger financing and management arrangements. On the other hand, with the exception, for example, of national health insurance markets in which contracts are arranged with major national or international corporations, the market for health insurance is essentially local. This is because integrated health insurance and delivery systems will primarily be governed by the markets in which health services are distributed, which are effectively local [24]. The need to offer prospective clients "local systems" of delivery will force insurance companies to establish formal ties with local health care organizations (for example, local multihospital systems and networks of primary care centers or physician groups), so that the insurance companies can compete more effectively at the local level and facilitate the control of health care costs.

History and tradition. The organizational and political dimensions of medical practice at the local level are well-rooted in local tradition and history. Many local hospitals have long-established constituencies and local physicians have enduring and significant linkages, carefully cultured as a necessary dimension of practice development. These firmly cemented professional relationships, values, and constituencies represent major barriers to organizational change, especially if the source of that change appears to be some distant corporate headquarters. These factors add to the environmental complexity with which health care organizations of all types must deal and thus give added impetus to the focus of organizational strategy at the local market level.

Local system development is clearly the product of health care firms' adapting to a changing environment, but within the constraints of a complex webbing of structures (including those effectively preserving the traditional autonomy of physicians) designed to provide for diverse and unpredictable patient needs. Local factors thus can be expected to have a major impact on the restructuring of the delivery system, a point developed repeatedly below.

Successful strategic adaptation in the future will be determined by both the innovative and efficiency-directed adaptive responses of health care organizations. Complex environmental changes in the field have created pressures for health care organizations to adapt in equally complex and often contradictory ways. Rising health care costs have forced improvements in the efficiency of health care delivery. Simultaneously, the increasing complexity of and intensity of rivalry in local delivery and insurance markets have caused health care organizations to innovate in their design of product and service offerings, some of which may ultimately increase the costs of health care [25,26]. The conflict in objectives can be traced to the significant diversity, from one area to the next, of the needs of local populations and to the diversity of demands placed on health care organizations by insurance companies, employers, government agencies, and providers of care. Emphasis on innovation may even accelerate with time, especially if the incentives of market and reimbursement mechanisms produce needed efficiencies. To the extent that this occurs, quality will emerge as the overriding determinant of business success. This conclusion is especially justified, given the critical nature of need and the consequent signaling value of quality in the health care marketplace.

Horizontal expansion, the dominant strategy of the late 1970s and early

1980s, will give way to a combined strategy of vertical integration of insurance and delivery systems at the local level and horizontal expansion of such systems at the national level. This conclusion is a direct extension of all that has been discussed thus far. Horizontal expansion by health care organizations served a purpose at a time of growing rivalry and threat and when delivery and payment systems still functioned relatively independently. However, increasingly intense competition in local insurance markets has produced great pressures for delivery and insurance organizations to integrate vertically to assure coordinated systems of delivery. An expected tendency to resort to formal rather than more purely market mechanisms for achieving such coordination is attributable not only to changing expectations of cost- and quality-conscious private industry and governmental organizations, but, again, to the complexity of patient needs and systems of care. It is not clear whether horizontally expanded delivery systems will be more or less effective in producing vertically integrated delivery and insurance systems at the local level. What can be argued, however, is that vertical integration is emerging as the dominant strategic approach to survival in a less predictable health care industry.

Structure

Health care organizations, regardless of size, will rapidly adopt divisionalized structures (either product based or geographically based) to facilitate complex strategies of product diversification. The trend toward divisionalized and away from functional structures is already well under way [27]. What is surprising about this trend is the pace at which it is occurring. The shift can be explained, in part, by new, combined vertical and horizontal growth strategies being adopted by health care organizations and by an orientation, possibly stimulated by the constraints of regulation, toward growth through acquisition rather than internal development and expansion [28,29].

It can also be explained, at least indirectly, by the inability of health care organizations to achieve growth without accommodating diverse claims on autonomy that accompany movement into new areas of service. The historically fragmented structure of the health care industry, both within and between major service sectors, is not likely to be easily overcome. Health care organizations are thus more likely, perhaps, than equivalent-sized firms in other industries to adopt at early stages of growth a divisionalized organizational structure. This particular structure also is consistent with the patterns of local strategic development predicted above.

Better-performing health care organizations will be those whose struc-

tures are relatively decentralized. To meet the demands of different markets and to remain responsive to changes in those markets, multiproduct health care organizations will rely upon decentralized decision-making structures. Compared to most other industrial organizations, the large health care organization is more limited in its ability to centralize decision making if flexibility in meeting consumer and physician demands is to be maintained. This applies even to centralization of the functional area of strategic planning. As a result, we would speculate that small, geographically concentrated health care organizations will, in the long run, be able to outperform large, geographically dispersed ones in spite of the economies of scale the larger organizations can bring to many activities.

The interorganizational contract (between physicians as collectivities and other health care organizations) will be the primary mechanism for integrating physicians into health care organizations. A number of the new organizational forms that have recently emerged in the health care field actually represent variations in the structure of contractual relationships among the various participants in the field, for example, independent practice associations (IPAs), PPOS, and HMOs. The intricate contractual web being spun among many historically independent elements in the field is the logical byproduct of a system continually adjusting to the prerequisites of need. The contract essentially preserves the many bastions or zones of autonomy, legitimized over time by independently exercised claims of "medical emergency," however current those claims may be. It is likely that such zones will erode very slowly, despite the powerful force of the new economics.

Physicians will continue to move into larger and more formal organizational forms as they attempt to buffer their professional work from an increasingly threatening and uncertain external environment. A corollary to the discussion of the contract is the probability that physicians will evolve consolidated medical practices for purposes of structuring referral and consultation linkages and managing growing complexities in the areas of payment, malpractice, regulation, and interorganizational relations. Consistent with traditional and continuing claims on autonomy, these organizations will primarily be controlled by and designed to serve the interests of the physicians who become their members. To survive in the new health care environment, however, such organizations will assume a greater bureaucratic form than they have in the past and will engage in more strategic and competitive behaviors. Many of these organizations will be internal to other health care organizations (for instance, physician staff organizations within HMOs and multihospital systems). Nevertheless, as suggested above, the structure of such relationships will be defined more through contractual mechanisms than through standard employee-employer arrangements.

Culture

The need to build collaborative relationships between physicians and major health care organizations (particularly hospitals, insurance companies, and HMOs) will require such organizations to be highly innovative in the creation of facilitating organizational cultures. Attempts by health care organizations to be both efficient and innovative to survive in the current environment will certainly challenge them to find ways to gain the cooperation and support of physicians. It is unlikely that the old strategies of cooptation as, for example, utilized by hospitals to encourage physicians to admit patients, will work as effectively in the future as they have in the past. New structural arrangements will help, though the degree to which they produce sufficient unity to facilitate strategic realignments will depend upon the effectiveness with which an accommodating organizational culture is also produced [30]. The health care organization must recognize physicians' need to protect the autonomy and financial viability of their practice while they participate in new programs and other innovations.

Ties to local community cultures will continue to be important in the effectiveness of health care organizations. Traditionally, hospitals have been expert at fitting in with their communities; a benevolent external environment allowed "community service" efforts to exist and be financed at relatively high levels. Hospitals have been institutional "pillars" of their communities, reflecting and engendering community values. Those institutions that can continue to mesh with community values, particularly values reflecting the concept of need, will prove more effective in the long run than those that ignore community norms in the interest of short-term profits or efficiency. Balancing community ties and efficiency will be a tough act for health care organizations. But as ong as local health care markets exert a strong influence—and we have argued that they will—adherence to the community service norm will be a prerequisite for effective performance.

As health care organizations aggregate into larger organizational forms, integrating the different organizational cultures into one unit will be a growing concern. The hospital in the recent past had a relatively cohesive set of norms and values that its employees shared, but this may no longer be the case. Managing organizational culture in today's health care organizations is not a simple job, nor will it become more so. The integration of organizations providing differentiated services and products or serving different market segments will require greater organizational attention to creating shared norms across the organization, by the use of such activities as those outlined in Theory Z management and the corporate culture literature [31,32]. Efforts toward cohesion will need to be tempered by recognition of the uniqueness of each of the components of the organization.

These are only a few of the adaptive responses that can be expected of health care organizations and professionals. Again, at the heart of these responses is the continuing challenge to manage complex patient needs, complicated by dramatically changing organizations, patterns of demand, and governmental systems of control.

GOVERNMENT RESPONSE

If our speculations about continuities in the field of health care are correct, we can anticipate that the role of government policy will shift in at least two major areas: public assistance and regulation. We briefly comment on these, as they have implications for the strategic management of health care organizations in the 1990s.

Disenfranchisement of those not covered by either private health insurance or public assistance programs and the trend toward a separate system for the poor will continue, producing new calls for public involvement in the payment for health services. The pressures that led in the early 1970s to widespread proposals for the implementation of a national health insurance system will build once again as the side effects of the current revolution in health care organization take their course. However, while the need for all citizens to receive adequate health care will remain unchanged, the mechanisms proposed for addressing that need may differ from those put forward in the early 1970s, when an apparent consensus had been reached that some form of national health insurance was needed. Proposals gaining national attention will be less likely to focus on middle to upper income populations, groups already reasonably well covered by private health insurance programs, than on much narrower population segments, particularly the "uncompensated care" groups who find themselves inadequately covered by the growing private insurance system (see Sloan, Blumstein, and Perrin [33]).

State and federal governments will expand their regulatory roles as they attempt to protect the patient in a health care industry increasingly responsive to the new corporate consumer. As corporations direct health care dollars to insurance companies and insurance companies funnel patients to hospitals and physicians, commitment to the traditional consumers — physicians and their patients — will erode. The patient, once the purchaser of services, is becoming the user of a network of services arranged through a four-step structure of negotiations and contracts: physicians to hospitals, hospitals to insurance companies, insurance companies to benefits officers in corporations, and finally corporations to employees (who become patients).

While it is too soon to determine the full consequences of this fundamental shift in market structure, it can be deduced, given the force of a rapidly changing environment, that a happy patient may be far less critical to the economic welfare of a health care organization or provider than will a satisfied corporate consumer. From a marketing point of view, of course, the happiness of the former may be directly tied to the satisfaction of the latter. However, the distance between the patient and the benefits officer making choices among health insurance systems may be so great that the markets will fail to be valid mechanisms for protecting the interests of patients per se. It is in this context that state and federal governments may need to intervene (through facility and human resources regulation) to assure that the quality of care delivered to the populace remains uniformly high.

This possibility does not contradict the points made earlier that quality will be increasingly emphasized as efficiencies are achieved and that markets will give greater priority to qualitative differences (differentiation) among health care organizations. As reasoned above, markets cannot be expected to be effective regulators of quality, despite the importance quality may play in future market decisions. While the purchasers of insurance may discriminate heavily according to qualitative differences among health delivery and insurance systems, it is doubtful that they can be relied upon to assure true quality. Thus we predict a greater government role in assuring the quality of health care.

These points and many others not discussed are logical responses to and by an industry delegated the role of making critically important clinical (and often economic) decisions for sick people. This role, a derivative of the concept of need, must be protected, especially in an era in which the traditional business model appears to be shaping organizational strategic behaviors and governmental policy.

IMPLICATIONS FOR CURRICULA IN HEALTH ADMINISTRATION

A changing industry clearly calls for thoughtful reassessments of curricula in health administration programs. As stated earlier, we suggest that particular attention should be given to assessing the role and teaching of strategic management in health administration curricula. This is because health care organizations are forced to undergo major organizational transformations, in both their structures and their guiding organizational strategies, in the face of an unprecedented revolution in the health care industry. Certainly, general management issues may need further attention in health administration curricula. However, it is the strategic area that is most likely to be underemphasized, given the relative recency of significant environmental change. Future leaders of the field must be equipped with useful, intellectual frames of reference if they are to labor for the survival of their organizations in a world of uncertainty and threat.

A first point is that, in teaching health care strategy, we should not assume that insights gleaned from the study of firms in other industries can readily be applied to the health care industry. Uniquenesses in industry structure, firm behavior, and the general environment, particularly as observed at the local level, make it essential that the concepts of strategy be fully assessed, modified, and tailored to fit the distinctive needs of the field. Before private-industry models of strategic behavior are integrated into teaching, faculty should: (1) carefully assess whether or not any of the vestiges that may once have distinguished the health care industry from the others remain, and (2) determine the significance of any such remaining distinctions for the teaching of health care strategic management.

Specifically, we suggest that faculty give considerable emphasis, both in teaching and in the development of innovative course content, to the areas of strategy, industry and competitor analysis, and the design of complex organizations. The major challenge facing health care strategic managers is to forge new organizational arrangements and strategies that take into account the complexities of local environments, delivery modalities, governmental regulations, and public expectations and the problems of managing organizations heavily influenced by powerful health professionals.

Care should be taken, however, to assure that purely descriptive material and increasingly outdated concepts (e.g., HMO, IPA, PPO, multi-institutional systems, alternative health systems) are not presented in the guise of strategic concepts. The pace of change and the intricacies of organizational forms in the health care industry guarantee the speedy obsolescence of such material. Instead, students must be exposed to the analytic techniques and conceptual frameworks that would enable them to assess industry, market, and organizational change. The needed conceptual and analytical skills fall under the general label of "strategic thinking" [34]. Strategic thinking requires that students be able, for instance, to internalize and use models of organizational adaptation that are developed in the disciplines of industrial economics and organizational theory (for an example, see Yasai-Ardekani [35]). Such models help to clarify and generalize the interdependencies that exist among organizational strategy, structure, and culture, between focal and other organizations, and between organizations and their environments. Encouraging strategic thinking is a bit like encouraging creativity and "blue-sky" thought, but with a strong grounding in basic management sciences.

Second, given the uniqueness of the health care industry, faculty should take care, in teaching strategic management, to integrate into the training practical examples and experiences. Unfortunately, the field appears to be advancing far faster than the knowledge base of faculty or the supporting literature. We have already argued that the standard examples derived from other industries may not fit situations in the health care industry. Therefore, there is an additional need to develop current case material to support the teaching of strategic management within health care organizations, and this material must be updated, modified, and revised with frequency. The field is evolving so rapidly that last year's cases may no longer reflect current realities.

Faculty also need to identify a cadre of leaders in the field and encourage them to come into the classroom and contribute to teaching within programs in health administration. A wide range of individuals must be so identified to assure coverage of key disciplines and unique organizational forms and product and market strategies. Particular attention needs to be given to seeking those practitioners who represent the organizational forms taking shape at the local level of health care delivery as well as those who bring a national perspective on the developing health care sector.

Third, a clear distinction must be made in the classroom between more traditional marketing and planning content and evolving content relating to strategic thinking, new venture development, and entrepreneurialism. The evolving content draws more on synthesizing didactic and experiential content than on learning procedures and memorizing terms. To assure that sufficient focus is given to these more creative areas of health administration training, it may be necessary to offer a whole course in strategic thinking or entrepreneurialism.

Fourth, specific areas of uniqueness in the health care field must be properly analyzed for their curricular implications. It may be necessary for a new paradigm to replace the older medical care organization (MCO) framework which emerged in the 1960s as the hallmark of health administration education. MCO became the integrating content area that assured that the traditional values associated with equal access and equity would be reflected in characterizations of the health care field. Those traditional values, we have argued, are still operative. However, they appear now to be operationalized more around problems of strategically and structurally orienting organizations that are able both to compete and to serve community needs. The old and new paradigms reflect differences not only in a national versus a local focus on issues, but in a private versus a public orientation to how the needs of society are to be met. The conceptual incompatibilities between the two paradigms need to be identified and associated ethical issues fully explored.

Finally, and related to several of the foregoing points, elevating the didactic role of strategic thinking might require that relatively less attention be given to the process and techniques of strategic planning in courses on strategic management. This is because the elements of health organization strategy are more likely to be uniquely linked to the distinctive features of the field than are the techniques of decision making, which themselves should be relatively generalizable across industries. This implies, of course, that the health care field is not only distinctive, but that its distinctiveness is sufficient to justify the search for strategic elements that may be unique to health care organizations. In a complex and rapidly changing health care environment, strategic thinking becomes a more vital skill than the ability to carry out "rationally" the traditional planning process. The requirement that organizations create feasible options that balance pressures to contain costs yet preserve physician autonomy and equal access to care clearly is not an ordinary task of the typical business organization. It is one which, if not undertaken with considerable forethought, could result in serious damage to an industry facing the challenge of its modern life.

REFERENCES

1. Quoted in Punch, L. Investor-Owned Chains Lead Increase in Beds. *Modern Healthcare* (June 20): 126–36, 1985.

2. Bernstein Research. *The Future of Health Care Delivery in America.* New York: Sanford C. Bernstein & Co., 1985.

3. Hofer, C.W. Toward a Contingency Theory of Business Strategy. *Academy of Management Journal* 18: 784–810, 1975.

4. Pauly, M., and M. Redish. The Not-for-Profit Hospital as a Physicians' Cooperative. *American Economic Review* 63: 87–99, 1973.

5. Lee, M.L. A Conspicuous Production Theory of Hospital Behavior. *Southern Economic Journal* 38: 48–58, 1971.

6. Boulding, K.E. The Concept of Need for Health Services. *Milbank Memorial Fund Quarterly* 44: 202–21, 1966.

7. Parsons, T. Definitions of Health and Illness in the Light of American Values and Social Structure. In *Patients, Physicians, and Illness*, ed. E.G. Jaco. Glencoe, IL: Free Press, 1958.

8.   Gallagher, E.B. Lines of Reconstruction and Extension in the Parsonian Sociology of Illness. *Social Science and Medicine* 10: 207–18, 1976.

9.   Arrow, K.J. Uncertainty and the Welfare Economics of Medical Care. *American Economic Review* 53: 941–73, 1963.

10.   Pauly, M.V. Is Medical Care Different? In *Competition in the Health Care Sector: Past, Present, and Future*, ed. W. Greenberg. Rockville, MD: Aspen Systems, 1978.

11.   Arnould, R., and L.M. Debrock. Competition and Market Failure in the Hospital Industry: A Review of the Evidence. *Medical Care Review* 43: 253–92, 1986.

12.   Freidson, E. *Profession of Medicine: A Study of the Sociology of Applied Knowledge*. New York: Dodd, Mead, 1970. p. 118.

13.   Harris, J.E. The Internal Organization of Hospitals: Some Economic Implications. *Bell Journal of Economics* 8: 467–82, 1977.

14.   Smith, H.L. Two Lines of Authority are One Too Many. *Modern Hospital* 84: 59–64, 1955.

15.   Starr, P. *The Social Transformation of American Medicine*. New York: Basic Books, 1982.

16.   Davis, K., and C. Schoen. *Health and the War on Poverty: A Ten Year Appraisal*. Washington, DC: Brookings Institution, 1978.

17.   Jain, S.C. Policy Concerns and the Changing Role of Government in Personal Health: A Perspective. In *Policy Issues in Personal Health Services*, ed. S.C. Jain and J.E. Paul. Rockville, MD: Aspen Systems, 1983.

18.   Daniels, N. Equity of Access to Health Care: Some Conceptual and Ethical Issues. *Milbank Memorial Fund Quarterly/Health and Society* 60: 51–81, 1982, p. 72.

19.   Freidson, E. The Reorganization of the Medical Profession. *Medical Care Review* 42: 11–36, 1985.

20.   Chandler, A.D. *Strategy and Structure*. Cambridge, MA: MIT Press, 1962.

21.   Kimberly, J.R., and E.J. Zajac. Strategic Adaptation in Health Care Organizations: Implications for Theory and Research. *Medical Care Review* 42: 267–302, 1985.

22.   Meyer, A.D. Adapting to Environmental Jolts. *Administrative Science Quarterly* 27: 515–37, 1982.

23.   Luft, H., J.C. Robinson, D.W. Garnick, R.G. Hughes, S.J. McPhee, S.S. Hunt, and J. Showstack. Hospital Behavior within a Local Market Context. *Medical Care Review* 43: 271–51, 1986.

24.   Luft, H. See number 23.

25.   Porter, M.E. *Competitive Advantage: Creating and Sustaining Superior Performance*. New York: Free Press, 1985.

26.   Lawrence, P.R., and D. Dyer. *Renewing American Industry*. New York: Free Press, 1983.

27. Alexander, J.A., and M.L. Fennell. Multihospital Systems as Divisionalized Forms. Paper presented at the 1984 meeting of the Academy of Management, Boston, 1984.

28. Alexander, J.A., B.L. Lewis, and M.A. Morrisey. Acquisition Strategies of Multihospital Systems. *Health Affairs* 4: 49–66, 1985.

29. Pitts, R.A. Strategies and Structures for Diversification. *Academy of Management Journal* 20: 197–208, 1977.

30. Shortell, S.M., T.M. Wickizer, and J.R.C. Wheeler. *Hospital-Physician Joint Ventures*. Ann Arbor, MI: Health Administration Press, 1984.

31. Ouchi, W.G. *Theory Z*. Reading, MA: Addison-Wesley, 1981.

32. Kilmann, R.H., M.J. Saxton, R. Serpa, and Associates. *Gaining Control of the Corporate Culture*. San Francisco: Jossey-Bass, 1985.

33. Sloan, F.A., J.F. Blumstein, and J.M. Perrin, eds. *Uncompensated Hospital Care: Rights and Responsibilities*. Baltimore: Johns Hopkins University Press, 1986.

34. Hickman, C.R., and M.A. Silva. *Creating Excellence*. New York: New American Library, 1984.

35. Yasai-Ardekani, M. Structural Adaptations to Environments. *Academy of Management Review* 11: 9–21, 1986.

American College of Healthcare Executives Code of Ethics

Introduction by
Duncan Neuhauser

INTRODUCTION

The American College of Healthcare Executives (formerly the American College of Hospital Administrators) was organized in 1933. Today it is the foremost professional association of health managers and, in particular, hospital administrators. From the outset, the College was concerned with the ethical conduct of its members. In 1938 a special committee was appointed to develop a code of ethics. After this committee had struggled with the code for some time, its members determined that an administrator's code would not logically be separated from a code applying to all hospital workers, so a joint committee was established with the American Hospital Association (AHA).

Since the subject matter was ethics, the viewpoints of religious hospital associations were taken into consideration. The drafting committee was careful to include influential members of major religious groups. It was not until June 1941 that the code received final approval by both organizations and was published.

THE 1941 CODE

According to the 1941 code, the primary objective of the hospital was to render care to the sick and injured. Financial concern and other inter-

Introduction based on Duncan Neuhauser, *Coming of Age* (Chicago: Pluribus Press, 1983).

ests were of secondary consideration. Another duty of the hospital was to advance scientific knowledge and the education of all participating in the work, and to take an active part in the promotion of general health. This was an obvious but profound statement of the central values of the hospital field.

The trustees had the duty to determine policies and to provide equipment and facilities consistent with community needs. The requirement to plan for community needs preceded the Hill-Burton Act of 1946, the growth of voluntary regional planning organizations, and the Federal Health Planning Act of 1966. The trustees were also responsible for seeing that proper professional standards were maintained for the care of the sick. Over the years, many court decisions have held the trustees responsible for delivering a reasonable standard of care.

No member of the hospital's board of trustees was allowed to profit by connection with the hospital. The trustee's voluntary commitment to the hospital was emphasized. Today's code has been amended to allow for proprietary (private) hospitals.

The 1941 code stated that, to ensure that "the medical staff be properly organized," medical records should be complete and adequate. Keeping adequate medical records was a chief concern of the American College of Surgeons, which managed the hospital accreditation program from 1918 until 1956; today, it is the concern of the Joint Commission on the Accreditation of Healthcare Organizations (JCAHO).

According to the 1941 code, "there should be no solicitation for patients by a hospital or by any person connected with it." Of course, this stance has been changed by the Federal Trade Commission's opposition to professional limits on advertising, and the rise of marketing as a legitimate activity for hospitals.

Hospitals "should bear to each other a spirit of friendly cooperation and interest." Whenever possible, unnecessary duplication of facilities in competing institutions was to be avoided. Competition between hospitals did not become a legitimate view of hospital relationships until the late 1970s.

"Hospitals should refrain from participating in contracts with companies, organizations, municipalities, governments or other bodies at rates which are obviously unfair to other hospitals in the community." Such contracts included those that paid the provider a fixed amount of money per person cared for; they were analogous to today's health maintenance organizations (HMOs). This policy continued through the 1947 and 1958 codes, but it was not part of the 1973 code.

Today's HMOs were once bitterly opposed because, both in the United States and in England, a company would seek the lowest bid from a doctor to provide medical care for its employees. In an era before the 1910 Flexner reforms made doctors scarce, hungry doctors were willing to bid very low prices and provide minimal care. The lowest bidder might have been the worst and hungriest physician.

"All hospitals operated by a church organization and for all patients who are members thereof, it is expected that the Moral Code of that denomination be observed." By 1980 this statement had become the following: "Health care institutions, wherever possible and consistent with ethical commitments of the institutions, should ensure respect and consideration for reasonable accommodation of the individual religious and social beliefs and customs of patients, employees, physicians, and others." The specific ethnic and religious focus that was common in many hospitals in earlier decades has been replaced by an ecumenical emphasis in recent years.

Recruiting nurses from other hospitals by holding teas or open houses was considered an unethical practice in 1941. In addition, an administrator was criticized for sending out large numbers of resumes in a shotgun approach to job hunting; this was seen as diminishing the dignity of the member and the College.

The joint committee of the American Hospital Association and the American College of Healthcare Executives continued its work on the code, publishing revisions in 1947, 1957, and 1963. In 1966 the College began to use the code more actively as a basis for disciplining unethical behavior. (The issue of adjudication contributed to the eventual division of the code in 1967.) The College went on to develop and publish a formal grievance procedure, which allowed any College member whose behavior was under review to present evidence in his or her own defense. In the early days, a working definition of ethical conduct was summarized as follows: "If you can stand to have that story printed on the front page of your local paper, it's probably okay." Unethical behavior included personal aggrandizement, recruiting employees of other neighborhood hospitals, and actively seeking to take a job away from a fellow administrator.

TODAY'S COMMITTEE ON ETHICS

In 1967 the decision was made to separate the College's ethical code for administrators, which would be used as the basis for disciplinary action, from the AHA's code for hospitals and health care institutions. The College first published its own code in 1970. Today, College members are expected to adhere to the Code of Ethics with the understanding that the ultimate punishment for unethical behavior is expulsion from the College. The Committee on Ethics focuses on serious ethical violations such as kickbacks, stealing, sexual harassment, and misappropriation of funds. This is not to imply that the ethical standards of health care administrators have deteriorated. There is no evidence that their standards have changed, for better or for worse, over the last 50 years.

AMERICAN COLLEGE OF HEALTHCARE EXECUTIVES CODE OF ETHICS*

PREFACE

The Code of Ethics is administered by the Committee on Ethics, which is appointed by the Board of Governors upon nomination by the Chairman. It is composed of nine Fellows of the College, each of whom serves a three-year term on a staggered basis, with three members retiring each year.

The Committee on Ethics shall:

- Review and evaluate annually the Code of Ethics, and make any necessary recommendations for updating the Code.
- Review and recommend action to the Board of Governors on allegations brought forth regarding breaches of the Code of Ethics.
- Refine the Code of Ethics to specific applications and to relate the Code to several membership classifications as compared to the Code for hospitals as institutions.
- Prepare a report of observations, accomplishments, and recommendations to the Board of Governors at the annual reporting session, and such other periodic reports as required.

The Committee on Ethics invokes the Code of Ethics under authority of the ACHE *Bylaws*, Article II, Affiliation, Section II (b), Termination of Affiliation, as follows:

Affiliation may be terminated by action of the Board of Governors as a result of violation of the Code of Ethics, nonconformity with the Bylaws or Regulations Governing Admission, Advancement and Recertification or conduct unbecoming an affiliate, as determined by the Board of Governors. No such termination of affiliation shall be effected without affording a reasonable opportunity for the affiliate to consider the charges and to

---

*Reprinted from *1988–1989 Annual Report* (Chicago, 1989), pp. 39–42, with permission, The American College of Healthcare Executives.

appear in his or her own defense before the Board of Governors or its designated hearing committee, as outlined in the "Grievance Procedure," Appendix I of the College's Code of Ethics.

PREAMBLE

The purpose of the code of Ethics of the American College of Healthcare Executives is to serve as a guide to conduct for affiliates. It contains standards of ethical behavior for healthcare executives in their professional relationships. These relationships include members of the healthcare executive's organization and other organizations. Also included are patients, clients or others served, colleagues, the community and society as a whole. The Code of Ethics also incorporates standards of ethical behavior governing personal behavior, particularly when that conduct directly relates to the role and identity of the healthcare executive.

The fundamental objectives of the healthcare management profession are to enhance overall quality of life, dignity and well-being of every individual needing healthcare services; and to create a more equitable, accessible, effective and efficient healthcare system.

Healthcare executives have an obligation to act in ways that will merit the trust, confidence and respect of healthcare professionals and the general public. To do so, healthcare executives must lead lives that embody an exemplary system of values and ethics.

In fulfilling their commitments and obligations to patients, clients or others they serve, healthcare executives function as moral agents. Since every management decision affects the health and well-being of both individuals and communities, healthcare executives must evaluate the possible outcomes of their decisions and accept full responsibility for the consequences. In organizations that deliver healthcare services, they must safeguard and foster the rights, interests and prerogatives of patients, clients or others served. The role of moral agent requires that healthcare executives speak out and take actions necessary to promote such rights, interests and prerogatives if they are threatened.

I. THE HEALTHCARE EXECUTIVE'S RESPONSIBILITIES TO THE PROFESSION OF HEALTHCARE MANAGEMENT

The healthcare executive shall:

A. Uphold the values, ethics and mission of the healthcare management profession;

B. Conduct all personal and professional activities with honesty, integrity, respect, fairness and good faith in a manner that will reflect well upon the profession;

C. Comply with all laws in the jurisdictions in which the healthcare executive is located, or conducts professional or personal activities;

D. Maintain competence and proficiency in healthcare management by implementing a personal program of assessment and continuing professional education;

E. Avoid the exploitation of professional relationships for personal gain;

F. Use this code to further the interests of the profession and not for selfish reasons;

G. Respect professional confidences;

H. Enhance the dignity and image of the healthcare management profession through positive public information programs;

I. Refrain from participating in any endorsement or publicity that demeans the credibility and dignity of the healthcare management profession; and

J. Refrain from using the College's credential or affiliation with the College to promote or endorse external commercial products or services.

II. THE HEALTHCARE EXECUTIVE'S OBLIGATIONS TO THE ORGANIZATION AND TO PATIENTS, CLIENTS OR OTHERS SERVED

A. Commitments to the Organization

The healthcare executive shall:

1. Provide healthcare services consistent with available resources and assure the existence of a resource allocation process that considers ethical ramifications;

2. Conduct both competitive and cooperative activities in ways that improve community healthcare services;

3. Lead the organization in the use and improvement of standards of management and sound business practices;

4. Respect the customs and practices of patients, clients or others served, consistent with the organization's philosophy; and

5. Be truthful in all forms of professional and organizational communication and avoid information that is false, misleading, and deceptive or information that would create unreasonable expectations.

B. Commitments to Patients, Clients or Others Served

The healthcare executive shall:

1. Assure the existence of a process to evaluate the quality of care or service rendered;
2. Avoid exploitation of relationships for personal advantage;
3. Avoid practicing or facilitating discrimination and institute safeguards to prevent discriminatory organizational practices;
4. Assure the existence of a process that will advise patients, clients or others served of the rights, opportunities, responsibilities and risks regarding available healthcare services;
5. Provide a process which assures the autonomy and self-determination of patients, clients or others served; and
6. Assure the existence of procedures that will safeguard the confidentiality and privacy of patients, clients and others served.

C. Conflicts of Interest

A conflict of interest may be only a matter of degree, but exists when the healthcare executive:

- is in a position to benefit directly or indirectly by using authority or inside information, or allows a friend, relative or associate to benefit from such authority or information.
- uses authority or information to make a decision to intentionally affect the organization in an adverse manner.

The healthcare executive shall:

1. Conduct all personal and professional relationships in such a way that all those affected are assured that management decisions are made in the best interests of the organization and the individuals served by it;
2. Disclose to the appropriate authority any direct or indirect financial or personal interests that might pose potential conflicts of interest;
3. Accept no gifts or benefits offered with the expectation of influencing a management decision; and
4. Inform the appropriate authority and other involved parties of potential conflicts of interest related to appointments or elections to boards or committees inside or outside the healthcare executive's organization.

III. THE HEALTHCARE EXECUTIVE'S
RESPONSIBILITIES TO COMMUNITY
AND SOCIETY

The healthcare executive shall:

A. Work to identify and meet the healthcare needs of the community;
B. Work to assure that all people have reasonable access to healthcare services;
C. Participate in public dialogue on healthcare policy issues and advocate solutions that will improve health status and promote quality healthcare;
D. Consider the short-term and long-term impact of management decisions on both the community and on society; and
E. Provide prospective consumers with adequate and accurate information, enabling them to make enlightened judgments and decisions regarding services.

IV. THE HEALTHCARE EXECUTIVE'S DUTY TO
REPORT VIOLATIONS OF THE CODE

An affiliate of the College who has reasonable grounds to believe that another affiliate has violated this Code has a duty to communicate such facts to the Committee on Ethics.

APPENDIX I
AMERICAN COLLEGE OF HEALTHCARE
EXECUTIVES GRIEVANCE PROCEDURE

1. To be processed, a complaint must be filed in writing to the Committee on Ethics of the College within three years of the date of the alleged incident; and, the committee has the responsibility to look into incidents brought to its attention regardless of the informality of the information, provided the information can be documented or may be a matter of public record. The three-year period within which a complaint must be filed shall temporarily cease to run during intervals when the affiliate is in inactive or suspended status, or when the affiliate resigns from the College.
2. Specifics of the complaint must be sent to the respondent, preferably by certified mail, by the staff of the College.
3. Upon receipt of the complaint, the Committee on Ethics shall refer the matter to the Regent of the area in which the respon-

dent presently is employed. The Regent shall make inquiry into the matter and in the process the respondent shall be given an opportunity to be heard.

4. Upon completion of the inquiry the Regent shall present a complete report in writing to the Committee on Ethics. In the report, the Regent may make recommendations regarding the disposition of the case.

5. Upon receipt of the Regent's report, and following the Committee's review and action, a copy of the report shall be sent promptly to the respondent.

6. If the respondent wishes to appeal, he may do so formally by a written request. This request must be filed with the Committee within sixty days from the date of the Regent's report.

7. If a respondent so requests, or if the Committee on Ethics or the complainant wishes to pursue the matter further, then the Committee on Ethics shall recommend to the ACHE Chairman the appointment of an ad hoc committee to hear the matter.

8. This ad hoc committee shall consist of three Fellows from the region of the respondent's area of employment at the time of the alleged infraction of the Code of Ethics. Adequate notice of the formation of this committee, notice of the hearing date, with an opportunity for representation, shall be mailed to the respondent. Notice of the ad hoc committee and the date of the hearing shall be given to the complainant. At least thirty days notice of the hearing date shall be given to all parties concerned. Reasonable requests for postponement shall be given consideration.

9. The ad hoc committee shall give the complainant and respondent adequate opportunity to present their cases and to be represented, if they so desire. At the close of the hearing, the ad hoc committee shall write a detailed report with recommendations to the Committee on Ethics.

10. A copy of this report shall go promptly to the respondent. If the respondent wishes to pursue the matter further, he may request, within sixty days of the date of the ad hoc committee's report, an appearance before the Committee on Ethics. The Committee shall give the respondent opportunity to state his case. Following this appeals hearing, the Committee on Ethics shall make its decision and provide the respondent with a copy of its report to the Board of Governors.

11. If the respondent wishes to pursue the matter further, he may request, within sixty days of the date of the Committee on

Ethics report, a review of the case by the Board of Governors. Following a review by the Board of Governors, the Board shall make its decision and provide the respondent and complainant with a copy of its decision. The decision of the Board of Governors shall be final.

APPENDIX II

Once the grievance procedure has been initiated, the Committee on Ethics may take any of the following actions based upon its findings:

A. Dismiss the grievance complaint.
B. Issue a letter of advice.*
C. Issue a letter of admonition.
D. Recommend censure.
E. Recommend probation.
F. Recommend suspension.
G. Recommend expulsion.

APPENDIX III
AMERICAN HOSPITAL ASSOCIATION
GUIDELINES ON ETHICAL CONDUCT FOR
HEALTH CARE INSTITUTIONS†

Introduction

Health care institutions, by virtue of their roles as health care providers, employers, and community health resources, have special responsibilities for ethical conduct and practices. The broad range of patient care, education, public health, social service, and business functions they undertake are essential to the health and well-being of their communities. In general, there is public expectation that they will conduct themselves in an ethical manner that emphasizes a basic community service orientation.

These guidelines are intended to assist members of the American Hospital Association to better define the ethical aspects and implications of institutional policies and practices. They are offered with the understanding that individual decisions seldom reflect an absolute ethical right or wrong, and that each institution's leadership in making policy and

---

*This is not an opinion letter, but rather one to inform affiliates of a change in the Code of Ethics of which they should be aware.

†Approved by the American Hospital Association Board of Trustees on November 19, 1987.

decisions must take into account the needs and values of the institution, its medical community, and employees and those of individual patients, their families, and the community as a whole.

The governing board of the institution is responsible for establishing and periodically evaluating the ethical standards that guide institutional practices. The chief executive officer is responsible for assuring that hospital medical staff, employees, and volunteers and auxilians understand and adhere to these standards and for promoting an environment sensitive to differing values and conducive to ethical behavior.

These guidelines examine the hospital's ethical responsibilities to its community and patients as well as those deriving from its organizational roles as employer and a business entity. Although some responsibilities also may be included in legal and accreditation requirements, it should be remembered that legal, accreditation and ethical obligations often overlap and that ethical obligations often extend beyond legal and accreditation requirements.

Community Role

- Health care institutions should be concerned with the overall health status of their communities while continuing to provide direct patient services. This principle requires them to communicate and work with other health care and social agencies to improve the availability and provision of health promotion and education and services as well as patient care and to take a leadership role in enhancing public health and continuity of care in the community.

- Health care institutions are responsible for fair and effective use of available health care delivery resources to promote access to comprehensive and affordable health care services of high quality. This responsibility extends beyond the resources of the given institution to include efforts to coordinate with other health care providers and to share in community solutions for providing care for the medically indigent and others.

- All health care institutions have community service responsibilities which may include care for the poor and the uninsured, provision of needed services and educational programs, and various programs designed to meet the specific needs of their communities. Not-for-profit institutions, in consideration of their community service origins, Hill-Burton obligations, and tax status, should be particularly sensitive to the importance of providing and designing services for their communities.

- Health care institutions, being dependent upon community confidence and support, are accountable to the public, and therefore their communications and disclosure of information and data related to the institution should be clear, accurate, and sufficiently complete to assure that it is not misleading. Such disclosure should be aimed primarily at better public understanding of health issues, the services available to prevent and treat illness, and patients' rights and responsibilities relating to health care decisions.
- As health care institutions operate in an increasingly competitive environment, they should consider the overall welfare of their communities and their own missions in determining their activities, service mixes, and business ventures and conduct their business activities in an ethical manner.

Patient Care

- Health care institutions are responsible for assuring that the care provided to each patient is appropriate and of the highest quality they are able to provide. Health care institutions should establish and follow procedures to verify the credentials of physicians and other health professionals, assess and improve quality of care, and review appropriateness of utilization.
- Health care institutions should have policies and practices that support the process of informed consent for diagnostic and therapeutic procedures and that respect and promote the patient's responsibility for decision making.
- Health care institutions are responsible for assuring confidentiality of patient-specific information. They are responsible for providing safe-guards to prevent unauthorized release of information and establishing procedures for authorizing release of data.
- Health care institutions should assure that the psychological, social, spiritual, and physical needs and cultural beliefs and practices of patients and families are recognized and should promote employee and medical staff sensitivity to the full range of such needs and practices.
- Health care institutions should assure respect for and reasonable accommodations of individual religious and social beliefs and customs of patients whenever possible.
- Health care institutions should have specific mechanisms or procedures to resolve conflicting values and ethical dilemmas among

patients, their families, medical staff, employees, the institution, and the community.

Organizational Conduct

- The policies and practices of health care institutions should respect the professional ethical codes and responsibilities of their employees and medical staff members and be sensitive to institutional decisions that employees might interpret as compromising their ability to provide high-quality health care.
- Health care institutions should have policies and practices that provide for equitably administered employee policies and practices.
- To the extent possible and consistent with the ethical commitments of the institution, health care institutions should accommodate the desires of employees and medical staff to embody religious and moral values in their professional activities.
- Health care institutions should have written policies on conflict of interest that apply to officers, governing board members, physicians, and others who make or influence decisions for or on behalf of the institution. These policies should recognize that individuals in decision-making or administrative positions often have duality of interests that may not ordinarily present conflicts. However, they should provide mechanisms for identifying and addressing conflicts when they do exist.
- Health care institutions should communicate their mission, values, and priorities to their employees and volunteers, whose patient care and service activities are the most visible embodiment of the institution's ethical commitments and values.

APPENDIX IV
AMERICAN COLLEGE OF HEALTHCARE
EXECUTIVES

*Statement of Principles for Students**
(Supplement to the ACHE Code of Ethics)

"The life of the health administrator is dedicated to the achievement of the highest possible level of performance in the competent and humane

---

*These guidelines were developed originally in 1973 by the Special Committee on Ethics and the AHA Council on Management and Planning. They were delivery of health services, and in education and research conducted in the interest of healthcare."

—Council of Regents, ACHE

Students of health administration have the opportunity to participate in the building of a worthy, purposeful, and progressive profession. This opportunity, however, is not without obligation, for the viability of the profession will rest on the integrity as well as the capability of its members. It is necessary, therefore, that the individual's behavior be ethical as a way of life in the conduct of personal and academic affairs. In pursuing this objective the student shall:

1. Conduct self at all times in a dignified, exemplary manner.
2. Abide by the procedures, rules, and regulations of the educational institution.
3. Respect the guidelines prescribed by each professor in the preparation of academic assignments.
4. Be objective, understanding, and fair in academic performance and relationships.
5. Strive toward academic excellence, improvement of administrative skills and expansion of other professional knowledge.
6. Encourage and assist colleagues in the pursuit of academic excellence, improvement of administrative skills, and expansion of other professional knowledge.
7. Encourage, aid, and teach others in the principles and practices of health services administration.
8. Not denigrate the work of colleagues.
9. Neither engage in, assist in, nor condone cheating, plagiarism or other such activities.
10. Foster and support sound programs of education and research to assure the proper direction of the profession.
11. Contribute interest, support, and leadership toward the overall improvement of the community, with special emphasis

---

approved by the Board of Trustees in 1974 for publication by the American College of Healthcare Executives (ACHE) in its pamphlet entitled *Code of Ethics*. In view of the increasing accountability of healthcare institutions to their communities, the guidelines were revised and updated in 1980 by the Council on Management and approved by the General Council. As of October, 1987, a proposal is being considered by the General Council to revise the Guidelines on Ethical Conduct and Relationships for Healthcare Institutions.

on delivery of healthcare, health education and related objectives.
12. Respect and protect the rights, privileges, and beliefs of others.

4 | Viewing the Health Care Manager

Anthony R. Kovner

ORGANIZATIONAL ACTIVITIES

Robert Allison et al. developed a list of 46 organizational activities that are performed by managers of hospitals, nursing homes, group practices, and HMOs. In their survey of six chief executives in each type of organization (24 in all), 32 of the 46 activities were determined to be crucial by one or more of the four types of executives.*

In figure 4.1, I have grouped these 32 activities into four role sets: motivating others, scanning the environment, negotiating the political terrain, and generating and allocating resources.

MOTIVATING OTHERS

Managers spend a great deal of their time recruiting and retaining managerial and supervisory staff and in making decisions about their rewards and promotions, work procedures, and development and training. To carry out these activities, managers use communications and analytical skills. Managers assist their subordinates in doing what is required and in doing what subordinates want to do, within organizational limits. This can be difficult if managers have not recruited their subordinates. Even when managers have recruited subordinates (and recruitment is more of an art than a science), an excellent winning percentage may be more like .600 than .850.

An example of motivating others is managerial development and

---

Excerpted from "Health Services Managers," in Anthony R. Kovner, *Really Trying: A Career Guide for the Health Services Manager* (Ann Arbor, 1984), 48–56, with permission, Health Administration Press.

*It is curious to note that "advocating for patients and consumers" is not one of the 46 critical managerial activities.

FIGURE 4.1

Allison et al.: 32 Crucial Activities, Grouped by Role Set

Motivating Others
  — Recruiting professionals and physicians
  — Decisions regarding professional and managerial salaries
  — Devising work procedures for professionals
  — Devising work procedures for nonprofessionals
  — Promoting and rewarding professionals and managers
  — Employee and management development and training
  — Disciplining professional and managerial employees
  — Motivating and directing immediate subordinates
  — Dealing with personal and interpersonal problems

Scanning the Environment
  — Market research
  — Product research
  — Long-range planning
  — Developing criteria systems to control quality
  — Decisions regarding financial and management information systems

Negotiating the Political Terrain
  — Public relations
  — Lobbying
  — Labor negotiations
  — Establishing agreements with other organizations
  — Negotiating with powerful external organizations
  — Creating and changing professional job units
  — Decisions regarding changes in decision making and authority structure
  — Influencing decisions of Board or Owners
  — Influencing decisions made by medical staff
  — Arbitrating between internal units and departments
  — Arbitrating between policymaking groups

Generating and Allocating Resources
  — Determine buying procedures
  — Obtain long-term capital
  — Obtain working capital: collections
  — Decisions regarding maintaining building and equipment
  — Decisions regarding charges and prices for services
  — Decisions regarding new construction
  — Decisions regarding housekeeping

Source: Robert F. Allison, William L. Dowling, and Fred C. Munson. "The Role of the Health Services Administrator and Implications for Education," in *Education for Health Administration*, vol. 2 (Ann Arbor: Health Administration Press, 1975), 147–84.

training. Managers in new organizations or in new positions in existing organizations must be developed and trained by their new or existing supervisors. Such development and training can shorten the subordinate's learning process. Managers can aid those who work with them by identifying the skills that must be learned and the information that must be acquired for effective performance in the new position. Seniors can also help juniors become more aware of their own values, how they are perceived by others, and how the values of others affect their job performance.

SCANNING THE ENVIRONMENT

Effective managers scan or search the environment for potential problems and targets of opportunity. Scanning activities include market and product research, long-range planning, and quality assessment. The development of management information systems may be essential for effective scanning. In large health services organizations, scanning activities are usually performed by special units of marketing, quality assessment, development, and planning. In smaller organizations, managers may scan the environment themselves or with the assistance of subordinates or colleagues. Information about what similar organizations and managers do is available from journals, books, newsletters, and advertisements. Managers attend continuing education and trade association meetings, where colleagues and experts discuss organizational and managerial opportunities and problems. Managers visit similar organizations to learn at first hand about possible ways to improve effectiveness and efficiency. Openness to such visits is characteristic of public and not-for-profit health services organizations.

NEGOTIATING THE POLITICAL TERRAIN

Effective managers maintain trust and build alliances with groups and individuals. A positive political climate contributes to effective decision making and implementation. New managers must find out "who is doing what to whom" in their organization; or, put another way, "What is the ballpark in which I am playing, who are the players, and what are the rules?" Managers learn the informal organizational power structure by reading and listening. The operative rules are not always easy to ascertain—they vary by organizational setting, and they depend on the issue being discussed. Decision makers establishing a joint laundry are different from those who decide to establish a renal dialysis unit.

Activities which the manager undertakes in the area of negotiating the political terrain include public relations, lobbying, labor negotiations, influencing decisions made by governing boards and medical staffs, arbitrating between internal units and departments, and negotiating with other organizations.

GENERATING AND ALLOCATING RESOURCES

Effective managers spend a great deal of time analyzing organizational efficiency and finding ways to increase revenues and decrease expenses. In doing this, managers must consider past performance in their organization, performance of like organizations, and industry standards.

Effective managers attempt to improve financial performance by making decisions about buying procedures, ways of securing long-term and working capital, building and equipment maintenance, price changes, and new construction. Effective managers attempt to understand whatever special circumstances may influence preferences among alternative standards and strategies, and they listen closely to explanations and analysis by subordinates and clinicians.

To be effective, managers continually have to make decisions about generating and using resources. This occurs as part of the budgetary process and in response to emergency or extraordinary requests. Less tangible resources, such as staff time, must also be allocated, as must resources that are less amenable to negotiation, such as space.

SKILLS

The manager uses communications and analytical skills in performing functions. Communications skills include reading, writing, speaking, and listening. Analytical skills include judging and deciding.

COMMUNICATIONS SKILLS

Most of most managers' time is spent communicating rather than deciding. Communication skills are probably underemphasized, relative to analytic skills, in graduate programs of health services management. As Urmy indicates:

> Hospital administration is not about sitting in your office with a calculator. . . . about ten percent of the job is pushing paper, bureaucratic work. . . . Although I may have gone to six meetings and put in a ten-hour day, sometimes I feel I didn't get anything done. . . . the primary function of a hospital administrator is to provide integration and coordination within the hospital. . . . this means meetings and talking with people.

Although communicating and deciding can take place simultaneously, lengthy communication often takes place before decision making and during implementation.

Managers receive stacks of written material and have to prepare similar stacks. Some managers compensate for limited reading and writing capability by doing most of their work in person or by phone. Reading, of course, includes analyzing numbers as well as concepts or service plans. Being able to interpret numbers critically is an important skill for health service managers.

Reading and writing skills can be learned. Managers should have learned them as part of their elementary and high school educations, but unfortunately some of them have not. Many colleges and graduate schools have instituted special remedial writing courses and workshops. Speedreading courses are widely available as well.

Listening and speaking effectively are even more important for health service managers than skill in reading and writing. Many managers are not even aware that listening and speaking skills (other than public speaking) can be learned. Yet managers can learn to make focused yet personal phone calls. They can learn to conduct meetings that accomplish goals yet make attendees feel that their points of view have been listened to and their feelings have been adequately taken into account.

Listening and giving the appearance of listening are important. In a primer on consulting skills, Stanley Klion and John DeRusso attempt to teach managers how to listen better. They list the following as reasons for poor listening: lack of practice; preoccupation with one's own ideas and opinions; preoccupation with other matters; time lag (people think four times faster than they talk); and lack of common ground for understanding (people fully understand only 25 percent of what they hear).

The authors go on to list several approaches to improving listening and understanding skills. These include continually recapitulating what one is told, numbering in importance the respective points, maintaining eye contact to avoid distraction and to show interest, asking oneself how to show genuine interest, and reacting with related questions.

ANALYTICAL SKILLS

Perhaps more clearly identifiable than reading, writing, speaking, and listening as managerial skills are the analytical skills of judging and deciding. Ray Brown has defined judgment as knowledge ripened by experience. Many managers feel that skill in judging and deciding can only come from experience, that it cannot be taught in school. Others argue that by analyzing and responding to managerial situations as structured cases or simulations, with students taking parts or playing roles of different participants, judgmental and decisional skills can be assessed and improved.

Before managers can judge or decide, they must, of course, be able to define a problem, gather data, structure alternatives, and calculate advantages and costs for each alternative. Each step of this problem-solving approach involves judging and deciding. For example, how valid is the manager's definition of the problem relative to key clinical chiefs' definition of it? How much time should the manager spend gathering what data?

Computational skills are also required, for example in making decisions regarding appropriate scheduling of patients for appointments, discounting the value of money over time to assess the true cost of capital financing, or pricing services to different payers so that revenues can be maximized.

PERSONA

The effectiveness of managers is determined as much by who they are and how they do things as by what they do. Managerial persona includes demographic characteristics, beliefs, style, and personality.

DEMOGRAPHIC CHARACTERISTICS

Managers are likely to think that how they manage rather than what population group they belong to affects how others view their contribution. However, managers tend to feel more comfortable with, and more trusting of, persons whom they see as similar to themselves.

Individuals sometimes react to managers primarily in terms of "Is the manager one of us or is he part of some group whom we dislike or fear?" The group practice administrator in a coal-mining community in Western Pennsylvania may have great difficulty gaining the trust of a union-dominated governing board of Italians and Poles when he is himself well-educated, Jewish, and from a wealthy suburb of Philadelphia.

BELIEFS

People trust one another partly because of what they think others believe. "If he believes in the same things that I do, perhaps it doesn't matter so much whether I like him. I can trust him because he is likely to do what I think he should do in a particular situation for his own reasons."

Registered nurses distrust managers who they believe are interested only in "money" and who they think have little or no commitment to providing high-quality patient care. They may see managers in general as holding such beliefs. Such distrust can usually be overcome only over time, as managers' beliefs become more apparent by what they say and how they behave.

STYLE

Managerial style is subjective, elusive, and difficult to generalize about. Some managers adopt different styles depending upon whom they are talking to. Style can be defined as the way managers perform their functions or roles and what they disclose about themselves in communication with others. Style can be learned by observing effective managers and adapting their styles to different organizational situations. The appropriateness of such adaptation depends upon the situation and the individual. Although management style may be easily differentiated and distinctly perceived by others, managers themselves may be the last to know that they are perceived as crude or overly polite, as dressing fashionably or behind the times.

Personal appearance is an aspect of style. In most organizations, physicians and nurses distrust or show little respect for a manager with a shaggy mustache, uncombed hair, no tie, and loose-fitting clothes. On the other hand, in a free clinic, such a managerial style may make performance more effective.

Formality in speech is another aspect of style. Does the manager address others initially by their first names? Does the manager initiate or encourage conversations on personal matters such as marital problems? Does the manager stand when someone enters the office? Does the manager have an open-door policy to all employees? Does the manager receive phone calls routinely during a meeting with physicians? Is the manager's desk cluttered or uncluttered? Is the manager's office formally and richly outfitted or simple and plain?

I believe that style can be learned and that it can help or hurt a manager in the performance of his or her duties. Some of my own style changes have included: more conservative dress, less talking and interrupting in meetings, and more courtesy shown to those meeting with me when I accept an important telephone call.

Managers vary in their willingness to listen at length and respond to non–work-related conversation from physicians, nurses, and employees and to listen and seek out the work and personal problems of department heads and other employees. Some managers prefer to deal with employees through the chain of command, routing personal inquiries to others unless these are from immediate subordinates. Other managers keep their doors open and welcome frequent interruptions and shifts in attention.

Some managers prefer opulent or cluttered offices; others, bare or sparsely furnished ones. Some managers place a large desk between themselves and visitors and sit in an oversized swivel chair while their visitors have low seats. Others have a work table and no desk and meet with visitors in armchairs around a low coffee table.

There is generally no right or wrong answer to a question of managerial style. Within a wide range of the acceptable, style may not significantly affect managerial job performance. Certain styles fit better in certain organizations. It is safe to assume, however, at least in most large health services organizations, that managers should dress conservatively, show courtesy to physicians and nurses, listen, and give the appearance of listening when addressed by persons who think they have higher status. Different stakeholders in an organization expect managers to behave in different ways, and managers should attempt to understand such expectations. Many managers tune in to others' needs unconsciously and have often been selected for their jobs in part because their style fits the expectations of those who have done the selecting.

PERSONALITY

Managerial personality is an important aspect of the way managers are perceived, of whether they are trusted. Personality can have a significant impact on managerial effectiveness and survival. Of course, different people have different ideas about what is important or good.

One of my bosses had tremendous ability and intelligence, was friendly, cheerful, enthusiastic, open, and witty. Yet he had an enormous ego and was dishonest, hot-tempered, and inconsiderate. This manager read all my mail and insisted that I never close my office door. He inspired in me a determination to do only what he specifically requested — and nothing more — and to look out for myself rather than for his interest or the organization's. Yet this man was a successful manager in meeting the demands of superiors and in attracting and retaining competent staff.

Another of my bosses was able, friendly, cheerful, open, witty, honest, considerate, intelligent, and calm. If he had a big ego, he concealed it from me in our everyday relations. He obtained for me the resources necessary to accomplish my work and was always available to help with a job-related or personal problem. My response was to do anything this manager asked of me and to give much higher priority to his concerns and to the organization's. Yet this manager was perceived by some subordinates and colleagues as cold, ruthless, and insufficiently concerned with the rights of others.

It is difficult for some managers to see themselves as others see them. Sometimes only friends will be appropriately critical. Friends may be wrong about a question at issue, but they are less likely to be wrong about how others perceive the manager. Generally co-workers, especially subordinates, do not volunteer negative criticism, because they have an interest in saying what they think the manager wants to hear. Some wait for the manager to be in a relaxed mood before sharing their concerns. If the manager is always on the go, they may never see the manager in such a mood. They may feel unsure of their assessments, as assessments are often necessarily based on impressions rather than facts. Managers need to elicit from subordinates and co-workers their feelings and perceptions prior to meetings on important issues with physicians and officials upon whom managers and the organization depend.

Managers should not attempt to change themselves merely because they think some other style may be more effective or in order to please others. Often such change is not possible and, if forced, leads to worse or different results than are intended. Managers should know themselves, however, and what it is about themselves that pleases or displeases others. In this way managers can adapt better to the demands of a situation, take advantage of their natural assets, and allow for or minimize their weak points.

SOURCES

Klion, Stanley R., and John J. DeRusso. Consulting Engagement Skills, mimeograph. Peat, Marwick, Mitchell & Co., 345 Park Ave., New York, NY 10017.

Urmy, Norman. Interview by Anthony R. Kovner, 13 May 1981.

5 | The Proper Way to
Live: Remarks on
the Teaching of
Hospital
Administration

John R. Griffith

> Our conversation is not about something casual, but about the proper way to live.

— Socrates

Technology of all kinds contributes to the successes of the twentieth century. From the advances in motive power to the subtler changes in advertising, the substitution of scientific and technical thinking for early approaches has brought great rewards. The spread of technology and technical thinking is itself speeded by communications technology so that the process has become self-sustaining. Technology supports thinking, which develops more technology. The success has led quite naturally to a heavy emphasis on technology in education. From the concern with elementary school math teaching to the emphasis on scientific publication for university faculty, scientific philosophies and technological concepts dominate the educational establishment. This is as true in general management education as in any other professional field. It is rapidly becoming true in education for health administration as the field increases its emphasis on statistics, finance, computers, and empirical research.

It is wise to examine any rapidly proliferating trend because all such

Reprinted from *Journal of Health Administration Education* 1 (Winter 1983): 27–36, with permission, Association of University Programs in Health Administration.

trends (so far) have eventually slowed. What will happen after we have computerized health care, quantified planning, and constructed empirically designed finance mechanisms? Is it possible that these noble goals are not fundamental, but derivative? If so, from what are they derived? Consideration of these questions over a period of years has led me to conclude that the fundamental questions of hospital management are not scientific. These remarks review what those fundamental issues are and how they affect hospital management education. I believe that many of the conclusions I have reached apply to some degree to the larger field of health care management education, but I leave the interested reader to work the applications out.

THE LIMITATIONS OF SCIENCE AND HOSPITAL MANAGEMENT

The important questions of life are never fully addressed by science or by technology derived from science. The proper way to live involves such value questions as how we worship, whom we marry, and what kind of work we do. My thesis is that what kind of hospitals there are is a value question. It must be answered first as part of the proper way to live. Further, I argue that the value questions involving the intimate relationship between hospitals and the way we live are the justification for the field of hospital administration, and therefore of hospital management education.

If the value questions were not important, hospital management education would have little reason to exist. The empirical research could be pursued in various university departments, and the teaching in the business school. It is the values that distinguish us and that require a unique focal point. Values are often beyond empirical assessment; one of our obligations is to clarify, select, and reinforce certain values relating to the health care system. I believe a hospital administration faculty is obligated to have answers to value-laden questions, to develop those answers responsibly, and to support them vigorously.

The faculty's principal market is hospital managers. The uniqueness and strength of the role of hospital managers are their willingness to address value questions in health care and their ability to work directly with physicians on these issues. No profession outside health care administration makes any significant effort to do either of these tasks. Therefore, faculty activities in teaching, research, and service should enhance or support this effort. Other skills are necessary to hospital managers as well, particularly in increasing their ability to relate effectively to other management professionals. We should assist our market with these skills, but the priority should be kept clear.

The key questions of managing a hospital are "What does it do?" "Whom does it serve?" "How does it run?" and "What does it cost?" These are questions which are illuminated by science but not answered by it. They are questions on which hospital managers and hospital administration faculty should have informed opinions.

WHAT DOES A HOSPITAL DO?

As for what a hospital does, the functional definition I believe most useful, and which I now teach my students, is:

A hospital is a capital and human resource used by a community to assist in providing personal health services.

This definition deliberately makes no reference to beds. While hospitals usually provide inpatient service, they also usually provide a great deal more. The definition is deliberately flexible because community hospitals have great latitude. There is no personal health service or, indeed, any related personal service they cannot provide if they choose.

The criterion governing the application of hospital resources is to improve community satisfaction with the process of health care. The resources may be applied to recruit certain kinds of physicians, or to discourage cigarette smoking, or to run an ambulance service, or to stimulate capitation payment systems, as well as to provide for surgery or for psychiatric care. (Many leading community hospitals perform these or a similarly broad set of activities.) A broader concept than the traditional three D's of medical care—death, disease and disability—is necessary to encompass the desirable functions of the community hospital. I suggest an encompassing fourth D—dissatisfaction. In other words, a hospital is a collection of capital and human resources, and it uses those resources in any reasonable way to improve the community's satisfaction. Recognizing the breadth of this opportunity is one of the first tasks of hospital management and, therefore, of teaching faculty. The opportunity is a great deal broader than purely technical functions such as surgery or inpatient care, and it introduces many more avenues to find the proper way to live.

WHOM DOES A HOSPITAL SERVE?

Hospitals serve communities of people. They are more egalitarian than many of our social institutions. Although they often fail to meet the needs of the poor, most hospitals make some effort in that direction. This effort—the spirit of altruism that is widespread in hospitals—is a contribution in its own right and a very important one. The desire to help one's fellow man is the thread that forms the fabric of civilization. It is one of the distinctions between humans and animals. That desire gets concrete expression in hospitals in important and unique forms related to the sick and dying. In a very real sense, through the expression of altruistic instincts hospitals serve us all, rather than simply those of us who are in discomfort.

If hospitals are to serve communities as well as sick individuals, the word "voluntary" is an important concept that permits them to do so. The notions of sanctuary and samaritanism are an essential part of the proper way to live.

It is currently popular to look at the narcissism of people, in hospitals and elsewhere. One talks of greedy doctors, revenue-maximizing trustees and administrators, self-promoting health professionals, and so on. Much of this is true, but it co-exists with nobler motives. Most of us are selfish and altruistic by turns, or possibly even simultaneously. To emphasize the selfish aspects of mankind and to diminish the altruistic is a self-fulfilling prophecy. It will eliminate the altruistic aspects of hospitals and make the fabric of civilization that much weaker.

HOW DOES A HOSPITAL RUN?

How a hospital runs is a complex question including both decision structures and operational decisions, that is, who decides and what they decide. Clearly, a hospital should be run as the law and the Joint Commission indicate, and clearly it should strive to be efficient in its operations. The central concept of these criteria is one of equity—avoiding the inequitable distribution of resources that might occur by error, inefficiency, omission, or fraud.

Somewhat more controversial is the notion of hospitals as a local resource, beholden to local groups. Local communities do not differ much in disease, that is, in strict epidemiological measures of pathology, but they do differ in attitudes toward treating disease and using hospital resources. I am inclined to believe that diverse viewpoints are valuable and possibly essential in sustaining an altruistic commitment. I see no advantage, and some possibly serious disadvantages, to schemes that place capital and human resources beyond the control of the local community. Because personal health service is so intimate, intangible, and diverse, local control has an intrinsic benefit. Neither federal nor absentee ownership structures are likely to perform as well. In part, this is because such structures encourage escape from the responsibilities to the sick. A local community governance structure is part of the proper way to live.

HOW MUCH SHOULD WE PAY FOR HOSPITALS?

My first professional publication more than 20 years ago dealt with the cost of hospitals.[1] In it, I noted with some puzzlement that the share of consumer expenditures devoted to hospitals behaved as a luxury rather than as a necessity. The relative expenditures on necessities — food, clothing, and shelter — tend to go down as income goes up; expenditures on luxuries go up. When measured for the United States as a whole, health care has behaved like a luxury.

I now understand the situation more clearly. Luxury spending is discretionary. In an important sense, the sense of discretionary hospital care is truly a luxury. The need for hospitals is relative, like the need for companionship. Little about hospitals is directly involved with lifesaving. Much about them is related to common economic trade-offs based on utility considerations. The point is reflected empirically in the enormous range of actual use of hospital care. Within the North Atlantic community, use ranges fourfold, from less than two occupied beds per 1,000 population to more than eight.

If hospitals are a luxury, or at least a discretionary activity dealing in satisfaction, then the answer to the question of how much we should spend on them is simply "as much as we want." The only serious issue is the mechanism by which consensus is found. I find that many of my colleagues in hospital administration misunderstand this point. They seem to believe they are entitled to funds, possibly because they believe hospitals principally deal with preventing death and curing disease. In reality, because hospitals do not, in fact, principally prevent death or cure disease, they are entitled to funds on the same basis as the local art museum or local whiskey dealer — namely, that the expenditure will be the proper way to live.

The teachers of hospital administration must keep this point clearly in front of our students, and we must accept it as a premise in our research. Such a premise does not rule out productivity-related research or even research in improving financial performance. It does clarify the objective function of hospitals: their income and expenditures — their costs — are set by the purses of their community. The function of all kinds of productivity is more opportunity for relieving dissatisfaction and for exercising altruistic motives — for a given a level of expenditures. The function of productivity research is never to cut costs.

One may disagree with the selection of these four questions or with the answers I have offered. It is not desirable that all faculty members agree with me, but simply that each holds an informed opinion, conveys it to his/her students, and uses it in research and in consultation. These questions or something very like them cannot be dismissed out of hand; despite the unconventional nature of my answers, they are at least partially correct. The key questions of hospital management require more than just science if we are to find the proper way to live.

I want next to discuss very briefly the process by which one might determine the proper way to live and then to move on to some specific obligations that acceptance of this line of thought implies.

THE PROCESS FOR DETERMINING THE PROPER WAY TO LIVE

My thesis subsumes rather than displaces scientific work. Although we can rely on scientific approaches to decisions, we must be prepared to go beyond them into questions of ethics. Frankena's popular text on ethics maintains that these kinds of questions are ethical ones relating to what is called "nonmoral goodness."[2] The author argues that ethical questions can be addressed by calm reflection, by rational dialogue, and by developing a body of values or standards over a period of time. He cautions, however, that the solutions to these questions cannot be found in the law because, among other reasons, these are the questions that determine the law. He also notes that the questions at their most fundamental level must be answered by individuals rather than by consensus. He reiterates in his approach the importance of careful and thorough empiricism and full evaluation of the consequences. That, of course, is where a research-oriented faculty makes its biggest contribution.

Utilitarian values prevail in most of the collective activities of the United States. That is, issues are decided for the most part on the basis of the balance of good over harm. I suspect that this criterion guides most research. More important, Frankena's process for resolving ethical questions reminds us of a number of teaching and research obligations which follow to the extent that my thesis is accepted.

Let me turn now to some obligations of teaching faculties that I consider to be of particular importance. I have divided them into three groups: our obligations as leaders, our obligations as researchers, and our obligations as teachers.

IMPLICATIONS FOR FACULTIES

OBLIGATIONS AS LEADERS

It is clear that faculty members have two obligations as intellectual leaders: 1) to supply the best possible empirical information; and 2) to join others in acting as guardians of the process of decision making. We have not always done well in honoring these obligations. We have now learned two lessons about the medical care system, but only after some unfortunate decisions were made. One lesson concerns the economic implications of the definition of hospitals. I wish now that I had spoken less tentatively in 1960 about hospital care as a luxury good. Twenty years ago the prevailing view was that hospital care was a "right." This view neglected the subtle and complex distinctions between need and demand. It was part of the basis of a headlong rush to argue the virtues of first dollar coverage of hospital cost and for some to argue for national health insurance. It may also have contributed to our national fascination with high technology as the proper solution to health care problems.

A second and perhaps clearer lesson is in the payment mechanisms we have selected for providers. Although a few faint voices warned against the folly of per diem reimbursement, and a few more spoke out against usual customary and reasonable fee schedules, they did not prevail. In particular, those people who had the foresight to detect the impact of Medicare on credit and capital formation could have guided us to a much more satisfactory way to live.

Where might we best honor these obligations as leaders in the future? One answer might lie in pursuing and making explicit an understanding of hospital care as a luxury good purchased for satisfaction. This perception has a number of implications in our views of the question of access, protection against the cost of illness, and emphasis on prevention. In particular, it should lead us to address the troublesome question of the cost of dying. Large fractions of our hospital expenditures are being consumed by people with only modest and sometimes very immediate life expectancies.[3,4] The implications of spending thousands of dollars on people in their final months of life cannot be ignored. It is a faculty obligation to make the implications clear and to propose alternatives. Part of the proper way to live includes addressing the question of the proper way to die. It may be wise to "go gentle into that good night" rather than to "rage against the dying of the light."

OBLIGATIONS AS RESEARCHERS

Most of our obligations as researchers are things we know well—the need for accuracy, for thoroughness, for conservatism, for a rich dialogue of criticism. The decision process itself is a fair subject of empirical research. Some of the empirical evidence from the Michigan Community Hospital Service Measures Project indicates that some communities may have been much more successful than others in their decision-making processes, but we do not know the mechanisms by which this has occurred.

A less obvious series of obligations stem from the utilitarian criterion as applied to research. This criterion comes into play most clearly at the outset of research thought when the topics are being identified and the projects designed. We select and stimulate not only our own research projects but those of our colleagues. The criterion of utilitarianism is more important for hospital administration faculties than it is for many university departments. While one might justify research in music or mathematics on the grounds of esthetics or pure thought, these nonutilitarian justifications are inconsistent with our role. We never apply such a justification directly. At an indirect level, however, the selection of research is influenced too much by the traditional arts and sciences taxonomy of research. We classify and try to judge both the product and the worker according to this taxonomy. The taxonomy itself, however, is not framed around the utilitarian criterion. Thus it has an inherent danger to lead us astray. The criterion of the "fit" of our research and our researchers within the traditional taxonomy is occasionally in conflict with the utilitarian criterion. Because of this, the taxonomy should always be secondary in importance.

In a similar vein, we do not listen enough to our customers, the practitioners. A significant number of any faculty should always be addressing the question "What is utility?" They should be led by the issues themselves, not by the guidelines of some academic department of the arts and sciences college. The practitioners in the world of hospital care are better placed to find out what these issues are.

OBLIGATIONS AS TEACHERS

Teaching is the central and essential activity of any hospital administration faculty. My view diminishes but in no sense dismisses the importance of research. We cannot teach well unless we do research; however, we cannot do utilitarian research unless it is applied. We must first teach the people who apply it. One cannot use an admissions scheduling and control system in a real hospital unless the hospital has a trained manager who understands first the values and reasons that make it appropriate to use and, second, the technical issues involved in its implementation. Our success in teaching makes our research more useful. It multiplies our contribution because it permits its translation to widespread application.

Part of our teaching obligation is in student selection. Managers first and foremost are leaders: we should look for leadership potential in selecting students. Our students must also be able to appreciate utilitarian concerns and translate them into practical decisions. We include these areas in our selection process, but we overlook them more than we should. Specifically, we have an obligation to look for evidence of previous leadership appropriate to the age of the applicant and to include it in our final evaluations. Second, we should continue to weigh heavily evidence of a practical commitment to service and to altruism. Third, we should place more weight on the ability to handle complex and value-laden ideas. Experience in writing and speaking on complex issues and a grounding in history and philosophy are essential for leaders who are seeking the proper way to run hospitals.

So far as curriculum content is concerned, the important point is that we are not producing technicians. We must identify the problems involved in selecting the proper way, that is, in dealing with value questions, in understanding the dangers of analogy, in grasping the limits of empiricism, and in recognizing the importance of independent thought and individual opinion.

We sometimes hesitate at certain parts of our obligations as teachers. A utilitarian criterion implies that we should teach those who can best use our education. If they happen to be older or in a position that requires continuing or nontraditional education, we should view our obligation and the opportunity independently of those facts. And, of course, if attention to job placement and a strong alumni association helps our graduates use their education, that is a full and sufficient justification for these activities. It is also full and sufficient justification for us to appropriately reward time spent on this activity.

SUMMATION

I have argued that health care is an intimate part of the proper way to live, and that as a result the justification of special education for the management of hospitals lies partly in the realm of values beyond the realm of science and technology. While science and technology are the major areas where an academic faculty contributes, they are never sufficient in themselves, either for the faculty or for the world of health care. The role of the faculty must always include something more. The mandatory additional element is the explicit recognition and consideration of the proper way to run hospitals. The framework for the question is utilitarian. "The proper way" maximizes the balance of good over harm. The faculty role includes obligations as leaders, teachers, and researchers, but the teaching obligation is central.

These obligations are demanding, and we have not always fulfilled them well. The principal dangers are incompleteness and the selection of inadequate analogies. It is seductive to assume that hospitals are like something else. Perhaps no such analogy should be accepted without formal reference to how hospitals are *not* like the thing in question. Incompleteness is another, more difficult problem. Perhaps it yields best to dialogue: to find the proper way it is important to collect a variety of knowledgeable and skillful people and to review the issues with them. Also, dialogue may be the best way to uncover the weaknesses of analogies.

How can we strengthen ourselves? I can think of only a few steps. We should be sure that faculty membership is open to all who are qualified, in both a formal and an informal or participative sense. Students and practitioners have a great deal to say to us, but we seem to have difficulty hearing them. Certainly our faculty selection should prize what our student selection seeks: a combination of intellect, motivation, and leadership ability. We should never lose sight of the fact that our work as a group is more important than our efforts as individuals, and that the value of the group effort depends on its completeness as well as on the rigor of its components. The issues of finance, law or engineering are never as important as the leadership skills of our graduates. The specific measures of a hospital's performance are never as important as the general question of how well it serves its community. At least, I hold, these beliefs are part of the proper way to live.

REFERENCES

1.   Griffith, J. R. Hospital care is still a bargain. *Hospitals*, November 16, 1960. Reprinted in *Trustee*, January 1961.

2.   Frankena, W. K. *Ethics*, Second Edition. Englewood Cliffs, N.J.: Prentice-Hall, 1973.

3.   Zook, C. J., F. D. Moore. High cost of medical care. *New England Journal of Medicine*. 302: 996–1002, 1980.

4.   Menzel, P. T. Pricing life: Reflections on the cost of health care. *Hospital Progress* (January): 46ff, 1982. See also Responses (April 1982) and Letters (May 1982).

II

Control

You may regard as a Utopian dream my hope to see all our hospitals devoting a reasonable portion of their funds to tracing the results of the treatment of their patients and analyzing these results with a view to improving them. You may prefer to ponder over the voluminous discussions now appearing in our journals and in the lay press about the pros and cons for state medicine and who is to pay the cost of medical care. I read these discussions, but they seem to be futile, until our hospitals begin to trace their results.

—E. A. Codman, 1935

ILLUSTRATION II

Information Needed for an Effective Quality Assurance Program

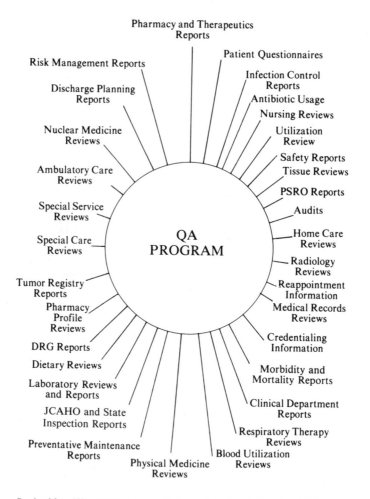

Pharmacy and Therapeutics Reports

Patient Questionnaires

Risk Management Reports

Infection Control Reports

Discharge Planning Reports

Antibiotic Usage

Nursing Reviews

Nuclear Medicine Reviews

Utilization Review

Safety Reports

Ambulatory Care Reviews

Tissue Reviews

PSRO Reports

Special Service Reviews

Audits

QA PROGRAM

Special Care Reviews

Home Care Reviews

Radiology Reviews

Tumor Registry Reports

Reappointment Information

Pharmacy Profile Reviews

Medical Records Reviews

DRG Reports

Credentialing Information

Dietary Reviews

Morbidity and Mortality Reports

Laboratory Reviews and Reports

JCAHO and State Inspection Reports

Clinical Department Reports

Preventative Maintenance Reports

Respiratory Therapy Reviews

Blood Utilization Reviews

Physical Medicine Reviews

Commentary

Anthony R. Kovner
Duncan Neuhauser

What is control? Is it good or bad? Does it work? Webster defines control as "power or authority to guide or manage."[1] Managers try to control the behavior of others, the use of scarce organizational resources, and the perceptions of others both inside and outside of the organization.

Systems of control include five elements: (1) accountability, which concerns the appropriateness of the control system; (2) governance, the evaluation of performance relative to expectations; (3) objectives or performance expectations; (4) information used to measure performance; and (5) incentives to influence performance.

Some of the problems with control systems are that they often measure the wrong things; they may need frequent updating or revising; incentives are often too weak to influence behavior; and control can be too costly relative to benefits.

GOALS AND OBJECTIVES

A goal is a broadly stated intention or direction—to improve the quality of care, for example. An objective is a measurable intention, such as lowering the infection rate. Organizational goals are determined by the preferences of individuals with power over a set of issues. Organizations are collectivities of people. Collectivities of people do not have goals; individuals do.

Goals are important because they provide organizational focus. They provide a long-term framework for dealing with conflict and they encourage commitment from those who work in an organization. Goals are implemented by individuals working together on budgets, allocation of functions, and the authority structure.

Organizations may have objectives for production, inventory, sales, profit, and quality. Managers determine unit or organizational objectives by reading formal official goal statements or by observing what is happening in an organization. These observations may reveal shifts in resources or decision-making power among units or individuals, what types of individuals are leaving or being recruited to the organization, and what the organization is not doing and which populations it is not serving.

Many large corporations expend a lot of effort in goal specification. However, some health care organizations do not specify objectives. They might find that dealing with intangibles provides greater motivation or that is it easier to accommodate diversity or change directions than to meet a goal. It may also be easier to avoid accountability and maximize discretion. Specifying objectives is also difficult because it involves negotiating a definition of health and agreeing upon desirable levels of goal attainment. Those in power sometimes prefer the status quo, and heavy costs in time and energy may be involved in the goal-specifying process.

What happens if health care organizations do not specify objectives? Organizations may lack focus in their programs and may be less likely to abandon products and services that are neither effective nor efficient. The powerful and their short-term interests will tend to be favored over the weak and the long term; there will be less adaptation to the environment; fewer decisions will be made by the governing body; and there will be a greater tendency to retain the status quo.

Health care managers should determine their organization's operative objectives. Official goals may not always provide reliable guidelines for managerial behavior. When those in power go against what a manager sees as the long-range interests of an organization, the manager should be careful, speaking out only if he or she is willing to pay the price and is certain about the facts.

GOVERNANCE

Governance is the process of making important decisions; it includes the structures and functions of decision making. The people who govern on any decision are determined by the nature of the decision. Governance is also affected by sponsorship of the organization. Sponsors include physicians, cooperatives, business corporations, unions, philanthropists, investors, church groups, and government. Each sponsor has different objectives that affect decision making.

There is little agreement as to which type of sponsorship works best. The debate has not been settled by empirical tests of differential cost and quality and access to public, not-for-profit, and investor-owned hospitals. Another unresolved issue is how much autonomy local health care organizations should have relative to regulators and which decisions they should make.

The functions of governing boards include selecting the chief executive officer (CEO), exercising direct control during periods of crisis, reviewing managerial decisions and performance, co-opting external influencers, establishing contacts and raising funds, enhancing the organization's reputation, and giving advice.[2] Boards pay limited attention to a limited number of issues and they have considerable power to determine what those issues will be.

INFORMATION SYSTEMS

Health care managers must obtain information about service volume in key product lines, the quality of care, service and production efficiency, market share, system maintenance, and the health status of the population served. They use the following measures to assess performance: cost per case, cost per visit, cost per day, profit, fixed and variable costs, market share, capital expenditures as a percent of sales, days of receivables and payables, top admitting physicians and their characteristics, staff turnover and overtime, sick time, and disability and fringe benefits costs.

The following directions for the next few years have been suggested for expanded capability of information systems in health care: revenue control with breakdown by services rendered, payor and employer, and insurance group; budgeting and variance reporting; clinical review, with automated medical records and larger and more detailed patient abstracts that are integrated with cost and revenue data, and concurrent review for quality of care; final product cost accounting, with data on homogeneous final-product patient groups at alternative levels of demand; and risk management, from incident reports to all untoward incidents, which are then aggregated and analyzed.[3]

INCENTIVE SYSTEMS

Incentives are stimuli to affect performance. Adoption of incentives is usually based on the answers to the following questions: Does the incentive contribute to desired results? Is the incentive the most efficient way to get the desired results? Is the incentive acceptable to those workers whose behavior managers wish to affect? Would implementation of the incentives produce other dysfunctional consequences (e.g., rewards for cutting costs might also reduce the quality of care)?

Organizations use both positive and negative incentives. Managers can attempt to influence individuals' perceptions of themselves; and they can change allocations of money, privileges, discretion, job security, and access to superiors. Although negative incentives do affect minimum performance, they do not unlock energy and innovation on the job. Negative incentives are most suitable for routine, measurable work.

There are also problems with implementing positive incentives. Is the incentive more costly than necessary to achieve the desired result? Is the incentive great enough to produce the desired result? Will it actually produce the desired result? Although promises of a raise in pay and higher status might motivate managers and others to work harder, such promises do not always produce the desired effects.

In business organizations, often 50 percent of the top manager's compensation, and 10 percent to 25 percent of middle managers' compensation, is based on meeting targets. This is not the case in most health care organizations, perhaps because fewer of them operate under for-profit auspices. Another explanation is that it may be more difficult in these organizations to agree upon standards and to measure performance. In addition, many of these organizations have not had to compete and grow to survive, as have for-profit firms.

PERFORMANCE REQUIREMENTS

A mechanistic analogy to an organizational control system is the household thermostat. Actual temperature is compared with a desired standard. If the actual temperature is below the desired level, the furnace goes on. The effect of this commanded activity is fed back to the thermostat on an ongoing basis by measured changes in the actual temperature. This analogy has its limitations, however. Managerial control is concerned with many unclearly defined and interacting activities and only approximately accurate standards. The manager should not take the control system as a given but should define and redefine it as circumstances change.

Broadly defined, the organizational control system can be seen as encompassing a large part of the manager's work. The literature on control tends to focus more narrowly on the measurement of organizational performance against standards and the way this information is fed back to decision makers. Because of this very broad concept and this narrow focus of attention, the use of the word "control" varies widely. Table II.1 shows how each of the chapters in Section II addresses the four performance requirements discussed below.

TABLE II.1

Perspectives on Performance Requirements and Control

Readings	Goal Attainment	System Maintenance	Adaptive Capability	Values Integration
Griffiths	Setting expectations	Performance indicators	Incentives	Cooperation
Kovner	Role of the board		Focus and energize the board	Support management
Owens et al.	Target setting	Indicators of performance for monitoring events	Relating data to management decisions	
Finkler	Budgeted targets	Analysis of variance	Priorities for management	
Craddick	Quality assurance	Professional liability warning system	Monitoring exceptions	Physician commitment to quality assurance
Neuhauser	Quality as the goal	High quality will ensure survival		Involve everyone in quality

GOAL ATTAINMENT

The organization's information system is the vehicle for measuring the degree of goal attainment and the basis for improving performance. Particularly in health services organizations, the central issue is the degree to which the information so generated is an accurate measure of goal attainment. Costs are easier to measure than quality of care. As goals shift, new information is needed. Overall goals must be articulated with divisional and departmental objectives. This articulation is not always easy to achieve. For example, costs and quality of care cannot be separated from each other. Higher quality often requires increased expenditures. When this occurs, decision makers must reconcile the desire for higher quality with the desire for cost control.

SYSTEM MAINTENANCE

Organizations can be viewed as a set of equilibriums that must be maintained by the manager. Revenues must balance expenses; in the long run, revenues must *exceed* expenses. The skills and knowledge of personnel must be maintained despite personnel turnover. Equipment and facilities must be added or replaced as the existing stock becomes obsolete. Outsiders who provide organizational support and revenues must be satisfied that they are getting their money's worth from organizational output. Each member of the organization must personally believe that his or her satisfaction with the organization is at least equal to his or her effort expended. The information system must monitor all these balances and be the basis for maintaining them.

ADAPTIVE CAPABILITY

Control systems that are routine, ongoing, quantitative, and computerized become inflexible and costly to change. Short-term informal controls based on observation are flexible and can be readily redirected and refocused. The routine, ongoing collection of information can be used to compare performance over time and to project future trends. One must be concerned not only with the trade-offs between flexibility and stability of the control systems, but also with the systems' ability to track and signal important changes in their own performance and in the external environment.

VALUES INTEGRATION

The collection of information, the specification of procedures for organization members, and the feedback of more information as a basis for corrective action are at the core of an organizational control system. All such controls are based on the assumption that matching the desires of members with organizational rewards results in appropriate behavior.

Workers' desires vary greatly and are only imperfectly known by the manager, so rewards can never perfectly match desires. In addition, organizational performance is inadequately measured in health care, so one can never precisely define appropriate behavior. Even though perfection cannot be obtained, managers should promote the development of mutually agreed-upon values, such as commitment to the organizational goal of good patient care. Monetary rewards are a partial answer to motivation for health care workers.

THE READINGS

Griffith focuses upon setting organizational expectations. He discusses cooperation, conflict resolution, comprehensiveness, clarity, and monitoring performance and incentives. He presents a classification of measures of hospital performance and criteria for selecting measures.

Kovner details four problems with the governing board's performance in hospitals: inability to specify objectives, ineffective and inefficient decision making, lack of corporate strategy, and conflict over board functions. He then recommends four solutions to these problems: integrating medical leaders into hospital governance; streamlining decision making, supporting management in the process of change, the focusing and energizing the board.

Owens, Fairchild, Pierce, and Goldberg describe the basic cost and volume measures that an internal management information costing system can generate.

Finkler reviews the contribution of variance analysis to organizational performance. Variance analysis is a financial management technique in which budgeted expenses are compared with actual results. Finkler reviews causes of variance, incentives, motivation, and variance analysis, suggesting that variance reports provide managers with useful information for determining where specific efforts are needed to control costs.

The problem of malpractice litigation has gone through several cycles in the last 40 years, and we are now at the crest of a new wave of concern. Larger and more frequent awards to plaintiffs have led to higher and higher malpractice premium rates. Craddick calls for instituting a preventive, ongoing quality-review mechanism. Quality assurance programs are now drawing together activities formerly located in various parts of the hospital organization, providing a focus for managerial attention.

Neuhauser looks at Edwards Deming's efforts to help Japanese industry develop high-quality products and applies Deming's theories to health care. He summarizes Deming's 14 points as a way of "putting everyone in the organization to work to accomplish a transformation." Neuhauser asks whether quality is adequately discussed at board meetings in health care organizations. He suggests that a superb product will be easy for health care organizations to sell and that financial solvency will follow.

ADDITIONAL TOPICS OF INTEREST

Accountability is discussed in Section VI of this book. Readers may be interested in exploring other related issues that are not directly addressed in the readings, such as the governance of health care organizations other than hospitals, the costs and benefits of information systems, and difficulties in implementation and criteria for evaluating hardware and software. More literature is needed on the impact of new incentive systems on managerial performance. The selected bibliography below provides suggestions for useful sources on the issue of control. Readers should also refer to the annotated bibliography at the end of the book.

NOTES

1. *Webster's New Collegiate Dictionary*, 9th ed., s.v. "control."

2. Henry Mintzberg, *Power In and Around Organizations* (Englewood Cliffs, NJ: Prentice-Hall, 1983), 67–95.

3. John R. Griffith, *The Well-Managed Community Hospital* (Ann Arbor, MI: Health Administration Press, 1987), 329–74.

SELECTED BIBLIOGRAPHY

Anthony, Robert N., and David Young. *Management Control in Nonprofit Organizations*. 3d ed. Homewood, IL: Irwin, 1984.

Austin, Charles J. *Information Systems for Hospital Administration*. 3d ed. Ann Arbor, MI: Health Administration Press, 1988.

Berwick, Donald. "Continuous Improvement as an Ideal in Health Care." *New England Journal of Medicine* 320, no. 1 (1989): 53–56.

Cleverly, William O. "Strategic Operating Indicators Point to Equity Growth." *Health Care Financial Management* 42 (July 1988): 54–62.

Cochrane, Archibald L. *Effectiveness and Efficiency*. London: Nuffield Provincial Hospital Trust, 1972.

Cohen, David I., D. Breslau, N.V. Dawson, N. Breslau, H.I. Goldberg, C.O. Hershey, J.C. Lee, C.E. McLaren, and D.K. Porter. "The cost Implications of Academic Group Practice." *The New England Journal of Medicine* 314, no. 24 (1986): 1553–57.

Delbecq, Andre L., and Sandra L. Gill. "Developing Strategic Direction for Boards." *Hospital & Health Services Administration* 33 (Spring 1988): 25–35.

Donabedian, Avedis. *Explorations in Quality Assessment and Monitoring*. 4 vols. Ann Arbor, MI: Health Administration Press, 1980–82.

Glandon, Gerald L., Michael Counte, Karen Holloman, and James Kowalczyk. "An Analytical Review of Hospital Financial Performance Measures." *Hospital & Health Services Administration* 32 (November 1987): 439–55.

Griffith, John R. "Voluntary Hospitals: Are Trustees the Solution?" *Hospital & Health Services Administration* 33 (Fall 1988): 295–310.

Grimaldi, Paul, and Julie Micheletti. *Prospective Payment: The Definitive Guide to Reimbursement*. Chicago: Pluribus Press, 1985.

Hancock, Walton M. "Dynamics of Hospital Operational Control Systems." *Hospital & Health Services Administration* 21 (Summer 1976): 23–42.

Kaluzny, Arnold D., D. Michael Warner, David G. Warren, and William N. Zelman. "Control and Evaluation." In *Management of Health Services*, 239–350. Englewood Cliffs, NJ: Prentice-Hall, 1982.

Mottaz, Clifford J. "Work Satisfaction among Hospital Nurses." *Hospital & Health Services Administration* 33 (Spring 1988): 57–74.

Smith, Howard L., and Norbert F. Elbert. "An Integrated Approach to Performance Evaluation in the Health Field." *Health Care Management Review* 25 (Winter 1980): 59–67.

Starkweather, David. "Hospital Board Power." *Health Services Management Research* 1 (July 1988): 74–86.

Stevens, Barbara J. "Nursing Division Budget: Generation and Control." *Journal of Nursing Administration* 4 (November–December 1974): 16–20.

Walton, Mary. *The Deming Management Method*. New York: Dodd, Mead & Co., 1986.

Wennberg, John. "Dealing with Medical Practice Variations: A Proposal for Action." *Health Affairs* 3 (Summer 1984): 6–32.

Williamson, John W. "Formulating Priorities for Quality Assurance Activity: Description of a Method and Its Application." *Journal of the American Medical Association* 239 (February 1978): 631–37.

6 | Controlling Hospital Organizations

John R. Griffith

USING THE CYBERNETIC MODEL

SETTING EXPECTATIONS

Intuitively, many people think that setting clear and complete expectations for each member of the organization reduces job content and freedom. They fear that overspecification may interfere with quality of work life; however, if expectations and policies describing work activities are truly well designed, the opposite can occur. Many of the constraints and frustrations of hospital work have to do with the integration of different tasks and work groups. Doctors frustrate nurses, nurses frustrate admitting doctors. The key to minimizing these frustrations is specifying and completing the individual tasks effectively, because the conflicts often arise from incomplete, ambiguous, and competing expectations. The result of improved specification is twofold: opportunities for confusion between units are removed, and opportunities to improve internal performance are increased.

The parts of cybernetic systems are a chain that is formed by expectation setting. Obviously, expectations may be set unrealistically high. Other potential errors which are frequently just as serious include ambiguity, conflict, impracticality, irrelevance, and redundancy. Expectation setting is a complex, ongoing process that is unique to each hospital. It is an important test of organizational design and managerial effectiveness.

A checklist for managing under cybernetic systems can be remem-

An excerpt from the chapter in John R. Griffith, *The Well-Managed Community Hospital* (Ann Arbor: Health Administration Press, 1987), 70–87, with permission, John R. Griffith.

bered by its four Cs: cooperation, conflict resolution, comprehensiveness, and clarity. The key to the process is an organization of open, two-way communication. The best goals are set by a wide-ranging process of discussion and debate, carried on essentially continuously at all levels of the institution. Discussion is foreclosed by conflict, and unresolved conflict eventually disables expectation setting. Thus procedures for conflict resolution are an important part of the overall expectation-setting process.

Cooperation: Participation in Setting Expectations

A well-designed goal-setting process becomes comprehensive by developing goals simultaneously throughout the organization. Goal setting occurs neither from the bottom up nor from the top down, but in both directions. In a well-designed system, unit managers are encouraged to think of improvements in their current goals. At the same time, planning and marketing staffs, financial staffs, and board-level committees are encouraged to consider what the outside environment demands. The board coordinates the effort by maintaining a mission statement and a long-range plan, concise but comprehensive documents indicating as clearly as possible who the exchange partners are and what services can be provided them. . . . The chief executive officer (CEO) also coordinates expectation setting by translating certain key environmental demands into quantitative expectations. An overall profit expectation, a total cost expectation, and expectations for a few major demand aggregates are often set by a board committee at the start of each budget cycle. . . .

When expectations are developed simultaneously, the role of the various levels of middle management is a coordinating one. Individual unit expectations must be coordinated with broader needs, and units must be integrated with each other. Effective middle managers carry out this task by encouraging participation and communication of differing viewpoints rather than by disposing authoritatively of conflicting views. Through discussion, each participant is encouraged to see the perspectives of others.

The process is not in any sense democratic, because the objectives of the organization prevail. The ultimate determination of an organization's expectations is the view of its most powerful exchange partner, almost always its customers. Members, that is, employees and doctors, are also important exchange partners. Their views must somehow be incorporated in the final expectations. The process of communicating, understanding, and integrating these views is a complicated and time-consuming one.

One perspective of a hospital organization is that it has an entire set of committees, conferences, task forces, and retreats solely for the purpose of gaining widespread participation in expectations setting. That broad group of organizational activities is called the **collateral organization** in this text. . . . The collateral organization always works well in a well-managed hospital. It permits the views of lower-level members to be heard by governing board and top executives and at the same time it permits members of the organization to see the exchange demands being imposed by customers and government. Thus attending physicians see the interests of other specialties and nursing, plant managers see radiology's needs for imaging services, human resources learns of changing needs for employment benefits, while all discover growth opportunities for the organization as a whole. Over time, knowledge and respect for various views lead the participants to grow together, rather than apart.

Resolving Conflict among Members

Conflicting views among participants are natural, and it is inevitable that in the process of setting expectations some participants will be disappointed. Each participant, after all, is rewarded for rigorously pursuing his or her specialty—whether nursing, cardiology, or cost control. It is useful to think of these conflicts as having two parts. One part, the process part, involves the discussion itself. The other part, conflicts over resources, involves the final decision. Well-run hospitals recognize, accept, and deal constructively with process conflicts by:

— Creating an open process of debate and decision, so that everyone who is interested understands each position
— Managing the debate in ways which emphasize content rather than rank and which do not tolerate personal attacks
— Establishing clearly the central governing board's authority to make the final decision
— Making the decision in a manner that demonstrates, if not wisdom, at least good faith and consistency

Conflicts over the resources themselves must also be resolved by process. Well-run hospitals follow these guidelines:

— The process for resource allocation is rigorously followed in order that every member has the opportunity to understand how, where, and by whom the decision will be made.
— The governance structure deliberately assists members in requesting resources. . . .
— The criteria for a resource allocation decision are specified in the

mission, the long-range plan, and the long-range financial plan and are well publicized.
— There is sufficient participation in the resource allocation process that any member can assure himself or herself of consistency and equity.
— In cases of severe disagreement there is a well-understood and respected appeals process.

Conflict is avoided and resolved by open processes, candid discussion, clear criteria, and well-understood decision and appeal mechanisms. Conflict can be seriously disabling, and the hospital which uses secrecy, ambiguity, and expediency is not well-managed.

Comprehensiveness: Tying Expectations to Goals and Exchanges

In the open systems processes, community wants and available resources must be identified, translated into organizational goals, qualified, and expanded to specify what outcomes are expected. . . . A variety of errors occurs when the outcome expectations are not carefully coordinated with each other and with exchange needs. Omission of important exchange needs may be a fatal error. Redundancy or duplication of activities creates inefficiency. The error known as *suboptimization* can be avoided by paying attention to the hierarchy of expectations within the organization. Suboptimization occurs when a unit increases its achievement in a direction not consistent with the whole. The X-ray department, for example, may reduce its costs by reporting results of examinations once daily instead of twice daily. If the slower reporting is out of phase with the activities of attending physicians and if the doctor waits for the X-ray report before initiating the next phase of care, increased length of stay can result. Errors similar to suboptimization occur when one unit is organized for more or less comprehensive service than another that feeds it. A cardiology unit may expect a great volume of referrals, but the internal medicine and family practice unit may be too small to provide these referrals.

Clarity: Sources of Expectations

Vague and ambiguous expectations divert workers' attention from their work to an effort to understand their limits. These probings to clarify expectations frequently create general adversarial conditions between workers and management (or doctors and management), causing relations to become highly dysfunctional. To paraphrase Robert

Frost, good expectations make good workers (and good managers). Often the clarity of an expectation can be improved by making it quantitative. Thus one of the efforts of the well-run hospital is to steadily quantify its expectations. The management record of hospitals since World War II has emphasized quantification of cost, demand, output, efficiency, and quality. As a specific expectation becomes more precise and more quantitative, managers try to gain a measurable, if small, improvement by changing the expectation with each budget cycle. So important is the quantification of measures in closed systems, it is a major theme in the balance of this chapter.

No matter what expectation-setting process is used, there are only four broad sources of inspiration:

1. *Subjective*—Subjectively, one can build an expectation on one's desires or philosophic commitments. ("Next year we will care for 2,000 poor people in our primary care clinics," or "Next year we will decrease our surgical mortality to half its current level.") An exchange partner may establish a subjective expectation and enforce it by the exchange requirements. ("Unemployment is so high we must care for 2,000 poor people next year," or "An additional family practitioner will require a $50,000 net income guarantee," or "The major employers in town insist that cost increases be held to 5 percent next year.")

   There need be no scientific support for subjective goals. Many important ones have been achieved on faith and willpower alone. Subjective external expectations are usually the result of considerations well beyond the health care field. Examples in the 1970s included sharp increases in fuel prices, higher standards for environmental health, and a "crisis" in malpractice liability insurance. In the 1980s, Congress's action limiting Medicare expenditures to a fixed percentage of the federal budget is a striking example with far-reaching ramifications.

2. *Historical*—The hospital's history is usually available and can serve as the source of expectations. Forecasts from history need not repeat last year's values; it is usually better if they carry forward past trends. ("Surgical mortality has been falling 10 percent per year for several years, so we expect it will fall 10 percent next year.") This is the *ceteris paribus*, or other things being equal, forecast. ("Our primary care staff can support a maximum of 1,500 poor people next year.") Even the best designed and best motivated changes often require time to

achieve, and thus the short-range expectations are a blend of history and the other sources of expectations.

3. *Comparative*—The achievements or expectations of others are often a guide. ("Average costs of laboratory tests in this area are $7.86.") In a competitive environment, it is occasionally necessary to consider the expectations of other hospitals. ("Crosstown Hospital has published a charge of $40 per emergency room visit, $10 lower than our charge.") It is not always necessary to match the expectations of others, even in a competitive situation. In fact, for a variety of reasons, this may be the least rewarding source of expectations.

4. *Scientific*—One may establish standards by careful, objective study, such as cost analysis, time and motion study, or the results of scheduling systems used as simulators. Willingness to investigate and use objective sources of expectations seems to characterize well-run hospitals. The science of others may suggest new expectations. ("Massachusetts General Hospital reported in the *New England Journal of Medicine* that it reduced intensive care unit usage by 22 percent using patient classification systems.[1] We should do that here.")

   Scientific and objective expectations should be adopted with care. In addition to allowing time to achieve a better position, management needs to consider its finite resources. Realistically, the profile of real achievement is almost always below what is the scientifically possible. Priority must be given to those deficiencies that most seriously impair exchange relationships — and they are not always the largest or most obvious.

Since the ultimate test of an expectation is not where it came from but how well it serves the organization in its exchange setting, there can be no ranking of these four sources of expectations. Expectations not subjectively accepted by participants are rarely achieved, but ideals uninformed by science or unaccepted by the customer are foolishness. A historical trend can be healthy or destructive. What others do is interesting, but it may not fit local history or exchange needs. Even exchange needs can be misinterpreted. Major employers who hold too rigidly to limited cost increases could find themselves with a shortage of doctors or labor strife.

The obvious answer is that well-run hospitals use all four of these sources of expectations, and crosscheck them thoroughly. Probably the best expectation is one that is a philosophic commitment, consistent with science and history and broadly shared in the local community. It need not be consistent with any other community or hospital; in fact, if it is truly innovative, it will be unique. On the other hand, a well-run hospital will note what other hospitals are doing to make sure no new advance escapes its attention.

MONITORING PERFORMANCE

Functions

An unmonitored system will drift unpredictably, even if expectations are clearly set. The functions of monitoring are as follows:

1. To provide unambiguous measures of achievement so that every member of the organization knows not only his or her own performance, but also that of relevant other members
2. To identify correctable errors or deviations from plan so that additional resources may be brought to bear
3. To provide an objective basis for rewarding members of the organization
4. To provide data useful in setting new expectations
5. To permit members to deal with the more complex and less well understood goals and problems of the organization

These functions can often be fulfilled by formal written reports, but it is wise to remember that the primary monitor's understanding is both quicker and broader than any possible formal reporting. Much of the organization's responsiveness depends upon unwritten and even unmentioned understandings. A sound view of closed system theory is that formal reports supplement rather than replace these understandings. Unambiguous expectations and formal reports permit members of the organization to focus their attention on the frontier of unresolved issues, the fifth and final function.

Components

In cybernetic theory, the monitoring reports are called *signals*, and the subsystems creating them, *signal detectors*. Because any real system contains a certain amount of *noise*, that is, variation that cannot be corrected with current technology, variations are assigned to two categories — *significant*, or likely to be correctable, and *not significant*. Significant variations can be called *error signals*. This terminology is not common in hospitals, but it pays to remember that noise does exist and that not all variations are worth correcting. A monitoring system has five parts:

1. *Signal detection*—collecting, entering, and processing the necessary information
2. *Signal evaluation*—comparing the signal to its expectation and its noise content to decide whether the variation is significant or not
3. *Analysis*—identifying possible causes and corrections
4. *Correction*—acting to reduce future variation
5. *Reporting*—integrating the preceding four steps to suggest revised expectations

Data Systems

Monitoring is principally a human activity, but automation has greatly increased the possibilities for control. The first two parts of the monitoring system are increasingly susceptible to automation. Speed, reliability, validity, and economy of operation are generally enhanced by using routine transactions in automated systems as the basis for monitoring and further using the computer to identify error signals. . . . The principal data systems that provide monitoring information are the following:

1. *Patient order entry or order communications systems*—These capture original entries into the accounts receivable system and identify the necessary descriptive characteristics of the patient (age, sex, disease, major procedures, residence, referral source, discharge destination, payment source, and treating physicians), the demand (specific service requested), and the service (location, time of completion). They are now automated for many inpatient applications.
2. *Patient medical records*—These are archival documents which are created in part by order entries and results, but which also contain other information. They are rarely automated, but increasingly detailed, electronically readable abstracts are being drawn from them for quality and utilization control.
3. *Departmental service and reporting systems*—These monitor all the internal activities of departments, including many aspects of detailed efficiency and quality control. They include patient scheduling and personnel scheduling. They also produce reports on patient services for clinical departments. Many are now partially automated, with laboratory and pharmacy systems leading in computerization.
4. *Accounts receivable systems*—These are fully automated and supply not only revenue information, but also counts of services used by each patient.

5. *Payroll systems*—These are fully automated for purposes of compensating workers and accounting labor costs. The better systems have been extended to report personnel usage to primary control units in both real and dollar terms and to provide a factual basis for analysis and control of other employment benefits.

6. *Materials management systems*—These monitor supplies, purchase costs, inventory levels, and usage. Automation progressed rapidly in the early 1980s, but few hospitals had current systems.

7. *Physical plant management systems*—These support maintenance, cost accounting, space assignment and planning, energy management, and equipment maintenance and replacement. Much automation has been through departmental or specialized systems. The static nature of the activity permits continued reliance on manual systems.

8. *General accounting systems*—These are usually fully automated to perform a variety of accounting and financial calculations, including cost accounting and financial analysis.

The output of each of these systems now meets its first objective, providing data for monitoring specific activities. Increasingly, output is also being summarized and fed to analytic and integrative systems developing clinical expectations at several levels, budgets, long-range plans, and long-range financial plans.

INCENTIVES FOR ACHIEVING EXPECTATIONS

Cybernetic systems involving human behavior must include rewards or positive incentives for desired behavior and sanctions for undesired behavior. Rewards yield better results than sanctions. It is theoretically possible to build some kinds of organizations on sanctions alone, but it is foolish to use them heavily in hospitals. There are three reasons for this. First, the sensitivity and variability of patient care is such that only those who seek to do it well will succeed. Second, rewards can be broader, longer lasting, and more flexible. Third, systems built on sanctions are inherently regressive rather than progressive. The attention of management is diverted from improvement to enforcement.

Well-managed hospitals assume that expectations will be met in the vast majority of cases. Even a few cases of failure require so much energy to investigate and correct that they endanger the entire system. Sanctions are a part of the well-designed system that is clearly understood but rarely used. Sanctions must be quickly and judiciously applied whenever necessary, but their basic purpose is to protect the organization from destructive behavior.

Incentives can be divided into two groups, those that are psychological, or *intangible*, and those that are monetary, or *tangible*. Although most individuals work for money, that is, they require a certain tangible compensation, well-run hospitals gain their distinction by more effective management of intangible incentives. They typically rely on a combination of tangible and intangible incentives which capitalizes on all of the following kinds of rewards and uses each as frequently as possible.

1. *Inherent satisfactions in treating the sick*—Both the caring role and the curing role are rewarded in human societies. Religious recognition is particularly strong. A surprising number of hospital workers at all levels feel God will reward them for their efforts or believe their work is part of a good life and therefore wish to do their jobs well.

2. *Acceptance by the work group*—Work is an important social event for most people, and the comradeship of the work group is an important reward. To use this reward for the benefit of the organization as a whole requires extensive socialization of the work groups, but it is not impossible. Hospitals have advantages over many kinds of commerce in that their professional groups already share a common socialization and in that they can attract people who share a Samaritan motive.

3. *Professional rewards*—The procedures for many of the activities occurring in hospitals are incorporated in professional education. Rewards may be recognition and honorary promotions in professional organizations. Merit pay increases or salary scale changes can reinforce these. The principal sanction is denial of access, as in loss of admitting privileges for physicians, or discharge for other professions.

4. *Job evaluations, promotions, and salary adjustments*— Promotion and merit increases may depend upon favorable evaluations. Ideally, these evaluations should be linked to the unit expectations; individuals who help units achieve their expectations should get a tangible reward. Tangible sanctions are rare, but the power of poor evaluations as an intangible sanction should not be underestimated.

5. *Prizes and special recognition*—Important intangible rewards can be achieved by special awards, such as Employee of the Month. Many employees expect praise and will work to avoid criticism. Cash bonuses, prizes, and other tangible rewards can

be added, but they are probably less important. There are no corresponding sanctions.

Tangible incentives in the form of salary adjustment, bonuses, and prizes are assuming increasing importance in hospitals but only as supplements to effective programs of closed systems management and intangible incentives. Formal wage programs such as piece rates and productivity incentive pay systems are rare, for several reasons. Incentive pay has had an equivocal effect upon production. The systems themselves are expensive; hidden costs in labor relations and grievances are frequently overlooked. They require extensive quality control and monitoring systems to be effective in complex activities. Hospitals' complex problems of coordination make attribution of improvement difficult, reducing the reliability of assigning rewards. Unit production incentives may draw a group's attention away from the need for cooperation with other units.

A number of very well-run hospitals exist without direct incentive pay systems. While many are interested in finding incentive pay systems, and there have been numerous experiments, it is accurate to say that no convincing model suitable for widespread application currently exists.

Limitations of the Incentives

The list of incentives available to hospitals has some notable deficiencies. There appears to be a wide variety of relatively weak but highly flexible rewards and a few sanctions, which seem to be mostly strong and irreversible. The natural result of having sanctions like dismissal and loss of privileges is that they will be used only sparingly. It is clearly a challenge to use the variety of incentives in an effective package, yet similar problems afflict other kinds of organizations, and on the whole, the hospital's list is as long and as powerful as that of many other complex organizations.

Hospitals that have difficulty motivating their personnel often have problems outside the incentives themselves. Lack of clear expectations and consensus on goals are probably the most common causes of disincentive. A feeling that the real rewards will be handed out on a basis other than achievement of the publicly stated goals may be the most destructive counterincentive. Boards and executive officers whose actions are unpredictable or inconsistent are in danger of generating this result. Cynical statements such as, "It's not what you do, but who you know," or "The doctors (or the surgeons, or the unions, or any other special-interest group) really run this place; they get what they want, and the rest of us get leftovers," reflect the alienation that causes cybernetic systems to fail. . . . The correction of many problems lies not only in incentives, but in the management structure itself.

Developing Measures for Closed System Performance

The closed system model will work better when as many expectations as possible are specified in quantitative terms. Although it is often necessary to substitute words and subjective judgments for quantitative measures, simply because a concept is too complex for measurement, the use of subjective measures increases the possibility of delay and dispute. Thus one dimension of effective hospital management is the constant search for ways to quantify objectives and performance.

Whether a quantitative measurement exists or not, any real activity must monitor all of the closed system elements. It is often easier to monitor a quantitative measure than one that requires study and subjective evaluation. Measurement and quantification help the monitor keep track of what is going on.

Substantial gains have been made in our ability to measure closed system parameters in the past several decades. The gains are the result of three major external forces: scientific advances in medicine and our understanding of the "right" thing to do for each clinical symptom or condition; improvements in general management applications of cybernetic models; and the development of computers that allow easy capture, storage, and recovery of voluminous quantitative information. There is every reason to think these three trends will continue.

Figure 6.1. classifies the measures used to quantify closed system expectations. Issues in the selection and design of measures are discussed below. . . .

MEASUREMENT AND SCALING ALTERNATIVES

The activities of health care rarely lend themselves easily to measurement. They are often continuous rather than discrete. Individual differences are important. No two patients or treatments are ever alike; two activities with the same name are quite different when performed on different patients. Quantifying the closed system parameters is a matter of continually searching for measures that usually evolve from crude, almost subjective beginnings. There are four measurement categories, or scales. All are useful, and measurement may evolve through several before reaching the most useful, ratio scales.

FIGURE 6.1

Classification of Measures of Hospital Performance

Demand Measures
    Counts
    Time distribution
    Market share

Outcomes Measures
    Outputs
        Counts
        Duration
        Intensity weights
    Efficiency
    Quality
        Statistical characteristics
            Attributes
            Variables
        Conceptual characteristics
            Outcomes
            Process
            Structural

Resource Measures
    Resource consumption
        Physical values
        Cost values
            Labor
            Supplies
            Plant and equipment
    Resource conservation
        Revenue
        Revenue proxies
        Profits

1. *Nominal scales* — These identify categories that represent reliable differences, such as sex, race, or specific diagnoses. Classifications for disease, procedure, and prescription drugs are all nominal scales underpinning health care computerization. (The International Classification of Diseases is now used almost universally to describe the illnesses leading to hospitalization. Often several categories are necessary to describe a real patient, and the order of these categories is also important.) Account classifications, both for functions and responsibility centers, are nominal scales.

2. *Ordinal scales* — These identify categories that move reliably in a uniform direction, so higher numbers represent consistently different situations from lower ones. (Nominal scales are assigned arbitrarily so that high numbers have no intrinsic meaning.) The five numerical classes of Papanicolaou smears, for example, indicate progressively more serious disease as the numbers get higher. Burns, respiratory distress, infant distress, and several other clinical characteristics are quantified by ordinal scales. In a recent application related to quality and appropriateness of care, intensive care units have been using an ordinal scale to determine necessity for admission.[2] Individual patients' daily nursing requirements are usually assessed with ordinal scales.[3] Satisfaction questionnaires use ordinal scales.

3. *Interval scales* — These are ordinal scales that have uniform values between entries (so that differences may be compared). The usual example of a scalar measure, temperature, is easily recognized, because two popular scales, celsius and fahrenheit, have two different, equally arbitrary zero points.

4. *Ratio scales* — A ratio scale fulfills all the requirements of interval measures but has in addition a nonarbitrary zero value. This permits the use of percentages. Height, weight, and percentile standing on comparative distributions are all ratio scales. In accounting, dollars are a ratio scale. Most outputs of closed system processes, such as discharges, patient-days, and treatments, can be processed as ratio scales, but nominal or ordinal scales must be used to group them into comparable sets.

The problem of too many measures is a serious one. Purely redundant or conflicting measures can be eliminated, and competing alternatives can be evaluated, as suggested by the criteria that follow. The problem of summarizing or aggregating multiple parameters in a single-dimensional concept of performance, in order to avoid an unmanageably large amount of data at high management levels, must also be addressed. For closed systems, multiple measures are a serious problem. Given two measures of different elements of closed system performance, any evaluation requires implicitly or explicitly weighting the two equally, or one of the two more heavily. In some cases, the weights are clearly understood. It is easy to aggregate costs and revenues, even for activities of very different character. Dollars serve as weights, for example, for radiologists' hours and raw food. Other dimensions of expectation and achievement aggregate badly because there is no agreed-upon weighting. One avoidable infant death and one failure to pursue preventive care in an elderly man do not clearly add to anything. Neither can one comfortably average "66 percent efficiency in the operating room" and "95 percent achievement of expected raw food costs."

Conceptually, there are three ways around the dilemma of multiple measures:

1. Rank the various measures by importance, and concentrate on a manageable number of the most important. Those omitted are not lost, they are just removed from the routine reports; they would still be available for special study and for setting future expectations. The ranking should follow the importance of the activity to the mission of the hospital.
2. Find acceptable weights to permit aggregation. There must be several of these because there are several different aggregation problems. Often an arbitrary weight is used, because the cost of more precise work exceeds the value of the measure.
3. Sample the measures, either at random or by identifying those that are representative of their group.

All three of these approaches are required, in combinations. Well-run hospitals are more aggressive and more ingenious than others in their pursuit of opportunities for condensing multiple measures. Most hospitals start with rank ordering, using weighting and sampling as adjunct tools. Although the actual rank order depends on the mission, suppose a criterion for assigning rank could be established for each of the major groups of measures. In some cases, this criterion would suggest the number and kind of measures as well. Then weighting and sampling or elimination of the measures could be decided on the basis of their importance as well.

CRITERIA FOR SELECTING MEASURES

One judges the acceptability of a measure by its value and its cost. Value is the measures contribution to performance. Value stems from systems of application, including the measure itself, expectations, and reporting. Selecting a measure, therefore, means selecting a measurement system. In most situations, the monitor is able to achieve some level of performance without a particular measure and a better level of performance with it. On the other hand, providing the measure involves certain costs. Conceptually, both values and costs must be measured against the mission of the organization. If the measure contributes more to achievement than it costs to maintain, it is desirable. Often there are several possible measurement schemes differing in reliability, validity, timing, and, as a result, both in costs and in value. Thus the design of a measurement system involves the selection of the best alternative.

Value

Measures are valuable because they assist the monitor in achieving control. If, for example, a given system for reporting budgeting and payroll costs allows the monitor to maintain operations while reducing labor costs by $5,000 per year, that is its value. Generally speaking, the more reliable, valid, and timely the measure is, the greater its value will be—up to the point where the monitor can change actual performance. As a result of this limit, the value of measurement systems is always constrained by a variety of other factors and characteristics of the organization.

Cost

The cost of a measurement system is a combination of two elements, the resources consumed in obtaining, processing, reporting, and setting expectations for it and the opportunity costs of incorrect reports. It is convenient to label the first group *accounting costs* and the second *hidden costs*. Thoughtful measurement design must always address both.

Accounting costs tend to increase with improvements in reliability, validity, and timeliness, but automation has generally permitted great reductions in accounting costs of measurement. Often accounting costs can be reduced at the same time the accuracy of the measure is increased, by a combination of automation and integration. If a large number of measures is generated from the same basic collection and processing system and the output is used frequently, the result is a relatively large number of accurate and inexpensive measures. Measurement system design, therefore, frequently involves seeking ways to integrate several different measures.

The cost of a measure can also be reduced by sacrificing accuracy and timeliness, although these sacrifices risk increasing the hidden costs. Hidden costs occur because of two possible incorrect interpretations of the error signal. *False negatives* occur when a correctable condition is not reported to the monitor, and therefore the monitor achieves less than he or she might. *False positives* occur when the measurement system reports a correctable situation when in fact none exists; the monitor must investigate the finding, and that investigation is costly.

Reliability

A measure is conceptually reliable if repeated application to an identical situation yields the same value. The repetition may be either in time, space, or detection system; test and retest and substitution of observers are frequently used to measure reliability. Lack of reliability impairs precision of measurement. Although reliability in excess of the monitor's ability to respond is valueless, it is also true that the monitor can only respond within the limits of the measurement's reliability. Allowance must be made for measurement error. If the goal is 200 units of output, but the reliability of the measure is only ± 10 percent, all values from 180 to 220 must be interpreted as achieving the goal.

Reliability is enhanced by clear definitions of what is to be counted or measured, good measuring tools, audits, and training of observers. A measurement that is used routinely is likely to improve in reliability because it is used frequently.

Validity

A measure is said to be valid if the reported value is true as defined by the exchange objectives. If an invalid measure is used in a cybernetic system, the energies of the unit can be directed toward achieving high scores on that measure rather than achieving the unit's true goals. The result may be a seriously disabling distortion of intended activity.

An anecdote may be the best way to illustrate the question of validity. A factory produced nails, and someone wished to improve its performance by setting output goals for the employees. So a goal was set at a certain number of nails per hour. After a short time, the goal was exceeded, but the factory was producing mostly tacks. So the goal was changed to a certain number of *pounds* of nails per hour. Again the goal was exceeded, but this time the factory was producing spikes. The moral is that validity of measurement depends upon what the goals are. If one wants a variety of nails, one's measures and expectations in cybernetic systems must reflect that.

Timeliness

There are two important criteria of timeliness: frequency and delay. Particularly at lower levels of the organization, the monitor must react quite quickly. The measurement system that reports too late for the monitor to respond is at best useless and at worst costly, because it generates hidden costs by prompting improper responses.

Measures also differ in how frequently they usefully can be reported.

Reports that are too infrequent allow correctable conditions to exist, yet reports can come too often. There is a finite time attached to a response cycle. Reporting more frequently than once per response cycle is not useful. In some of the complex issues of quality and efficiency the response cycles are quite long. For example, changing physical facilities may be possible only at intervals of many years. Interim reports on the cost of physical facilities will be of little value. Several dimensions of quality require extensive and careful responses and as a result tolerate infrequent measurement.

Special Studies

A special study is basically an infrequent, or nonrecurring measurement system. It is a relatively low-cost, useful means of evaluating and selecting measures. Using research techniques, measurements can be as reliable and valid as desired, within the limits of current technology. The results can be considered in terms of the monitor's ability to respond, the potential value of the response, and both the accounting and hidden costs of a continuing or more frequent measurement system. Special studies are useful for a variety of purposes, including verifying assumptions about improvement in performance, evaluating changes in systems, evaluating changes in measurement systems, and collecting very expensive performance measures. The most common examples of special studies in hospitals are measures of quality, because both their accounting and their hidden costs are frequently quite high. Surveys of doctor, patient, and community attitudes are another example. Special investigations of medical and nursing care of specific kinds of cases are yet another.

IMPORTANCE OF OUTPUT MEASURES

Although many closed system parameters can be measured, the extent to which hospital organizational units have a countable product or output is particularly critical in the design of cybernetic systems. Having countable outputs greatly simplifies the management task. Not only demand and volume, but efficiency, revenue, profit, and at least one measure of quality are easily quantified as a result. Efficiency, the ratio of output to inputs, is measurable only when output can be measured. Revenue can be posted only when a unit of service has been defined. The measurement of profit depends upon revenue. A pass-fail judgment on work by inspection of a sample of output constitutes a basic measure of quality.

Obstetrical deliveries and appendectomies are discrete, unambiguous events, archetypes of countable outputs. Complications are relatively rare and can be handled by establishing a separate, much smaller count. In contrast, many hospital activities are quite difficult to count. Clinical services such as psychiatry and social work and support services such as housekeeping are more continuous than discrete. Managerial support services with infrequent or intermittent end points, for example planning and marketing, essentially cannot be measured by output. There is no meaningful analogy in these departments to number of births.

Operating rooms, delivery rooms, clinics, kitchens, laboratories, pharmacies, laundries, and X-ray and physical therapy units all have measures of output and, as a result, measures of most of the closed system parameters. Continuous service activities such as medical care, nursing, housekeeping, and plant maintenance, require major adjustments. Counselling services (for example, personnel, social service, and psychology) present serious measurement problems that reduce the contribution of quantitative approaches. Such staff services as planning and public relations are very difficult to measure. The cybernetic process still works, but words and concepts must be substituted for measures and expectations. The clearer expectations can be made, however, the better the cybernetic process will work. . . .

NOTES

1.   D.E. Singer, et al., "Rationing Intensive Care — Physician Responses to a Resource Shortage," *New England Journal of Medicine* 309 (1983): 1155–60.

2.   W.A. Knaus, E.A. Draper, and D.P. Wagner, "The Use of Intensive Care New Research Initiatives and Their Application for National Health Policy," *Milbank Memorial Fund Quarterly* 61 (Fall 1983): 561–83.

3.   R.C. Jelinek, "An Operational Analysis of the Patient Care Function," *Inquiry* 6 (June 1969): 53–58.

7 | # Improving the Effectiveness of Hospital Governing Boards

Anthony R. Kovner

PROBLEMS WITH THE BOARD'S PERFORMANCE

Peters and Tseng note some common characteristics of boards of well-managed hospitals: the boards are active and working, they have a clear understanding of their own and management's responsibilities, and they are viewed by management as an ally in managing change.[1] There is, however, disagreement about what the board's contribution to hospital performance should be and even about hospital performance itself, other than avoidance of bankruptcy and retention of accreditation.

It is commonly suggested that boards evaluate their own performance.[2] This is a good idea, but, even if methodological problems could be overcome, the costs of effective evaluation might be too high. Self-evaluation is costly in terms of both the time the board would have to spend in reaching agreement on measurable hospital objectives and the opportunities to do other things the board would have to forgo. Self-evaluation is much less costly when hospital performance standards are set in advance each year, because board standards can then be set in relation to hospital objectives. Less frequently, the process of setting standards itself should be examined in order to make certain that what is being measured has remained critical to the hospital's ability to attain its goals.

In focusing upon the board's contribution, evaluators may look at the board as a whole, the individual members of the board, or both. Factors

An excerpt from the article in *Frontiers of Health Services Management* 2 (August 1985): 20–29, with permission, Health Administration Press.

that should be considered in evaluating the contribution of the board as a whole include:

- How well the board functions in relation to hospital bylaws, accreditation, and circumstances;
- How effectively the board reviews and approves hospital objectives and the processes by which they are set;
- The extent to which the board participates in the hospital's decision-making process and the effectiveness, timeliness, and appropriateness of its action on reports received;
- The extent to which the board uses the data it receives in reviewing managerial decisions and requests additional data, when appropriate;
- How competently the board evaluates management performance;
- How conscientiously the board monitors its structures, including continuing education for members and compensation for members.

Factors relating to the performance of individual members include:

- How carefully job descriptions for board members are written, followed, and updated;
- Whether the board member spends an appropriate amount of time on hospital business;
- The extent to which the member participates in the board's decision making;
- The adequacy of the member's boundary-spanning activities;
- How effectively the member generates resources;
- Whether the member generates support for the CEO.

There are four key problems in hospital governance: (1) board inability to specify hospital objectives; (2) inefficient and ineffective hospital decision making; (3) lack of corporate strategy and, therefore, lack of ability to implement strategy; and (4) conflict over the functions of the governing board. These are problems about which many boards can do something.

INABILITY TO SPECIFY OBJECTIVES

One of the chief advantages that investor-owned hospitals have is the clarity of their organizational objectives. Corporate financial policies and objectives of one such investor-owned multihospital system, Hospital Corporation of America (HCA), are as follows:

- A 60 percent – 40 percent debt-to-equity ratio;
- An expected after-tax return on average equity of at least 17 percent;
- An expected after-tax return on average capital of at least 11 percent;
- An annual earnings-per-share growth, after general inflation, of at least 13 percent;
- The maintenance or improvement of net profit margins;
- The maintenance of a dividend rate sufficient to meet HCA's capital needs and to provide a return on shareholders' investments.[3]

Presumably, if HCA hospitals or services in these hospitals cannot meet these objectives now or in the immediate future, HCA will either close them or change financial policies and goals.

Many hospital boards do not specify objectives, because board, management, and medical staff cannot or will not agree on either the objectives themselves or a desirable level of attainment. Conflict over objectives stems in large part, I believe, from the fact that the medical staff is only partially integrated into the hospital's organizational structure, and, as a result, it is unclear whose hospital it is. I assume that the hospital is the governing board's, either as external sponsor or as the representative of the community served. I believe also that it is in the board's interest for managers to set policy within a wide scope, subject to board review.

INEFFICIENT, INEFFECTIVE DECISION MAKING

There are several possible reasons for inefficient, ineffective decision making: the board may be too large; too many groups and individuals may be involved in strategic decision making; too many levels of groups may be involved; those who make strategic decisions may not be adequately informed; and it may be unclear which group at what level is supposed to make which strategic decision.

The following description of decision making in a teaching hospital is a good example of such ineffectiveness.

First, there are two boards that govern the hospital, each with different orientations and separate reporting lines and with few guidelines to determine how decisions are allocated between them. . . . Second . . . the hospital's director continues to be subject to the line authority of several functional vice presidents of the university. Third, the hospital director and the dean of the medical school share line authority over the same chiefs of the hospital's clinical services, who are also chairpersons of academic departments within the medical school. Finally, each line executive's bureaucratic authority is countered by a collegial body of subordinates who advise the executive in matters affecting their vital interests.[4]

Often CEOs are either not expected or lack the staff to develop and implement a strategic plan, with due consideration of alternatives, for board approval. Further, boards do not always either accept the plan or suggest changes for the chief executive to take into account for presentation at a subsequent meeting. Hospital decision-making processes may still be geared to earlier environments and missions for which they were more appropriate.

LACK OF CORPORATE STRATEGY

According to Ritvo, hospital boards are coping with actual problems rather than anticipating future issues. In identifying concerns, they rely heavily on internal data rather than on data regarding competitors.[5] In a study of 32 hospital plans, Kropf and Goldsmith found that, although "strategic planning, competition, marketing, and the use of sophisticated analytic techniques are constantly being called essential to the survival of hospitals, there was no evidence in a sample of plans that these concepts and techniques are being widely adopted."[6]

Key reasons for the lack of emphasis on corporate strategy are, first, that physicians are only partially integrated into the hospital's organizational structure and, second, that CEOs are not demanding rigorous staff work. In competing for physician services with other hospitals, boards and managers have tended to allocate resources to the acquisition of sufficient new technology rather than to the development of appropriate planning and marketing capabilities. Chief executive officers often lack skills in these areas; even when they have employed planning and marketing specialists, the specialists seldom work closely enough with physician leaders. Their plans and programs, often lacking in political reality, are then delayed, rejected, or watered down by the medical staff and are therefore not effectively implemented.

CONFLICT OVER BOARD FUNCTIONS

According to Dayton, "every time you find a business in trouble, you find a board of directors either unwilling or unable to fulfill its responsibilities."[7] According to Pfeffer, "corporations who fail to use their boards as links to their environments pay penalties in reduced profits."[8]

It must be clear what group in the hospital is supposed to make what decisions. Is the board to make the strategic decisions, with the help of management? Should the board review and approve management's making of the strategic decisions? Or is the board merely supposed to raise money to provide physicians with equipment and facilities for patient care?

It is difficult to make strategic decisions if there is conflict among board, management, and medical staff as to what each group is supposed to do. The board's responsibilities should be related to its functions at any particular hospital. Board functions, I believe, should be specified and agreed upon by contending or accommodating parties in order for the board to carry out its responsibilities effectively.

For example, if the board is to assume primary responsibility for strategic decisions, its members must be informed and willing to make such decisions. I reject this alternative because many hospital boards are not. If, on the other hand, the board is to review and approve management's decisions, management must be informed and willing, and the board must be able to evaluate the competence of management. I believe that boards can find or retain managers who are informed and willing and that boards can capably evaluate the competence of managers—that is why I urge this alternative. If the board is expected to provide financial resources to support the practices of individual physicians, it must be willing and able to generate funds to a much greater extent than is common now. I reject this alternative as well, because I do not think that most hospital boards are willing and able to do so.

RECOMMENDATIONS FOR IMPROVING PERFORMANCE

My focus has been on hospital adaptation through changes in governance. I am assuming that more hospitals are facing increased competition and a more rapid rate of change; that the trend toward fewer, larger hospitals will continue; and that management will have increasing power relative to boards and medical staffs in making strategic decisions. I am assuming that hospitals which cannot adapt successfully will close, merge, or lose their share of the market. In some cases this may be negative for hospital officials and positive for those who pay hospital insurance premiums. Even if my recommendations are adopted, some hospitals will have to close, merge, or lose market share, but they may be able to avoid more severe environmental jolts or adapt to them more easily than if present governance patterns were continued. Adapting to change can be traumatic, yet hospitals have substantial power to manage change.

In 1978, I developed a list of proposals made by others to improve hospital governing board performance. I have added to this list new proposals, shown in italics in Table 7.1. In 1978, proposals in the areas of internal board structure and function appeared to offer the most promise for improving board performance, and I listed several of them in the table.

Now I am focusing on specific proposals to improve board function and structure in order to improve hospital decision making and performance in an environment that is more threatening, rapidly changing, and risky than it was six years ago. Boards should (1) integrate medical leadership into hospital governance, (2) streamline the process of making strategic decisions, (3) support management in managing change, and (4) focus and energize the board itself.

INTEGRATE MEDICAL LEADERS INTO
HOSPITAL GOVERNANCE

Better medical staff integration is required if hospitals are to make and implement strategic decisions in the face of increased competition and limited inpatient reimbursement. Formal physician leaders should be recruited, retained, and held accountable by hospital managers, with board support.

Integration involves contractual obligations between the hospital and physician leaders who are at least partially salaried and who are selected and retained in part because of their competence as strategic managers.[9] Some of these physician leaders may also serve on the hospital governing board. They or other physician leaders may play a major role in considering joint hospital-physician ventures to protect market share.

Increasingly, the hospital may be competing with physicians for patients. As the hospital strengthens its affiliations with some physicians, its affiliations with other physicians will be weakened; these physicians will choose to compete with the hospital or to pursue other markets rather than respond to the influence of physician leadership.

Sufficient integration can be attained without a corporate form of organization. Physician chiefs will influence primarily physicians rather than other staff who provide patient care. Sufficient integration does not require employment of full-time chiefs of service or partially salaried chiefs for every service. It may require employment of a medical director who is in charge of physician services at the hospital.

STREAMLINE DECISION MAKING

Streamlining strategic decision making requires fewer members on the decision-making body (either the board as a whole or the executive committee), fewer layers of decision making, more informed board mem-

TABLE 7.1

Proposals for Improving Hospital Board Performance

Area	Proposal
Reduction of autonomy	Regulate hospital services provided Restrict fund raising Control rates Pool depreciation Approve line-item budgets and specified staffing *Merge with other hospitals* *Use management contracts* *Deregulate hospitals* *Develop trustee organizations across hospitals*
Accountability	Sanction board members for poor hospital performance Reduce hospital reimbursement for poor board performance Extend existing conflict-of-interest prohibitions Provide for elections of board members by the community *Restructure the hospital into several separate corporations* *Integrate physician leaders into the organizational structure*
Composition	Limit tenure (by years of service and age) Adopt business form of corporate organization Limit the size of governing boards Allow consumers to control hospitals Include staff physicians on boards *Include CEOs of other hospitals on boards*
Function	Require that hospital goals and performance standards be set Establish information systems to monitor compliance with goals and standards Establish control systems to evaluate performance relative to expectations Establish incentive systems to influence physician performance *Focus board planning and evaluation* *Support management in managing change*
Structure	Pay board members Hold open meetings of the governing board Publish minutes of board meetings Conduct longer, more frequent board meetings Require board involvement in resolution of complaints Mandate self-auditing and external auditing of governing board performance *Improve the board's education* *Appoint the CEO chairman of the board* *Appoint fewer and smaller committees* *Write job description for board members*

Adapted from Anthony R. Kovner, "Improving Community Hospital Board Performance," *Medical Care* 16 (February 1978): 79–89, with permission, J. B. Lippincott. This table has been revised; additions are in italics.

bers, fewer board committees and fewer members on those committees, and increased support from management in planning and marketing.

The object is to increase the quantity and timeliness of strategic decisions. This does not mean that strategic decisions should be made too quickly, that input from those affected by such decisions should not be solicited, or that reasons for moving ahead or not moving ahead in the face of sizable or deeply felt opposition should not be given.

Streamlining requires that more attention be paid to how decisions are made and by whom and to explaining to physicians and others how the process works. Streamlining requires a more active role for management in the decision-making process, with continued oversight and support provided by the governing board.

SUPPORT MANAGEMENT IN MANAGING CHANGE

There has been an increase in the turnover of hospital managers in the 1970s and 1980s. Often this has resulted from governing boards' unwillingness to support managers who were attempting to implement change opposed by medical staffs.

Managers need to become more active, to lead in the development and implementation of corporate strategy. Board members require the information and the will to effectively carry out a support function. Too many board members now are selected or retained without regard to their ability to support management effectively. For example, most board members are given too little information about competitors' characteristics and trends in the industry. Few board members have executive experience in hospitals or similar organizations. Recruitment and retention of capable board members are hampered by little or no compensation for members' time.

FOCUS AND ENERGIZE THE BOARD

Given my assumptions about the problems hospitals face, more boards should focus on long-range planning and evaluation of management rather than on hospital operations. Boards should approve and review corporate strategy rather than formulate it. Rather than managing hospitals themselves, boards should spend more time holding managers accountable and assuring that competent managers are trained for medical and other services.

An important aspect of the recent trend in corporate restructuring is its potential for focusing and energizing boards. Peters and Tseng cite the experience of Alta Bates Hospital in this regard:

In the corporate reorganization, the hospital realized that there were too many issues for the hospital board to handle and that it was necessary to reduce the time commitment and committee activity of trustees. In addition, there was a desire to diversify the board structure so that the talents of board members could be tailored to the needs of the different subsidiary corporations.[10]

Related approaches include the creation of a separate foundation for hospital fund raising and the use of board committees rather than the entire board to do most of the work on certain issues.

Creating different boards for different purposes poses problems of its own: the activities of the several boards must be integrated, and management must spend additional time providing support services and communicating with the members of the various boards. Restructuring is generally more useful when it moves in the direction of smaller, more informed boards and a stronger role for managers.

Effective managerial staff work can help focus and energize the board. Board members should receive, in advance, information about the issues to be discussed at a meeting. Subcommittee reports can be accepted unless there is dissent. New business can be referred to subcommittees. Much of the work now done by board subcommittees should probably be done by management. The CEO should make recommendations concerning most items on the agenda.[11] More of the board's attention should be focused on reviewing and testing long-range plans and on evaluating management.

IMPLEMENTATION OF THE RECOMMENDATIONS

Implementing change that does not work is probably worse than doing nothing—and "if it ain't broke, don't fix it."

There are more ways to enhance the decision-making and governance processes than those indicated here, and, of course, hospitals can successfully make decisions even if they do not implement these recommendations. For example, I have studied a very effective hospital governing board that has over 60 members, a senile chairman, no physicians (although the CEO is a physician), and numerous large committees. The board is successful because of the active involvement of 20 to 25 members, many of whom have managerial experience, some of whom are new to the board, and some of whom are in their 40s and 50s. These members commit the necessary time and have become informed about the hospital's business. Further, the hospital has capable managers who have been there a long time. I believe that governance of this hospital is effective *despite* its deviation from my recommendations rather than *because* of it.

The following constrain the implementation of these recommendations:

- Groups in power prefer the status quo;
- Some managers lack the necessary skills and competence to implement them;
- Physician leaders are unwilling or unable to lead or become integrated in hospital governance;
- Attending physicians are opposed to the desired changes;
- Board, management, and medical staff are in conflict over the hospital's mission.

The following present opportunities for implementing these recommendations:

- There is a greater sense of crisis or impending crisis in many hospitals because of increased local competition and new reimbursement ceilings;
- The supply of physicians is growing;
- Investor-owned corporations, whose board structure and function embody several of the recommendations made here, have been successful;
- Some boards, with the support of physician leaders, are focusing on better recruitment and retention of competent managers.

THE NEED FOR RESEARCH

I will not attempt to convince anyone that research on hospital governance is necessary and cost-effective, even though I believe it is. Boards and managers need to know what works in hospital governance, what does not work, and why. Research is one of the ways through which boards and managers can determine the following:

- In what ways do governing boards make a difference in hospital performance?
- What information do boards need to make better strategic decisions?
- What are the characteristics of effective and ineffective boards?
- What role, if any, should governing boards play in assuring high-quality care?

ACKNOWLEDGMENTS

I wish to thank Alan Altshuler, Jeffrey Alexander, John Griffith, Christine Kovner, Maureen Lowry, Stephen Shortell, Phyllis Virgil, and Bruce Vladeck for their comments on earlier drafts of this paper and Maureen Lowry for her research assistance.

NOTES

1.   Joseph P. Peters and Simone Tseng, *Managing Strategic Change in Hospitals*, (Chicago: American Hospital Publishing, 1983), pp. 59–63.

2.   Joint Commission on Accreditation of Hospitals, *Accreditation Manual for Hospitals*, 1984 ed. (Chicago: JCAH, 1983), p. 51.

3.   Hospital Corporation of America, *Annual Report* (Nashville, Tenn., 1984).

4.   Robert F. Allison and Jephtha W. Dalston, "Governance of University-Owned Teaching Hospitals," *Inquiry* 19 (Spring 1982): 11–12.

5.   Roger A. Ritvo, "Adaptation to Environmental Change: The Board's Role," *Hospital and Health Services Administration* 25 (Winter 1980): 23–27.

6.   Roger Kropf and Seth B. Goldsmith, "Innovation in Hospital Plans," *Health Care Management Review* 8 (Spring 1983): 7.

7.   Kenneth N. Dayton, "Corporate Governance: The Other Side of the Coin," *Harvard Business Review* 84 (January-February 1984): 34.

8.   Jeffrey Pfeffer, "Size and Composition of Corporate Boards of Directors: The Organization and Its Environment," *Administrative Science Quarterly* 17 (1972): 219.

9.   Anthony R. Kovner and Martin J. Chin, "The Participation of Physician Leadership in Hospital Strategic Decision-Making," unpublished.

10.   Peters and Tseng, *Managing Strategic Change*, pp. 127–28.

11.   John Griffith, personal communication, October 1984.

8 | Simplified Manual Systems for Clinical Management: The Internal Management Report

Richard Owens
Patricia Fairchild
Annette Pierce
Ronald Goldberg

Any health care service delivery system, whether it be a free-standing National Health Service Corps site or a large Comprehensive Health Center, requires information systems for tracking particular target groups, for monitoring particular events and management indicators, for auditing the service delivery process and for reporting project activities to government sponsors, boards of directors, service providers and project managers. The structure and format of these systems depend on project size, services provided, management structure, project procedures, state laws and so forth. Thus it is not possible to design a total system that will satisfy all the information needs of every project. It is always necessary to customize systems to fit a project's particular needs.

Most primary health centers, even small rural practices, are fairly

Reprinted from *The Journal of Ambulatory Care Management*, Vol. 3, No. 2, pp. 1–17, with permission of Aspen Publishers, Inc., © May 1980.

This project has been funded in part by DHEW Region X contract 290-77-0007. The contents of this article do not necessarily reflect the views or policies of DHEW.

complex systems. Management activities are often carried out by a number of people: the administrator, the medical director, the board chairperson, etc.; each has responsibility for different aspects of the system. Even if one person has overall responsibility, he or she cannot always know what is happening in all parts of the project. Even in the smallest project, a tremendous amount of data exists, ranging from simple financial data to service statistics to population demographic data. It is rare that any one individual can (or would want to) keep track of a significant portion of these facts.

For these reasons, it is desirable to have available in summary form a project's most important management information, for use within the organization. This article addresses the definition, collection and display of such information, in a form called an Internal Management Report (IMR). In general, the audience is assumed to be small- to medium-sized practices, for whom computer capability is unavailable, impractical or overly expensive. The following discussion addresses only management information that can be collected manually.

There are two major assumptions that dictate the content and structure of an IMR. The first is that only data that will actually be used for decision making by project staff or board members should be collected. The second is that to be usable, the data must be organized in a clear, concise form, here called management indicators.

CHARACTERISTICS OF MANAGEMENT INDICATORS

Stated simply, a management indicator is a number or a combination of numbers that can, for the purpose of management decision making, be used to represent a complex series of program activities.

There are several important considerations in the selection of such indicators. First and most important, as implied by this definition, is that the indicator must be related to decision making. For example, there is no point in knowing the number of medical care visits by age group unless consideration is being given to establishing specific programs for specific age groups. Second, an indicator must be sensitive enough to reflect the consequences of the decisions being made. The fertility rate, for example, changes very slowly, and for reasons that may be outside the health system. Therefore, fertility rate by itself is not an adequate indicator for measuring effectiveness of a family planning program. Last, a good indicator must be simple, clear and concisely displayed in a format conducive to the decision being made.

Thus a management indicator is a number that can be used for the purpose of management. It is not a health status indicator, although health status indicators are important. It is also not synonymous with funding criteria, although funding criteria can be management indicators.

Management indicators reduce drastically the amount of data that must be recorded and reported, and if they are well chosen, pinpoint information most important for decision making. Because managers cannot concentrate on everything at once, indicators should focus attention on aspects of the service system where performance is different than planned; an indicator should raise a warning flag whenever some portion of the delivery system requires management assistance. For example, one indicator in an ambulatory health care program is the number of encounters each month. Should this indicator decrease over time, program managers would be warned of a potentially serious problem.

It should be noted, however, that a management indicator normally only warns managers of areas where performance is worse or better than expected; it cannot explain why the difference has occurred. In the example given, the decrease in encounters could be due to scheduling problems, to a change in the types and lengths of encounters or to the more serious problem of patients leaving the system. It is impossible for an IMR to anticipate every possible cause.

Clearly, an IMR is a tremendous simplification of program activities. Its success as a management tool depends largely on the aptness of the management indicators chosen. Also important, however, is how to measure the indicators; this decision depends on the uses to which the information will be put. First, it is necessary to decide whether to use a cumulative measure. For example, year-to-date expenditures are most appropriate for comparison to an annual budget; however, encounters should be counted month by month for resource planning purposes. Second, it is important to display indicators in the most mathematically useful fashion. Encounters, for example, should be presented as an absolute number, whereas the ratio of charges to collections should be shown as a percentage. Third, some indicators should be displayed as a function of time, because it is the change over time that is primarily of interest. Encounter data fall into this category. Fourth, and most important, indicators should be presented in comparison to targets whenever such targets can be reasonably set. For example, total physician encounters against a program goal of x encounters per time period might be shown.

Use of Management Indicators

The simplest framework for categorizing decisions holds that managers engage in three activities: planning, implementation and evaluation. That is, they plan a program by setting goals and objectives, defining activities and targets and determining required resource inputs. They then implement this program, and as implementation progresses, they evaluate progress in relation to the plan. It is in planning and evaluation that the IMR is most useful.

One key to effective program management is the establishment of goals and priorities that can be quantified and measured. Lack of agreement among program managers regarding goals and priorities causes different groups to work in different, sometimes contradictory, directions, to compete for resources when cooperation would be more advantageous or to misallocate resources. Agreement can only be obtained when goals, objectives, and priorities are explicitly quantified and made available to all the managers involved.

This explicit quantification is usually called target setting. Examples of measurable targets are as follows:

- increase encounters per full-time equivalent (FTE) physician from 3,500 to 4,200 per year, and
- increase the ratio of new patients to total encounters by 4 percent.

Target setting, generally speaking, is what managers do worst. If explicit targets are set at all, they are usually set for long-term measures that will not change for years. The reason for this is not that managers are incompetent, but rather that target setting is very difficult, and baseline data needed to establish targets are usually lacking. Nevertheless, health programs continue to operate, in many cases quite satisfactorily, because program managers make decisions relative to targets that they hold implicitly. One purpose of planning is to make these targets explicit and open to discussion by all concerned.

The default method of setting targets is "last year's level plus or minus 5 percent." In this case the IMR provides baseline data for making such a calculation. If the program has been performing well, this method of target setting may work, although setting targets in relation to norms or standards is much more appropriate.

The mathematical expression of a target must be thought through carefully. For example, the target "300 total visits per month for the next year" is not appropriate if demand varies with the season. The target should either reflect this seasonal variation or be specified as "an average of 300 visits per month for the next year." Moreover targets are frequently set in terms of an acceptable range, as with a standard growth chart.

If measurable targets have been set in the planning process, then evaluation involves simply monitoring each indicator at appropriate intervals to see how performance compares to targets. In general, evaluation of progress can only be expressed in three ways: on target, above target and below target. However, for many decisions, the course of action is not obvious. Being either above or below target can be either good or bad, or it may mean that the target is inappropriate. Moreover, "good" deviations from target may also require action: someone should determine why the program is able to do better than anticipated.

In cases in which managers have not or cannot set such measurable targets, it may be possible to at least specify whether changes over time in a management indicator are good or bad. This type of evaluation is usually called "trend analysis." For example, if no population data are available, it may not be possible to set a realistic target for new patients. However, if the assumption is that health center services are good, then clearly more new patients are better than fewer. Thus an IMR that keeps track of new patients over time can be used to decide whether the program is doing better or worse than it did the previous year.

Thus it is necessary to select management indicators that are appropriate, concise and sensitive, and to establish targets and norms or appropriate trends for monitoring progress. It is also necessary to display these indicators in a usable format.

ORGANIZATION AND DISPLAY OF MANAGEMENT INDICATORS

Management indicators must be organized and displayed in a format that facilitates decision making. At a minimum, it should be easy to compare indicators to targets or norms and, where appropriate, to previous time periods.

For many people, an appropriate organization is one that also minimizes the amount of data displayed; a report that simply lists 10 or 15 items across a page may be too confusing to interest anyone who lacks a background in statistics. At the same time, it is desirable, especially in a manual system, to reduce the number of pages of data that must be kept organized. Thus, several displays of information may be required, depending on the audience. The simplest way to minimize problems of information display, again, is to minimize the amount of information; a list of 50 management indicators is probably useless, even if each indicator meets the aforementioned criteria.

It is also important to distinguish between collection of data and display of information. Most data in a manual system should be collected at least monthly; otherwise the collection effort is likely to become unmanageable. Larger projects may find daily collection more reasonable. However, the information may or may not be used on a monthly basis; for example, some measures might be used monthly by staff members and quarterly by board members. This timing also affects the formats in which information is presented.

Figure 8.1 presents one possible organization of an IMR that is suitable for monthly collection of data and for some trend analysis. Figure 8.2 presents a format that allows for a quarterly summary of the same data, and for comparisons to budget or target as well as previous year figures. Thus this arrangement assumes monthly collection but uses primarily quarterly analysis.

The first section of each report lists the most aggregate indicators of program performance, because it is assumed that many users will look no further if the aggregate indicators are satisfactory. More detailed indicators are organized according to functional areas by which a health center might be managed. Although a representative list of functions for a small health center has been used in the example, this organization, as well as the indicators, may change from project to project. The indicators may also change as problems are solved or as the project's environment changes; thus the IMR format should not be rigid.

For very small projects, these sample reports may be more complex than is necessary; for larger projects (e.g., ones with multiple sites), these samples are too simplistic. DHEW Bureau of Community Health Services projects will note that not all required Bureau Common Reporting Requirements (BCRR) indicators are shown in this example. To avoid duplicating this federally mandated collection system, only indicators which may be of interest on a monthly basis are included here.

Examples of Management Indicators

SUMMARY STATISTICS

This section of the IMR summarizes the most important and frequently used management indicators, as follows.

Total Encounters

The most aggregate measure of services provided is the total number of encounters for a given period. The absolute level of encounters is a useful number, when compared to target population figures, for judging project impact; it is also useful in resource planning, because variable resources (staff time, supplies) are expended in proportion to encounters.

FIGURE 8.1

Monthly Internal Management Report
(Calendar Year 19× ×)

Indicator	Jan.	Feb.	Mar.	Apr.	May	June	July	Aug.	Sept.	Oct.	Nov.	Dec.	Total
Summary statistics													
Total encounters													
Total operating costs													
Total collections													
Total cash													
Health center services													
Encounters by type													
medical													
prenatal													
dental													
New patients													
Year-to-date users													
medical													
prenatal													
dental													
New patient ratio													
Encounters per FTE staff													
MD													
MLP													
dentist													
team productivity													
Reception													
No-show rate													
At-visit collection rate													
Financial management													
Break-even ratio													
Charges ratio													
Self-sufficiency ratio													
Collection ratio													
Total net charges													
Net charges													
Medicaid													
Medicare													
other insurance													
private pay													
Total A/R at end of month													
A/R by source													
Medicaid/total													
Medicare/total													
other insurance/total													
private pay/total													
Months of A/R													
A/P at end of month													
Operating costs													
salaries													
other													
Cost per encounter													
Personnel management													
FTE staff													
medical													
administrative													
other													
Staff turnover rate													
provider													
other													

FIGURE 8.2

Quarterly Internal Management Report
(Calendar Year 19 × ×)

Indicator	January–March			April–June			July–September			October–December			Yearly Total		
	Target/ Budget/ Last Yr.	Current Period	% Change	Target/ Budget/ Last Yr.	Current Period	% Change	Target/ Budget/ Last Yr.	Current Period	% Change	Target/ Budget/ Last Yr.	Current Period	% Change	Target/ Budget/ Last Yr.	Current Period	% Change
Summary statistics															
Total encounters															
Total operating costs															
Total collections															
Total cash															
Health center services															
Encounters by type															
medical															
prenatal															
dental															
New patients ratio															
Financial management															
Break-even ratio															
Charges ratio															
Self-sufficiency ratio															
Collection ratio															
Total net charges															
Cost per encounter															
Personnel management															
Staff turnover rate															
provider															
other															

The trend in encounters is also important, as the most basic measure of whether a project is stable, growing or shrinking.

In projects that use a one-write registration and billing system, encounters can conveniently be tracked using one or more of the extra columns on the one-write daily tally sheet. A simple tally sheet maintained at the registration desk, or an encounter form, which might also be used for billing, could also be used.

Total Operating Costs

Most managers continuously track their total operating costs, for obvious reasons. On the one hand, costs that are consistently above projections or costs that are consistently rising raise critical questions about the long-term financial viability of the health center. On the other hand, costs that are lower than those projected may mean additional resources if revenue projections are on target. Monthly monitoring of these figures allows action to be taken before serious problems develop. Some managers choose to monitor monthly operating costs in more detail. However, for summary purposes it is best not to confuse the total with specific breakdowns.

Total Collections

Total collections include the cash coming into a health center from direct patient fees and third party reimbursement. Monitoring this figure closely is clearly important. Most budgets, for example, are based on a certain level of collections, but collections are the most variable component of project income. If collections fall below projections, there may be a need to cut back on some budget items.

Collections also vary considerably based on the billing and collection systems in place at a health center. By closely monitoring collections, weaknesses in these systems may become apparent, and action may be taken quickly. Information to determine total collections is easily retrievable from the cash receipts journal recap or the daybook summaries.

Total Cash

Total cash includes cash kept at the health center, cash in the bank or cash in investments. Whenever possible, this figure should equal at least three months' operating expenses, both to avoid problems with cash flow and to cover emergencies. If total cash is decreasing consistently, it is possible that health center costs are exceeding revenue. Total cash figures are derived from bank statements, petty cash balances and investment portfolios.

HEALTH CENTER SERVICES

These indicators measure the output of the health center, in terms of services provided. The examples measure services at an aggregate level; larger and more sophisticated projects may have more detailed objectives (e.g., outreach to particular age groups), and may therefore need more detailed indicators (e.g., age breakdowns of new patients).

Encounters by Type

Encounters by type simply break down the total encounters measure into more detail. The example in Figures 8.1 and 8.2 assumes that three programs are being tracked: medical, prenatal and dental. Alternatively, it might be useful to track encounters by type of visit (e.g., initial, annual medical and problem) or by provider (e.g., MD, midlevel practitioner [MLP] and other), depending on the management decisions a project faces. In a manual system, however, more detailed breakdowns may become prohibitively difficult to collect. Again, the data source is the one-write (or other) tally sheet or a more detailed encounter form.

New Patients

Another important indicator of health center activities is whether services are being expanded to reach new people. The indicator is new patients, where a new patient is defined as someone who has never been seen before for any reason. Note that this indicator is different from the users indicator. Also it does not measure the project's overall growth, as the dropout rate is not accounted for.

New patient data may be collected on the one-write or other tally sheet, by adding a data item to the encounter form, or by counting how many new patient numbers have been assigned.

Year-to-Date Users by Type

Of interest to many program managers is the number of unique individuals who have been seen by a project in a particular calendar year. For example, a program goal in a family planning project might be to provide services to a specific number of women in a certain age group, irrespective of how many visits each woman makes. This number is called "users." In the example given, users is broken down by type of program, for individual program monitoring.

The definition of a user is related to a specific time period (this year), rather than to the time period of the report; this causes some problems of data collection and interpretation. In particular, the number of individuals seen in the first quarter plus the number seen in the second quarter does not equal the total number of people seen in the first six months of the year. This is because a person seen in February and May would be counted once in the first quarter report of unique individuals, and once in the second quarter report, but would still be counted only once (not twice) in a six-month report. Moreover, the estimated number of users in a year is not twice the six-month figure, because a person is more likely to be counted at the beginning of the year than at the end. For these reasons, users should always be counted as a cumulative number from the beginning of the year. Thus the second quarter report includes all individuals from January through June, not just those from April.

User status can be determined at the time a patient enters the health center by asking the question: "Have you been here since January 1, 19xx?" or for a detailed breakdown: "Have you been here this year to see an MD or MLP?" or by referring to the patient chart.

New Patient Ratio

The new patient ratio is defined as the ratio of new patients to total encounters for a particular period; it is thus a measure of the percentage of all encounters that were provided to individuals who had never been seen before.

The new patient ratio estimates the stability of a patient population and gives some indication of continuity of care. In a well-established project with a fairly steady level of encounters, a high new patient ratio means a high dropout rate. This could be because the patient population is transient, but it might also indicate questionable quality of care. New projects should expect this ratio to be high initially and to decrease as the project approaches capacity or saturation. At any event, project managers who are worried about turnover in the patient population may find this indicator helpful. New projects should expect a very high patient ratio, but the ratio should decrease as the project stabilizes.

One can easily conceive measures that would address these issues more directly; common indicators are drop-out rate, continuation rate and active caseload. However, these indicators are much more difficult to collect, especially with manual systems, and it is questionable whether such information would be sufficiently more accurate to justify the extra trouble.

Encounters per FTE Staff

This indicator measures the average number of encounters seen per FTE for each type of staff person. Calculated by staff category, or for each staff member, it addresses issues of staff capacity, utilization and efficiency. Of course, care must be taken in use and interpretation of these figures. Higher ratios are not necessarily good, and lower ratios are not necessarily bad. Data for this calculation should be available in any project's personnel and financial records.

RECEPTION

This section summarizes two indicators that may be useful in measuring performance in the reception/front desk area. Other indicators might be developed for a particular health center.

No-Show Rate

The clinic no-show rate indicates the percentage of appointments that patients did not keep and for which there was no advance notice. The number of patients who do notify the center of their inability to keep an appointment may also be of interest but is not included in this indicator. No-show patients may have a severe effect on productivity and patient flow and are costly to the health center. Although there are no simple solutions to the problem, some changes can usually be made to improve the rate. A very high or continuously rising no-show rate may indicate problems either in quality of care or in patient education. Clinic no-show rates are extrapolated from the appointment book.

At-Visit Collection Rate

The at-visit collection rate divides the number of cash payments made at the time of visit by the total number of self-pay visits. This rate is a good indicator of the success of on-site collection efforts, which should represent a substantial portion of a center's self-pay collections. Information for this indicator is summarized from the daily log if a one-write system is used or from a comparison of daily cash receipts entries to daily encounters.

FINANCIAL MANAGEMENT

Indicators relating to the financial status of a health center are the most often used in internal management reports. Such indicators are important, but they should not be used exclusively to determine the well-being of a center.

Financial management indicators presented represent only a small fraction of the potential financial indicators; however, an attempt has been made to select a representative sample. Individual health centers should be careful to select the most appropriate indicators and to limit the number of items tracked.

Break-Even Ratio

The break-even ratio compares total revenue to total operating costs. Revenue here is defined as income from all sources, including fees, grants, donations and in-kind services. Costs are defined as all expenses incurred during the period involved. This indicator is of critical importance to all health centers; it should be monitored over time to see if the project has consistently higher costs than revenues or whether revenues are consistently sufficient to cover costs. When costs are generally higher than revenue, there is an immediate need to either increase revenue or decrease costs to avoid a shortage of resources. If revenue is generally higher than costs, plans may be made to utilize the excess revenues. The general ledger and/or monthly financial statements provide the necessary data to determine total operating costs and total revenues.

Charges Ratio

The charges ratio compares total gross charges (charges before any adjustments) to total operating costs. While it is expected that most health centers will not collect on the basis of gross charges, the ratio is useful in indicating whether the center's schedule of charges is designed to cover the costs of the center. If the ratio is below 90 percent, costs may be unreasonably high, utilization may be lower than required to support the center or the charge structure may be unnecessarily low, in which case the center is probably losing valuable income. The gross charges for a health center are retrieved from a summary of the daybook or from the one-write tally sheet.

Self-Sufficiency Ratio

The self-sufficiency ratio relates collections to total costs. Although sliding scale adjustments and nonreimbursable services make it unlikely that most grant-supported health centers will ever totally cover costs through collections, it is still important to monitor the percentage of total costs covered by collections. It is particularly important to monitor this indicator over time to determine whether dependency on outside resources is increasing or decreasing. Collections are determined from the cash receipts journal.

Collection Ratio

The collection ratio determines what percentage of the net charges are being collected. Net charges are defined as total charges minus sliding scale adjustments and contractual disallowances. Net charges represent the amount a health center should expect to collect with a very small additional allowance for bad debt write-offs. Consequently this ratio should be close to 100 percent, with anything below 95 percent considered unacceptable.

If the collection rate is below 95 percent, two potential problems should be considered. First, it is possible that the sliding scale adjustments are not being consistently applied to the gross charges so the net charge portion of the calculation is inaccurate. It is also possible that collection procedures are not adequate or that they are not being effectively followed.

Net charges, like gross charges, are determined through daybook summaries and collections from the cash receipts journal.

Total Net Charges

It is necessary to keep track of total net charges in order to compute the collection ratio. Furthermore, net charges reflect the amount a center should reasonably expect to collect in fees; thus it is important to be able to predict this figure with some certainty. It is useful to compare actual net charges to projected net charges to determine the accuracy of past projections. Information on net charges is obtained from the daybook summary.

Net Charges by Payment Source

Of more interest to many health centers than the total net charges figure is a break-out of net charges by payment source. This break-out may be simple, as in net charges to third-party versus net charges to self-pay patients, or more complicated, as in the example, with specific third party payers listed. In either case, by dividing net charges by payment source, a profile of the type of patient being seen can be developed. Furthermore, by comparing actual experience to past experience and to projections, trends in user types may become evident. The center may, for example, see an increase in the percentage of self-pay patients. This could mean that third-party resources are not being adequately identified during registration or that patients with third party payment are seeking care elsewhere. Net charges by payment source, like total net charges, should be available through the daybook summary.

Accounts Receivable at End of Month

It is essential to keep track of accounts receivable on a monthly basis to determine whether such accounts are decreasing, stable or increasing. Ideally, all health centers should attempt to decrease or at least stabilize accounts receivable. Consistently increasing accounts receivable indicate problems in the billing and/or collections systems and deserve immediate attention. These figures are available from the accounts receivable section of the general ledger.

Accounts Receivable by Source

By dividing accounts receivable by payment source, the site gains further insight into specific causes for overall trends. Thus a consistently increasing accounts receivable for self-pay patients might indicate problems with collections at time of service or problems with the sliding scale, whereas increasing Medicaid accounts receivable may be due to inefficient Medicaid billing. Additional information can be developed by comparing accounts receivable by payment source to the net charges by payment source. Medicaid, for example, may represent only a small portion of the total accounts receivable but may be a substantial portion of the net charges to Medicaid, in which case problems exist. Accounts receivable by payment source, like total accounts receivable, should be broken out in the accounts receivable section of the general ledger.

Months of Accounts Receivable

In attempting to determine whether the accounts receivable balance is reasonable, it is helpful to estimate how many months of charges are represented in the accounts receivable total. Thus this indicator takes total accounts receivable and divides by an average month's charges (usually the average of the last three months). The resulting figure represents the months of outstanding accounts receivable. Generally, if more than two months' charges are outstanding, cash flow in the center is constrained, and the effectiveness of the billing and/or collections system must be examined.

To compute this ratio, total accounts receivable are retrieved from the general ledger. Average charges are taken from the monthly summaries of the daybook.

Accounts Payable at End of Month

To assess the overall financial status of the health center, it is important to keep track of the accounts payable balance. A center may have sufficient cash to cover operating costs, but at the same time have a high or growing accounts payable balance. This could indicate future financial difficulties. Accounts payable balances are retrieved from either the open invoice file or purchase journal.

Operating Costs, Salaries versus Other

Total operating costs are almost always tracked by managers. What often is not tracked is the proportion of these costs that is taken up by various components of the health center. Such detailed breakdowns can be revealing. Reporting salary figures, for example, highlights how much of a center's resources are tied up in staff and may influence decisions on hiring or salary increases. Some centers may find it useful to track other cost components, such as administrative costs or indirect costs, on an ongoing basis. At any rate, it is often useful to detail operating costs in addition to tracking the total. A word of warning: it is seldom useful in a summary management report to track all budget categories or line items. Monthly fluctuations in categories or variances from projections are to be expected, and the detail involved in following the specific budget or cost items often obscures more important information.

Information in the general ledger can be summarized into various categories and into various areas of operating costs depending on the needs of the health center.

Cost per Encounter

This measure, which is determined by dividing total costs by total encounters, indicates to managers how much it is costing to provide services. It is most useful when trends are watched to determine if costs are increasing or decreasing. The indicator, however, is not without problems. In a comprehensive health center, for instance, services may vary considerably in unit cost. The gross measure of encounters to costs does not indicate whether one service is very costly and another very inexpensive. The gross measure, then, should only be used by health centers with a limited number of services. More complex programs may break out services by type, or rely on the other indicators to assess their financial stability. The information needed for this indicator can be obtained from the daily log or encounter forms for encounter totals, and from the general ledger for costs.

PERSONNEL MANAGEMENT

Two indicators are presented as examples here. In large projects, more attention to this issue may be appropriate; in very small projects, even the indicators shown here may be superfluous.

FTE Staff

This indicator tracks the size of the staff at a health center and may, over time, indicate growth or decline in total staff. Some health centers may find it useful to further categorize staff by type, such as medical, administrative, and other, or by part-time versus full-time staff. All information on staff should be available from payroll records.

Staff Turnover Rates

The staff turnover rate is a good indicator of other severe problems in a health center. Without tracking this indicator regularly, the frequency of staff turnover is not apparent. The rate is easily calculated from personnel records by taking new staff in relation to total staff; it may be useful to track turnover by type of staff such as providers versus others.

DEFINING AN INTERNAL MANAGEMENT REPORT

Few ambulatory health centers suffer from a lack of data for management purposes. Far more frequent is the problem of having too many data which are not organized in a fashion suitable for management decision making. One solution to this problem is condensing program data into a reasonable list of management indicators, and presenting those indicators in a usable format. Final definition of a project's IMR requires a clear understanding of both the audience of the internal management report and the management decisions to be made.

9 | Control Aspects of Financial Variance Analysis

Steven A. Finkler

Variance analysis is a financial management technique in which budgeted expenses are compared with actual results. This comparison represents the feedback portion of the organization's overall management control system.

MANAGEMENT CONTROL SYSTEMS

Management control systems are systematic efforts to ensure that the organization achieves, to the greatest extent possible, its desired results. The desired results are determined based on the organization's mission statement. This is usually accomplished by first developing a set of goals and policies. The goals provide objectives, and the policies set out the actions that may be taken to achieve the goals. Programs are then established to pursue the goals directly.

Decisions must be made by management concerning the organization's specific goals and policies. Decisions must also be made concerning the specific programs that will be undertaken to achieve the goals. And decisions must be made about the specific ways that programs are implemented and run on an ongoing basis. According to Anthony, Dearden, and Bedford,

> When these decisions have been completed, though they are reexamined continuously, management needs some way to assure that people in the organization do what they are supposed to do. *Control* is the process used to do this. It aims to assure that people in organizations do what management wants them to do. The management role in control is called "management control"; and the system used to do such things as collect and analyze information, evaluate it, and use it and other devices to control activities is a *management control system.*[1]

149

FEEDBACK

Feedback is an essential element of any management control system. It allows managers to determine whether or not things are working according to plan. A critical weakness in many organizations is that a wide variety of decisions are made, and actions are undertaken after time-consuming and expensive study, with no feedback system to allow for evaluation of the system.

The management control system is flawed if it does not require an evaluation of results. Only through an evaluation can successes be encouraged and failures be remedied. Variance analysis provides critical feedback in the management control process.

VARIANCE REPORTS AND THE NONFINANCIAL MANAGER

Variance reports are not the only type of feedback mechanism in management control systems. Quality assessment departments, for example, provide feedback on whether systems adequately monitor the quality of care provided. However, this discussion will focus on financial variance analysis and its role in the control process. Managers should not consider variance reports as a tool for financial managers. Financial managers act in a staff capacity only, generating reports for use by line managers. If some process is out of control, it is generally the operational managers who must rectify the situation.

Suppose that an operations study at a hospital determines that nurses are doing a substantial amount of drug reconstitution at the nursing station. Several years earlier this might have been reasonable. In light of a severe nursing shortage, however, it may be deemed advisable (both financially and in terms of quality of care) for the reconstitution to be done by pharmacists, allowing full-time nurses to devote their attention to other aspects of patient care, and reducing the hospital's need for agency nurses and nurse overtime. A new procedure therefore assigns all drug reconstitution to pharmacists. This is an example of the management control system at work; decisions are being reexamined and altered in order to improve the ability of the organization to carry out its mission.

However, people's habits are not changed as easily as are organizational policies and procedures. Nurses may continue to prepare drugs at the nursing stations. This will undoubtedly demand more nursing time and less pharmacist time than the budget allotted. If we fail to examine actual costs in comparison with budget on a frequent basis (usually monthly), we might not realize that the new plan is not being followed.

By the end of the year, we might accumulate substantial amounts of nursing overtime because of the unplanned work being done by nurses. At the same time, we might have high pharmacist costs because we are overstaffed in that area.

We must have an automatic feedback system in place to ensure that the management control system is able not only to implement decisions, but also to follow up on them. A variance report prepared by financial managers would show that nursing costs were rising above the budgeted amount. However, it is unlikely that the financial managers who prepared the report would be able to ascertain why variances were occurring in nursing or pharmacy.

The financial manager might not even be aware of the operational change that was made concerning drug reconstitution. Since variances might also be arising in radiology, dietary, medical records, laboratory, and throughout the hospital, much of the variance in each department would be attributed to causes related to providing services in that department. Financial managers cannot be experts in each hospital area.

It is the nonfinancial manager who has the key role in variance analysis. Generating the numbers is the easy part. The intellectual challenge of determining why variances occur is left to the various nonfinancial managers throughout the health care organization. Only through direct hands-on supervision and experience will a manager have the ability to evaluate a variance and determine, with a reasonable degree of accuracy, its likely cause.

The determination of the cause of a variance is a critical step. It completes the feedback portion of the management control system loop. The next step in the loop—also to be undertaken by nonfinancial managers—is to incorporate that information into a change in the way operations are carried out. Too often managers view the variance analysis process as a way for the organization to determine who has performed poorly, with the aim of punishing those individuals. In reality, the key focus should not be retribution. Variance reports are generated so that we can change the system to operate more efficiently in the future.

If nurses reconstitute drugs for one month, a small variance occurs (relative to the year-end variance if no monthly analysis is undertaken). The departmental managers, upon investigation of overtime variances, will review what nurses are doing, uncover the need to change the system according to the plan, and take prompt actions to make sure that the plan is implemented correctly. For the next 11 months (and for years into the future), they will not encounter variances due to this problem. The main reason for having a variance analysis is so that the information generated by this feedback mechanism will lead to changes that will prevent the problem from recurring. Control is primarily future oriented.

CAUSES OF VARIANCE

There are many possible causes for variance and many ways to categorize those causes. One of the most important distinctions is whether or not the variance is controllable. Simply spending more than the budgeted amount, and therefore having an unfavorable variance, does not mean that a manager or a department performed poorly.

For example, suppose that the silver market is cornered by a rich Texan. As the price of silver rises, the cost of x-ray film will rise dramatically. In turn, the radiology department will go over budget. The manager has done nothing wrong, nor have the various technicians in the department. This is simply an uncontrollable variance. It is unfortunate for the hospital, but there is no way around it. We need to take x-rays, and all x-ray film (let us assume) requires silver.

We need to investigate the excess costs in the radiology department to see the cause. Once the cause has been determined to be the price of silver, we must determine whether we could use a substitute for silver. If not, we must evaluate the long-term impacts on the hospital if the costs of the radiology department remain higher than predicted before the silver market was cornered. However, in the short run, no specific management action is required with respect to changing the way radiology operates.

At the other extreme is a department that is headed by a new manager who wants to be liked. The manager has allowed coffee breaks to lengthen on slow days from 15 minutes to half an hour. If a worker is occasionally late, and is a good worker, no note is made of it. After the manager's fourth month, the variance report indicates a substantial labor overtime variance. Investigation determines that coffee breaks average 30 minutes on all days, lunch breaks average 90 minutes on all days, and the average worker arrives 30 minutes late.

The variance report is the tool that will give the manager direct feedback on the implications of being so lenient. This is the classic example of a controllable variance. Without variance reports, the entire year might go by without any specific identification of a problem. The variance report forces the department manager to note the existence of a problem and to investigate it. The result is that the problem can be brought back under control through the implementation and enforcement of a strict set of work guidelines. These new guidelines, and the enforcement of them, represent a change in the management control system, which controls the behavior of people working in the organization. The change can only occur as the result of a strong feedback system that highlights the existence of a management control breakdown.

Not all situations are clearly controllable or noncontrollable. Suppose that a hospital is particularly good at treating an expensive illness that requires substantial fixed resources — open-heart surgery, for example. The hospital might make an effort to attract more patients who need that treatment. This marketing effort is a controllable activity. From an economic perspective, if we can increase heart surgery patient volume from 100 patients to 200 patients, the fixed costs of treating those patients will be more widely distributed. The cost to the hospital of a heart-lung bypass pump is the same whether it is used for 200 patients per year or for 100 patients per year. If the patients pay a flat diagnosis-related group (DRG) rate, then doubling the number of patients will double the revenue; but due to fixed costs, the total cost of treating twice as many patients will not double. This sounds like a pretty good deal.

However, due to inadequate communication, the departments with primary responsibility for treating those patients might not have been advised of the marketing program when they planned their budgets. The operating room, the recovery room, the intensive care units, the medical-surgical units, and the various ancillary departments could all go over budget as they provide extra services to these additional patients. The extra costs are not controllable by these departments. The hospital can control the costs by turning away patients, or at least not making a specific effort to attract them. However, the hospital does not really want to avoid those extra costs, because they are associated with even greater increases in revenue.

An unfavorable variance is not necessarily bad. Many departments will go over budget because of the additional patients, and therefore will report an unfavorable variance. However, the cause of the variance is the increased profitable volume, which is good for the hospital. "Unfavorable" simply means spending more than expected. It is quite possible for unfavorable variances to represent good events.

Similarly, favorable variances might represent unfavorable events. If, due to a staffing shortage, a nursing department lowers actual nursing care hours per patient day to a point substantially below the budgeted level, there will probably be a favorable labor variance. Quality may have deteriorated drastically (a bad event for the hospital), but the financial numbers will simply indicate that we have spent less than expected. Therefore, the variance is favorable.

Here, again, we see that line managers need to take a strong role in the area of variance analysis. Financial managers will tend to view lower spending as a good sign and higher spending as a bad sign. The actual departmental managers must view variances with a critical eye. Only by finding the underlying cause of the variance can we come to any conclusion about whether an individual variance, either favorable or unfavorable, is good for the institution.

Variances can be caused not only by changes in external prices (e.g., the cost of silver), quality (e.g., nursing care hours per patient day), patient volume (e.g., the number of open-heart surgeries), and efficiency (e.g., the length of coffee breaks) as discussed above, but also by a variety of other factors. For example, the introduction of new technology may change a variety of resource requirements. Availability of staff is another element that has a dramatic impact on the amount of overtime actually incurred as compared with the budgeted amount. Of course, another cause of variance is that budgeted expectations are simply unreasonable.

Sometimes we make plans that are not attainable, even by a very good manager who works very hard. One must remember that the management control process depends on human behavior. We want people in the organization to do what they are supposed to do. However, whether we can actually achieve that goal depends on the incentives to and motivations of those individuals.

INCENTIVES, MOTIVATION, AND VARIANCE ANALYSIS

It is likely that the goals and objectives of a health care organization and those of the individuals working for the organization will diverge. The management control system, and variance analysis in particular, must be designed to provide a set of incentives that motivate managers to act in the best interests of the organization.

GOAL CONGRUENCE

Most people do not go into health care professions to get rich. They have value systems oriented toward helping people. There is truth in the health care rhetoric suggesting that "we're all in this together," or "first and foremost is the well-being of the patient." However, people do want to be paid, and being paid more is preferable to being paid less. An organization, trying to provide as much health care as it possibly can, would like to pay everyone less so that it can do more.

Managers want bigger offices. Organizations hoard space. Managers want new furniture. Organizations find old desks and chairs from the storeroom. Managers want a large happy staff providing top quality care. Organizations seek to use the minimum staff possible to get the job done.

The management control system must develop ways to enable these divergent views to converge. Goal congruence occurs when we find ways to bring together the goals and desires of the organization and the workers. How can we make the individuals' interests contribute to the best interests of the organization?

We do not want to demoralize our managers and staff. Too often budgets are set at perfection levels so that staff can work toward a goal. That is an unfortunate policy. The result (since few of us are perfect), is that variance reports will consistently show that the objective was not achieved; therefore, failure occurred. How many times will managers work as hard as possible to achieve a goal, once they realize that they will always fail? If you are going to fail when you do your best, you might as well take it easy. Therefore, budgets should always be set at an attainable level.

To further encourage managers to keep control over their departments, and to make results meet up with expectations, we should make it clear that someone cares about whether or not the goals are met. Again, the nonfinancial managers have a key role in this process. In most institutions, managers must justify their variances, and the process usually ends there. However, suppose that managers were given a bonus for good budget performance.

Most industries have found that bonuses can be very good motivators. Why not health care? Some would answer that health care workers are interested in helping people, not earning bonuses. Why must the two conflict? There is concern that our incentives may cause a manager to be in a position in which reduced quality of care results in direct financial increases to the manager. If a manager were to receive 10 percent of any savings in cost, he or she might be tempted to cut essential services along with unnecessary services in order to boost the bonus. This creates a conflict that is undesirable. For that reason, bonuses should not be offered unless strong quality review is in place.

Bonuses are not the only way that an organization can demonstrate concern over budget results. One simple and underutilized approach is an annual letter from each superior to each subordinate discussing budget performance. A letter saying that "you did a good job in controlling the budget and I know it" can often overcome the fact that there is no financial reward for that good job. People will not undertake an unpleasant task unless they think there is a good reason to do it. Controlling costs by saying "no" is not a pleasant task. However, some indication that the individual's boss recognizes the effort that went into containing costs, and that the effort is important to the organization, can help to overcome the negatives involved.

SETTING RESPONSIBILITY
EQUAL TO CONTROL

We must also develop systems that ensure that managers feel that they are being treated fairly. A basic accounting rule is that responsibility should be equal to control. One of the biggest motivational mistakes made by health care organizations is that they often assign responsibility to individuals for costs that they cannot control.

For example, suppose that an emergency room (ER) department manager is responsible for all ER departmental costs. One element of costs is supplies. If supplies were budgeted at $30,000 for the month, and actual expenditures were $60,000, the manager has apparently done a poor job of controlling supply usage. In fact, if substantial amounts of supplies have been wasted, that may be a fair evaluation. Perhaps staff are opening several suture packages at the beginning of a procedure, but only one package is needed. The rest are no longer sterile and are thrown away. Perhaps poor control over supplies has resulted in a high theft rate. These are efficiency issues that the manager can control and for which the manager should be responsible.

On the other hand, perhaps the number of emergency room visits was exactly double the number expected. The doubling of volume would probably double the need for supplies, and therefore double the cost. The manager has no control over the number of emergency patients and should not be held responsible for that increase in cost. Similarly, the mix of patients may be different than anticipated and may be skewed toward patients who consume more supplies. In that case, the issue is whether the manager should have been able to anticipate the change in the mix of patients.

Another problem arises if the variance results from the price of the items purchased. We may have used exactly the supplies anticipated but find that the prices have doubled. Since supply cost is assigned to the emergency room, it is the ER manager who is held responsible for the supply variance. However, the supply costs were probably budgeted based on prices supplied by the purchasing department. In that case, the purchasing department has erred in its estimates.

A similar situation is created when overhead costs are assigned to departments. Most departments have no control over most of the overhead assigned to them (although some overhead costs are at least partly controllable). For instance, the laundry charge is based on the amount of laundry used. However, what if the laundry is poorly managed, and the cost per pound cleaned rises dramatically? A share of that increase, which is totally out of the control of the ER manager, will be assigned to the emergency room. It makes no sense to evaluate a manager based on assigned overhead costs that are out of that manager's control.

Overhead variance, changes in volume, changes in patient mix, and changes in prices all create the same negative impact as the use of the "ideal" or "perfection" budget. They may create animosity, a feeling of managerial impotence, and a great deal of resentment. These attitudes inevitably affect the entire performance of the manager and the department. These attitudes are not the fault of the manager; they represent a poorly designed management control system. The feedback portion of the system will only create ill will if we fail to follow the rule of setting the manager's responsibility equal to the manager's control.

MOTIVATING THE STAFF

It is unlikely that managers will succeed in controlling a budget unless they have found ways to pass on positive motivation to their staffs. Unfortunately, budgets are generally viewed in a negative light by health care employees. The budget is the enemy. It prevents the workers from being paid more, from having better working conditions, and so on. They see it as cause of their excessive hard work, and in some respects, they are probably right.

However, maintaining a negative attitude cannot help the organization in any positive way. The negative feelings about the budget should not be surprising. Most workers never hear anything about the budget unless something has gone wrong. When a variance report indicates that everything is going well, managers view it as a reward for their own hard work. However, when a very unfavorable variance report arrives, the manager is often quick to share the blame with the workers who have performed so poorly. Thus most workers only come into contact with the budget when things are not going well.

For a management control system to function most effectively, all workers need to be motivated to work to achieve the organization's goals. Conserving resources is one of those goals. Thus every worker must become aware that they are responsible for managing the use of resources. Many clinicians will reject this concept, suggesting that they are in the clinical professions to provide care to patients, not to manage resources. Health care organizations can no longer allow this philosophy. The individual clinician does decide what supplies to use for each patient. The clinician does make decisions about how much time to spend with the patient. These labor and supply decisions directly affect the resources used by the organization. Every employee is a manager of resources, like it or not.

Most managers should hold weekly staff meetings at which the budget is one of the topics on the agenda. The implications of going over budget should be discussed, but so should the benefits (to the department and the institution) of meeting the budget. An effort should be made to view the budget as a positive reinforcement tool, rather than a negative one. The constant attention to budget issues should make it clear to all employees that controlling the costs of running the institution is a part of their job, and that variance reports simply aid in determining specific areas that need attention.

Variance Analysis

Variance reports provide information for managers to use to determine where specific efforts are needed to assure that costs are under control. The better the variance information, the easier it is to avoid wasting time investigating uncontrollable items and to focus efforts on improving areas that can be improved.

Historically, variance reports have been generated by health care organizations for each department. Within the report for each department, information is generated for each line item, comparing the budgeted amount for that line item with the actual result. Information is usually shown for the results of the month just ended, as well as for the year to date. This information typically falls short in helping health care managers because it lacks sufficient detail and because it is often based on poor-quality data.

VARIANCE DETAIL: VOLUME, PRICE, AND QUANTITY VARIANCES

Since the beginning of the 1980s, more and more health care organizations have begun to recognize that substantial changes in volume inevitably result in variances that are not controllable. Increases in volume of patients require departments to use more resources in order to treat the additional patients. Conversely, reductions in volume should be accompanied by reductions in cost.

Variance reports have reflected this new focus by using a flexible budget. A flexible budget shows what the organization would have expected a department to spend, given the actual volume of patients. Actual costs for each line item are compared with the flexible budget rather than the original budget. Thus a department may have planned a budget for 20,000 patient days but find that there were actually 22,000 patient days. The variance report given to the manager compares the actual spending to a flexible budget for 22,000 patient days. This splits the variance for the line item into two parts. The volume variance reflects the increase or decrease in cost as a result of the difference between the actual and expected number of patients treated. This variance is generally not controllable by managers, and they should not be held accountable for it. The other part of the variance is caused by anything other than the change in volume. Managers are generally held accountable for that part of the line item's variance.

This growing trend is definitely an improvement over the more traditional approach of having one variance amount for each line item. However, there are some problems in the calculations. Department costs include both fixed costs (those that do not vary with the number of patients treated) and variable costs (those that do vary in proportion to the number of patients). If the actual volume of patients exceeds the expected volume by 10 percent, the costs will not all rise by 10 percent. The fixed costs will not rise when volume increases, nor will they fall when volume decreases.

Therefore, proper calculation of the volume variance requires an assessment of the fixed and variable costs in each department. This is often overlooked. A flexible budget is usually calculated by simply adjusting each line item in the original budget upward or downward by the percent change in the volume of patients. Such information can be quite misleading. As a result, the portion of the variance that is attributed to factors other than volume may be substantially over- or understated.

Another problem with this split in variance is that the manager is usually given very little direction with respect to the portion of the variance resulting from factors other than volume. For many decades, firms in other industries have taken that remaining variance and split it into two pieces: the part resulting from changes in the *cost* of each unit of input, and the part resulting from changes in the *amount* of input used to generate each unit of output.

The first of these two parts is referred to as the *price*, or *rate*, variance. It reflects changes in the price of supplies and equipment, or the hourly rate for labor. If a health care organization were to calculate this variance and determine that part of the line item variance was the result of changes in the price or rate, this information would be quite useful. Investigation of the variance might indicate that it resulted from the purchasing department paying a higher price for supplies than was included in the budget. This variance could not be controlled by the department using the supplies, and the manager should not be held responsible for it. However, the purchasing department might be called upon to explain why the price increase was not anticipated. On the other hand, the department manager may have changed the specifications of the supplies; in that case, the department manager, rather than purchasing, should be held accountable.

A rate variance might be the result of a union-negotiated contract, which lead to a higher-than-budgeted pay increase. Again, the department manager would have no control over such a variance and should not be held responsible for it. On the other hand, investigation might show that the department manager was hiring overqualified staff at an unduly high rate. We cannot automatically assume that rate variances are not controllable.

The second part of the variance remaining after the volume variance is split off is commonly referred to as a *quantity, use,* or *efficiency* variance. This portion reflects the amount of resources used to produce a given unit of product. If we expect to use 3.5 hours of nursing care per patient day, and we actually use 4.0 hours, the difference will result in a quantity variance. Note that we are not focusing on the use of more nursing hours because of more patients; that difference is reflected in the volume variance. Here the focus is specifically on the amount of resource used for each patient.

Although industry generally uses the term "efficiency variance," one should be cautious about applying that term to health care. A widget manufacturer may be able to measure their product with a great degree of precision. If they can make the exact same product using less input, they are being efficient. If a hospital treats a patient with fewer nursing resources, is it being efficient, or is it producing a product of lower quality? Because of this quality issue, it is more appropriate to speak of a "quantity" or "use" variance based on the average quantity of resources used to treat a patient.

The amount of information generated by the financial managers of a health care organization depends greatly on the value they place on the information. What benefit will the organization receive in exchange for the resources devoted to generating additional information? Before DRGs were a dominant force in hospital reimbursement, cost overruns were not as critical a problem as they are today. If a department spent more than their budgeted cost, it was likely that a fair amount of that excess could be collected from payers who reimbursed based on cost. Today, when the revenue generated by treating a patient is often independent of the cost of treating that patient, cost overruns are more serious.

Thus it makes more sense not only to produce a line item variance, but also to subdivide that variance into price, quantity, and volume.

Consider the problem that arises if volume starts to decline, and staffing remains unchanged. The amount spent for staff salaries and wages will come in right at the budgeted level. The decline in volume, which should actually lower costs, is matched by an increase in the labor cost per patient. This is because the same amount of staff is treating fewer patients. A labor line item comparison of budget and actual expenditures will show no variance.

A more sophisticated variance system would immediately highlight the favorable volume variance and the unfavorable quantity variance contained within the labor line. (Note that the volume variance is not favorable because treating fewer patients is good, but simply because seeing fewer patients implies spending less money, and accountants classify reduced spending as a favorable variance.) Once these variances are reported, a manager is much more likely to take immediate action to control costs by reassigning or reducing staffing. That is the key to variance analysis: the generation of information that will allow managers to focus their attention on where problems are arising and to take appropriate action to eliminate the problems.

The more sophisticated variance analysis represented by the use of price, quantity, and volume variances is also a great aid in resolving the motivational issue of responsibility and control. Subdividing the line item variance makes it much easier to identify the items that are beyond a manager's control. Once responsibility for those variances is accurately identified, the manager has a much greater incentive to control those items that are controllable.

VARIANCE DETAIL: ACUITY, WORKED VERSUS PAID, AND DIRECT VERSUS INDIRECT VARIANCES

Although most industries currently use price, quantity, and volume variance information to control their operations, the health care industry can actually go even further in the area of generating useful variance information. Specifically of interest are acuity, worked versus paid, and direct versus indirect variances.

It is widely assumed that the volume variance is not controllable and that the price variance is often not controllable. It is also assumed that the quantity variance generally is controllable. After all, long coffee breaks and inefficient modes of operation will show up in the quantity variance because they contribute to increased resources used per patient.

However, there are a number of factors that affect the quantity variance but that may not be controllable by a manager.

Patient severity is one such factor. If the mix of patients is more severely ill than expected, there will be a need for more resources, and a quantity variance will be generated. For example, most hospitals now have patient classification systems for their nursing units. These systems assign an acuity level to each patient. If the expected average acuity is 2.3, and the actual average acuity is 2.8, it is likely that more nursing hours will be needed and used by the unit. Unless we wish to allow quality of care to decline substantially, nursing inputs must be increased, even though the total number of patients or patient days is unchanged.

The increased resource use will result in an unfavorable quantity variance. However, the manager cannot control that change because it results from a change in the mix of patients treated. The quantity variance can be subdivided into the portion that is due specifically to the change in the mix of patients, and the remaining portion.

Paid versus worked hours is another area of concern. When we look at a line item variance for a labor category, we are comparing the total amount budgeted with the total amount spent. These amounts are for total paid hours, including hours not worked because of sick leave, vacations, holidays, and so on. When a quantity variance shows 4.0 actual hours per patient day, as opposed to 3.5 budgeted hours per patient day, we are referring to paid hours, not hours of direct care.

Suppose that a worker is injured on the job and goes on disability for three months. We will probably continue to pay the worker and also hire a replacement. The total paid hours will rise and there will be an unfavorable quantity variance, even though the number of worked hours for the department remains unchanged. Certainly, this is beyond the control of the department manager. It is possible for the accounting department to subdivide the remaining quantity variance into the portion attributable to an increase in paid hours, and the portion relating to hours that were actually worked.

In keeping with the idea of holding managers responsible for only those costs that are within their control, a subdivision of the quantity variance would help to identify its cause. We must exercise care, however, in subdividing these variances. An increase in the number of hours paid but not worked might result from a general increase in the level of absenteeism, reflecting a low employee morale. Such a problem would certainly be a controllable variance. Thus we are not eliminating the need for managers to investigate variances. The goal of a sophisticated variance system is to point out where the variances are occurring and to make it easier to find the underlying cause of the variance.

A final possible subdivision of the quantity variance is between direct and indirect work time. Ideally, we would define direct work time in terms of actual time spent on patient care, but that would be too expensive to measure accurately. Such measurement would require either that each worker maintain detailed logs (an inaccurate approach) or the use of one extra employee per worker to observe whether time is being spent on direct or indirect care (an accurate but extremely costly approach). Instead, we can think in terms of time worked in the employee's department, as opposed to work time spent on projects outside the department, such as educational programs.

Suppose that each employee is allowed to attend five days of educational programs per year, but that they typically take only an average of three days per year. We will probably budget for three days. If the actual average time taken is four days, we will have to replace the workers on the extra educational day taken, and we will go over our labor budget. By subdividing the quantity variance for direct work time versus indirect work time, we can eliminate indirect activities from the quantity variance. This does not mean that we are not concerned with monitoring the variance for an increase in indirect work time. We *do* want to track and investigate such a variance, but we would also like to separate that variance from the quantity variance, which assesses resource consumption per patient.

Thus the quantity variance can be subdivided into four elements. We can find the portion attributable to a change in the patient mix, the portion due to a change in the number of hours paid but not worked, the portion due to a change in the number of hours worked in the department, and a remaining quantity variance. This remaining variance contains unexplained factors such as changes in efficiency.

Is it worthwhile to generate all of these variances? The accounting departments could calculate them. A growing number of health care organizations have been calculating the volume variance, and a number are beginning to measure the price and quantity variances. The acuity variance is a new concept, but one that will probably receive attention and use. The paid versus worked, and direct versus indirect variances are concepts that are useful, but they have not yet been implemented. Each organization must determine how far to go in variance analysis, based on the expected cost of generating the information and the perceived benefits of that information.

One must always bear in mind that information costs money. Generally, we want information so that we can make decisions. In the case of variances, the decisions we make determine our future actions to avoid unnecessary expenditures. If the cost of generating the variances exceeds the expected savings from the use of the information, the variances become an expensive academic exercise. The amounts and quality of data generated must depend on their cost.

PROBLEMS OF VARIANCE DATA QUALITY

Regardless of the degree of detail used in calculating line item variances (whether just the traditional variance for each line, or subdivided variances), the quality of the data generated is critical to the usefulness of the variances. Unfortunately, both health organizations with simple systems and those with sophisticated systems have been calculating their variances using extremely poor raw data.

Health care accounting departments have focused largely on preparing reports for external users. It is only recently that there has been a growing focus on better information for management decision making. As a result, many managers are interpreting variances that are really meaningless. Consider, for example, the situation of a hospital that floats nurses from slow units to busy units. Which unit is charged for the float nurse? Conceptually, there is no debate. The unit that uses the nurse must be assigned the cost. If we intend to determine which units are consuming too many or too few nursing resources per patient day, we must have an accurate measure of each unit's resource consumption.

Some hospitals do a good job of assigning costs to the proper unit. Many hospitals, however, always charge a nurse's salary to the "home" unit, simply because it is much easier. After all, the cost is the same regardless of where it is assigned. That kind of rationalization is sufficient for getting reimbursed from Blue Cross, but it fails miserably if we are concerned with efficient resource management. Without accurate charging, we cannot measure productivity and can take no steps to improve it.

Taking another instance, let us assume that supplies are appropriately charged to the department that consumes them (an assumption that may not always be true). The budgeted amount for use of supplies by a department is based on careful estimates of the numbers of patients for each month and the average consumption per patient. The actual charges to the department should reflect the actual resource consumption. However, in health care accounting systems, supplies are often charged to the department when the invoice is received or paid, rather than when the supplies are used.

If the organization chooses to buy a three-month supply of an item to benefit from a quantity discount, the entire three-month supply will be charged in one month, with no charge for that supply in the two subsequent months. Given such distorted information, how can a manager make a reasonable investigation concerning the budgeted versus actual use of supplies?

It is costly to collect information, but in some cases it is clearly necessary. If we expect to hold managers accountable for supply costs, we must develop a system that collects appropriate information measuring actual monthly consumption. Otherwise, top management is simply deluding itself into thinking it has good information, and lower-level managers are frustrated by being asked to explain variances that are out of their control.

If we expect to hold managers accountable for labor variances, we must charge labor costs to the correct department, and for that matter, in the correct month. Year-end accruals of unused vacation time drive some managers crazy. All year long they receive variance reports showing favorable labor variances. At the end of the year, unused vacation time is charged in one lump sum, and the department has a tremendously unfavorable variance for the month, if not for the whole year. And at that point, managers are expected to explain why they used too much labor.

Variance reports are internal management reports, and managers must demand that they are generated using appropriate information for management analysis. Standard information generated for external financial reporting is simply not good enough.

CONCLUSION

Managers often think that strategic planning, followed by careful implementation, will result in a smoothly running organization. In reality, things go wrong. Sometimes something goes wrong and nothing can be done about it. Sometimes things go wrong and we can prevent them from continuing to go wrong. We must first know that there is a problem. Variance analysis provides a feedback mechanism to let managers know that a problem exists.

The level of detail of variance analysis varies from institution to institution. We are in a period of increasing sophistication in the use of variances to control operations. Managers must select a variance system that will allow for proper motivational incentives, that will generate adequate, accurate information for taking necessary actions to control the organization's costs.

REFERENCE

1.   Anthony, Robert, John Dearden, and Norton Bedford. *Management Control Systems*. Homewood, IL: Irwin, 1984.

ADDITIONAL READINGS

Finkler, Steven A. *Budgeting Concepts for Nurse Managers*. Orlando, FL: Grune & Stratton, 1984.

———. "Flexible Budget Variance Analysis Extended to Patient Acuity and DRGs." *Health Care Management Review* 10 (Fall 1985): 21–34.

———. "The Pyramid Approach: Increasing the Usefulness of Flexible Budgeting." *Hospital Financial Management* 12 (February 1982): 30–39. Reprinted in *HFM Readings*, Healthcare Financial Management Association, 1983.

Horngren, Charles T., and George Foster. *Cost Accounting: A Managerial Emphasis*. Sixth Edition. Englewood Cliffs, NJ: Prentice-Hall, 1987.

10 | The Medical Management Analysis System: A Professional Liability Warning Mechanism

Joyce W. Craddick

In recent years, systems for detecting and evaluating events that affect hospitalized patients have proliferated rapidly. The traditional concern of the medical profession for patient well-being has been augmented by interest, guidance, and massive funding from state and federal governments, licensing bodies, and other sources. Systems developed in response to this increased interest in evaluating the quality of hospital care have become so numerous that physicians and hospitals have sometimes expressed dismay at their number and cost and at the personnel, administrative activity, and space they require. Concern also has been voiced about the amount of physicians' time needed to conduct quality assurance (QA) activities, about whether these activities judge the quality of medical care fairly, and about the effect these activities have on staff morale and confidentiality of medical information.

Systems currently used to evaluate the quality of patient care vary widely in philosophy, sophistication, efficiency, and effectiveness. In some hospitals, several systems duplicate the same QA efforts. Multiple systems with only minor variations operate in the same institutions to

Reprinted from *Quality Review Bulletin* 5 (April 1979): 2–8. Copyright 1988 by the Joint Commission on Accreditation of Healthcare Organizations, Chicago. Reprinted with permission.

satisfy the demands of various sponsors that each assert an individual right to observe and assess the quality of care and services for which they pay. Although some systems are practical, others are too theoretical; many are overly complex, and almost all reflect idealistic goals.

In some instances, characteristics of the QA effort itself — its relative newness, the rapid proliferation of different systems, the diverse backgrounds of administrative personnel, and the variety of goals reflected in each system (e.g., goals related to the quality and cost of medical care or to political motives) — have led to chaos. Not all of the interest, guidance, and funding from the government and other parties have been welcomed enthusiastically by the medical profession, the hospitals, or the patients, who are the intended beneficiaries of the QA effort. In fact, few patients understand this activity, and some would not approve of it if they knew its costs. Other general criticisms of QA activities include charges that too much review activity is taking place and that review systems are becoming too complex and too rigidly organized. This complexity and rigidity may lead to rejection of the effort by health care providers or to superficial compliance only.

One partial solution to the problems caused by diverse QA methods, motives, and sponsorship may be found in giving medical care providers themselves more opportunity to solve these problems. Physicians and hospitals are confronted now more than ever with the economic losses that can result from their actions. A growing number of hospitals and physicians are self-insured; this fact creates a new and clearly understandable motive for providers themselves to inquire into the quality of patient care in hospitals. Any doubt in the minds of hospital administrators or medical practitioners as to the value and necessity of assuring quality care has been removed by the consequences they themselves incur when it is not provided. The insured are now also the insurers, and thus they will be highly motivated to solve medical care problems rather than allow them to continue at their own expense. One example of an attempt by providers to develop an improved system of health care evaluation is provided by the Medical Management Analysis System, which was developed following a study of hospital-incurred adverse events conducted in California.

The California Medical Insurance Feasibility Study

In 1976, the California Medical Association and the California Hospital Association sponsored the California Medical Insurance Feasibility Study (CMIFS) to determine whether it would be desirable to make financial recompense to patients for all negative outcomes associated with hospital care. For the study, techniques were developed to determine the types and severity of adverse events that occur in hospitals. A committee of physicians and medical audit experts devised 20 general outcome criteria that were used to retrospectively review more than 20,000 records from 23 California hospitals. This initial screening identified cases that did not meet one or more of the criteria; these cases were then reviewed by physicians and physician-attorneys to determine whether a potentially compensable event had occurred. Results indicated that 4.65% of patients hospitalized in 1974 (nearly one out of every 20) experienced an adverse event that was potentially compensable. Of these events, 20% were determined probably to be due to legally recognizable fault on the part of the provider.

The conclusions based on the results of the CMIFS were not totally unexpected: Given the current malpractice crisis, drawing more public attention to the occurrence of adverse events in hospitals would be ill-advised, and awarding financial damages to patients for every adverse event would certainly not be economically feasible. After much debate, the House of Delegates of the California Medical Association decided that if the study did nothing else, it illustrated the enormity and complexity of the problem of hospital-related adverse events.

An important difference was noted between data compiled by the CMIFS general outcome screening and data gathered by more traditional audit screening. General outcome screening was accomplished by using comprehensive criteria to compile data on the care given all patients and thus led to the detection of adverse events frequently missed by audit criteria pertinent only to specific diagnoses or procedures and used to screen a limited number of records. In addition, if general outcome screening were to be conducted while the patient was still hospitalized or immediately after his discharge, adverse events would be detected sooner than they would have been by a routine retrospective audit, and action to correct problems could be undertaken sooner. Thus, if properly used, general outcome screening could provide data that were more comprehensive, more current, and consequently, more practical than the data provided by most QA systems.

In one hospital, for example, while the coronary care committee was conducting a retrospective audit of the care given patients with myocardial infarction to determine whether nurses had instructed patients regarding proper diet, the same committee was unaware that six coronary care unit patients had suffered injuries because they had fallen out of bed. Incidents such as falls are often not detected by a diagnosis-specific audit; in this case, however, they would have been detected by a general outcome criterion that screened for *any* adverse event related to hospitalization (i.e., "hospital-incurred incidents including drug and transfusion reactions"). In another hospital, members of the obstetrics and gynecology audit committee spent an hour debating the value of urine cultures for catheterized patients, unaware that a gynecologist on the staff had recently transected three ureters while performing hysterectomies. Again, a general outcome screening criterion ("unplanned removal or injury or repair of an organ or part of an organ during an operative procedure") would have detected serious adverse events that were overlooked by a traditional audit.

DEVELOPMENT OF A PROFESSIONAL LIABILITY WARNING SYSTEM

During the course of the CMIFS, it was realized that the general outcome screening criteria devised for the study might be adapted for use in an early warning system that would detect potentially compensable adverse events occurring in hospitals. This concept was brought to the attention of the Physicians Professional Liability Division of Marsh & McLennan, Inc. an international insurance brokerage with offices in northern California. Marsh & McLennan agreed to sponsor adaptation of the CMIFS general outcome screening criteria for use in a professional liability warning system. The criteria were incorporated into a centralized patient care evaluation system known as the Medical Management Analysis System, which currently is being implemented and refined in a number of hospitals throughout the country. The system is also being used by two physician-owned professional liability insurance companies managed by Marsh & McLennan, both to evaluate the office practices of physicians who apply for insurance when underwriting problems are suspected and to evaluate and improve the practices of insured physicians who have had large or numerous claims against them.

THE MEDICAL MANAGEMENT ANALYSIS SYSTEM

The Medical Management Analysis System is a concurrent, continuous review system designed to provide early identification of hospital-incurred adverse events and patterns of substandard care. The system uses a set of specific, objective, outcome screening criteria adapted from the CMIFS (see Table 10.1). These criteria cover all aspects of hospitalization and are generally used to screen every patient record. The criteria set was tested during the CMIFS and found effective in identifying nearly all important adverse events that occur in hospitals. Nevertheless, the criteria should not be adopted without consideration of individual insti-

TABLE 10.1

General Outcome Screening Criteria Set for Hospitals

Elements	Standard 0%	Exceptions		Instructions for Data Retrieval
1. Admission for adverse results of outpatient management	X	1A. Prior medical care unrelated to this hospital's outpatient department (OPD) or did not involve any member of this hospital staff	1.	Check admission note, diagnosis, consult notes for complications, failure to treat or prevent or failure to diagnose†
2. Admission for complication or incomplete management of problem on previous hospital admission	X	2A. Complication or incomplete management occurred at another hospital 2B. Readmission for chronic disease, e.g., asthma, congestive heart failure, cancer and discharge plan and follow-up documented on previous admission	2.	Check admission note, diagnosis, consult notes; review discharge summaries on prior hospitalizations within 6 months
*3. Hospital-incurred incidents including drug and transfusion reactions	X	3A. None	3.	Check progress notes, nurse's notes, consult notes, discharge summary‡
4. Transfer from general care unit to special care unit	X	4A. Scheduled prior to surgery or other special procedure 4B. Intensive care unit (ICU) used as a recovery room	4.	Special care = ICU, coronary care unit, respiratory care unit; check orders, nurse's notes. Report reason for transfer and condition on transfer

continued

TABLE 10.1. Continued

Elements	Standard 0%	Exceptions	Instructions for Data Retrieval
5. Transfer to another acute care facility	X	5A. Mandatory transfer for administrative reasons 5B. Transfer for test or procedure not available in this hospital	5. Report name of facility, reason for transfer, condition on transfer
**6. Operation for perforation, laceration, tear or injury of an organ incurred during an invasive procedure	X	6A. None	6. Check operative note, progress notes, nurse's notes§
7. Cancellation of or repeat diagnostic procedure due to improper preparation of patient, technician error, or equipment failure	X	7A. None	7. See orders for repeat procedures, nurse's notes, progress notes, lab and x-ray reports, operative notes
8. Unplanned return to the operating room (OR) on this admission	X	8A. None	8. Planned return to the OR must be documented prior to first surgery
**9. Unplanned removal or injury or repair of an organ or part of an organ during an operative procedure	X	9A. None	9. Check operative note, consult form, preoperative plan, and compare with pathology report
**10. Myocardial infarction during or within 48 hrs of a surgical procedure on this admission	X	10A. Preop work-up included normal electrocardiogram (ECG) and enzymes and negative cardiac history	10. Check ECGs, progress notes, consults 10A. Check history, preoperative ECG, lab work

Criterion		Exception	Notes
		10B. Emergency operative procedure	10B. Patient operated on for life-threatening condition
11. Infection not present on admission (nosocomial)	X	11A. None	11. Instructions per infection control coordination; include wound infections
12. Neurologic deficit present at discharge which was not present on admission	X	12A. None	12. Check nurse's notes for seizures, loss of consciousness, impairment of special senses or motor functions, fecal or urinary incontinence, or intractable pain, cerebrovascular accident, stroke
13. Length of stay (LOS) $\geq$ 90th percentile	X	13A. Increased LOS due solely to nonmedical problems	
**14. Cardiac or respiratory arrest	X	14A. None	14. Assume arrest if code called or any resuscitation performed. Include newborn resuscitation for Apgar $\leq$ 4 in delivery room
**15. Death	X	15A. None	15. If death occurs, attach mortality review sheet to committee work sheet
16. Other complications	X	16A. None	16. List all not covered by criteria
**17. Subsequent admission for a complication or adverse effect of this hospitalization	X	17A. None	17. Check subsequent admissions history, final diagnosis, consult notes

continued

TABLE 10.1. Continued

Elements	Standard 0%	Exceptions	Instructions for Data Retrieval
18. Subsequent visit to emergency room (ER) or OPD for complication or adverse result of this hospitalization	X	18A. None	18. Check ER/OPD visits for unplanned returns for unexpected results

*Report immediately if severe

**Report immediately

†Clues to adverse results of outpatient management include delayed diagnosis (e.g., first admission for advanced tuberculosis, metastatic carcinoma; perforated appendix; severe diabetic ketoacidosis; shock; septicemia; any disease with systemic complications); any condition attributed to outpatient drug therapy (e.g., digitalis intoxication; hypokalemia while on diuretics; gastrointestinal bleeding while on aspirin, steroids, butazolidine, indocin; bleeding while on anticoagulants; parkinsonism while on tranquilizers; anaphylaxis, drug reactions); complications of procedures performed in the office, clinic or emergency room (e.g., malunion, non-union, or complications of fractures; irradiation burns; wound infections; physical defects; neurological defects; complications of physical therapy, x-ray, or laboratory procedures or other outpatient procedures); any disease for which immunization available (e.g., measles, mumps, polio, hepatitis, diphtheria, tetanus).

‡Incidents include medication errors, patient accidents, procedural errors, electrical shock or burn, intravenous errors, drug or contrast material reactions, transfusion reactions, and actual or attempted patient suicide.

§Invasive procedures include intubations (tracheal, esophageal, gastric, rectal); percutaneous aspirations (thoracentesis, paracentesis, pericardiocentesis, bladder aspirations); percutaneous biopsy of heart, lung, liver, kidneys, prostate, etc.; catheterization of bladder, heart, vascular system; x-ray procedures (arteriograms, renograms, ventriculograms, bronchograms, pneumoencephalograms); endoscopics (bronchoscopy, cystoscopy, sigmoidoscopy, esophagoscopy, mediastiinoscopy, peritoneoscopy, laparoscopy, culdoscopy, urethroscopy, ureteroscopy); pacemaker insertion; uterine sounding; enemas; and rectal temperatures.

Table 10.1 originally appeared in the monograph, *Medical Management Analysis, A System for Controlling Losses and Evaluating Medical Care*, published by Marsh & McLennan, Inc., 1978. Reprinted with permission.

tutional needs. For example, some hospitals might add criteria that relate to informed consent or patient dissatisfaction; others might delete criteria that are not particularly applicable to the institution or to a review focused on a specific service or area. Specialty hospitals might add criteria appropriate to their special focus (e.g., a psychiatric facility might add criteria to screen for suicide attempts or assault by one patient on another or on a staff member). However criteria are modified, each criterion should serve as a "liability sensor" designed to raise a warning flag when an adverse event occurs.

Application of the criteria and implementation of the Medical Management Analysis System should be flexible. Any system, however, should include certain essential characteristics: concurrent review of patient records to detect adverse events; immediate professional review of all serious adverse events; documentation of all adverse events in a manner that will help identify recurrent problems; centralization of responsibility for the collection and monitoring of all data; and centralization of responsibility for reporting activities and findings and for implementing and following up recommended actions. One possible implementation model is shown in Figure 10.1.

The coordination of data retrieval in the Medical Management Analysis System reduces and may even eliminate multiple, overlapping reviews of individual patient records. (Figure 10.2 illustrates coordination of the system.) Data retrieval coordination saves time for hospital personnel (medical records, medical audit, utilization review personnel, etc.) and medical staff (e.g., time spent on peer review activities and committee work). Total review to meet all QA and liability prevention requirements can still be accomplished by adding separate criteria for surgical case, transfusion, and antibiotic review and for record completeness to the general outcome screening criteria. Utilization review coordinators, nursing care coordinators, and medical audit personnel freed from retrospective abstracting can be employed in concurrent data compilation.

Follow-up of review findings requires sophisticated and sensitive claims management. Claims personnel who have been trained to review records for serious adverse events only and then to take retrospective action may need to be oriented to the purposes of concurrent review and to the need for immediate evaluation of events for potential liability. Immediate evaluation is necessary so that claims can be prevented by quick follow-up action. Initially, incident reporting should also be included in any system. Results to date have indicated that, until the Medical Management Analysis System is fully operational in the facility, incident reports are also necessary to ensure that all events are being detected and recorded.

FIGURE 10.1

An Implementation Model for the Medical Management Analysis System Shows the Steps in One Possible Version of the System

Medical Management Analysis System Implementation Model

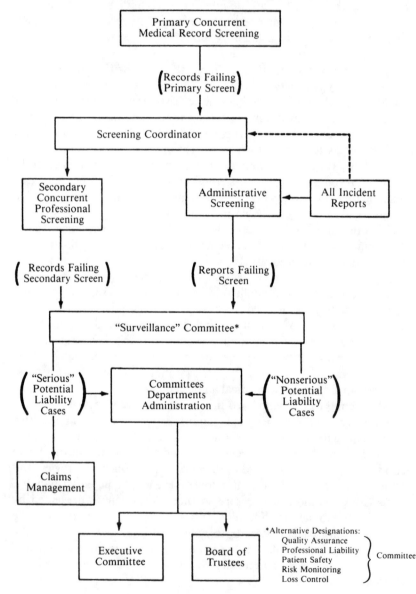

FIGURE 10.2

Concurrent, Coordinated, Centralized Data Collection on the Medical Management Analysis System Eliminates the Need for Multiple Review of Patient Records While Ensuring that the Data Needed for all Quality Assurance and Liability Control Activities Is Obtained and Distributed to the Appropriate Committees and Departments for Analysis

Medical Management Analysis System Data Retrieval Coordination

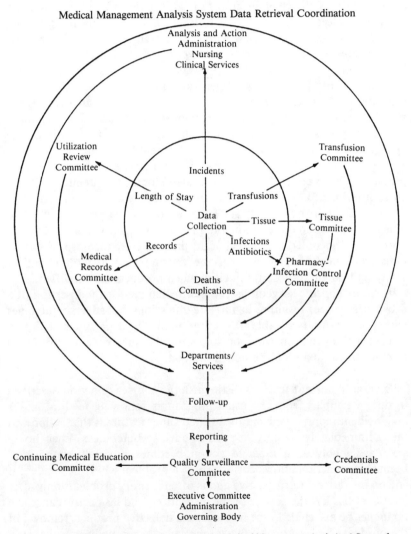

Figure 10.2 originally appeared in the monograph, *Medical Management Analysis, A System for Controlling Losses and Evaluating Medical Care,* published by Marsh & McLennan, Inc., 1978. Reprinted with permission.

Although it is too early to draw final conclusions, some selected examples of adverse events detected by the Medical Management Analysis System and of follow-up actions taken can illustrate benefits of the system. (Nonessential details of the examples have been altered or omitted to protect the identity of the institutions involved.)

• In one hospital, general outcome screening detected that, in one month, three of the chief surgical resident's patients had repeat surgery because of bleeding (see Table 10.1, criterion 8). Responsible staff conducted an immediate interview with the resident to determine the cause of the problem; the situation was resolved by counseling the resident and by changing his supervision.

• Review of the findings of general outcome screening in another institution revealed a pattern of medication errors (see Table 10.1, criterion 3). Immediate investigation determined that a nurse from a temporary agency was responsible. Follow-up action included notifying the agency and terminating the nurse's employment in the hospital.

• Review of a patient death revealed a connection between a defective product and the patient's having aspirated stomach contents (see Table 10.1, criterion 15). This had not been reported by a traditional incident report, although the nursing staff was aware of the problem and had independently altered the product to prevent further difficulties. Discovery of the incident led to removal of the product from the hospital and an intensive education program for the nursing staff regarding patient safety and potential hospital liability when products are modified.

• An orthopedic surgeon used a new technique for the insertion of a prosthetic device, resulting in three readmissions for adverse outcomes within one month (see Table 10.1, criterion 2). The department chairman discussed the situation with the surgeon, who subsequently concluded that he should abandon the new technique.

Several important features distinguish the courses of action described in these examples from the usual procedures following medical audits and incident reports. One major distinguishing feature is that action was taken immediately to prevent further adverse outcomes. When house staff are involved, immediate action becomes especially important, because such action allows correction of a problem while the resident is still on the service; retrospective audits often identify problems only after a resident has left the service or the institution, and his performance can no longer be affected. In the instance of a defective product, removal of the product would probably have taken place eventually, but the early action made possible by concurrent screening almost certainly prevented further injury and liability. Another feature of the actions in the examples given is that they sometimes occur in response to hospitalwide problems that would not be detected by most audits or incident reports. In the instance of the discovery of a pattern of medication errors, for example, medication errors had previously been reported as separate incidents, but no comprehensive analysis of time or location had taken place, so their cause had not been determined. Comprehensive screening of all patient records enables identification of patterns of substandard care that may not be related to one diagnosis or one service and probably would not otherwise be identified.

The Medical Management Analysis System has been in operation for nearly two years, and improvements in the system continue to be made. The enthusiastic cooperation of physicians and hospitals is largely responsible for the success of the system. The system is voluntary, flexible, and simple; it should remain so to continue to be effective in reducing adverse events, liability, and the cost of malpractice. Current results indicate that the Medical Management Analysis System has much promise as a tool for improving the quality and decreasing the cost of patient care.

11 | The Quality of Medical Care and the 14 Points of Edwards Deming

Duncan Neuhauser

Edwards Deming is best known for having advised Japanese Industry in developing high quality products. Although he is much less known in the USA and almost unknown in American health care, interest in his ideas is growing. Deming, in his book, *Out of the Crisis* (1982), summarized his ideas in 14 points, which this article reviews one by one. But before doing so, it is necessary to understand his basic statistical view of quality control. He starts with a production process which can be any repeated work activity. This could be drawing blood specimens, typing letters, reading x-rays, or hernia surgery.

A PRODUCTION PROCESS IN CONTROL

In the examples above, differences in performance are due to chance variation. The mean level performance is stable and individual performance measures vary randomly around this mean.

Imagine a hospital unit with 20 nurses, where the percent of medication errors per week are recorded for each nurse. The mean error rate is 5% and a 99% confidence interval of 0 to 10% errors. That is to say, any reported error rate less than 10% can be accounted for by chance. Week after week the mean error rate is close to 5% (also varying a bit randomly). One conclusion Deming derives from this is that these 20 nurses are doing their best, given the current means of production; therefore

---

Reprinted from *Health Matrix* 6 (Summer 1988):7–10, with permission, National Health Publishing.

there is no need to single out for praise or criticism any one of these nurses. The only justification for singling out any worker for special praise or correction is if it can be statistically demonstrated that they persistently fall above or below the band of chance variation.

A PRODUCTION PROCESS OUT OF CONTROL

When workers' scores fail to fit a bell-shaped distribution and the mean score fluctuates wildly, a production process is out of control. If these 20 nurses have an error rate this week of 5%; next week of 30%; next week of zero; this would be out of control. If 17 nurses were clustered closely around the 5% error rate, but three nurses have 80% error rates, the production process is out of control for these outliers. Under these circumstances, management needs to intervene to bring the production process back into control.

Deming uses three standard deviations to define inliers and outliers. This is a very generous cut-off point in that by chance only about .5% of observations will fall into the category of poor quality outliers by chance.

This approach suggests the need for a vast increase in the level of measurement in hospitals. Think of all the things that could be measured: telephone answering time for 15 switchboard operators; time for a meal to reach a patient; time between discharge and completion of medical records; turnaround time for lab test results; surgical infection rates; percent of appropriate patients receiving mammography. We could think of thousands of such measures, only a small fraction of which are being measured in any hospital today.

The concept of such extensive measurement, though simple on the surface, has profound implications. Consider the possibility of the Health Care Financing Administration (HCFA) reporting mortality rates hospital by hospital. The HCFA could publicly report mortality rates by hospital. Local newspapers could publish the list on the front page, rank ordering the hospitals from lowest to highest mortality. Reporters would call the top and bottom hospitals; in the former hospital, the administrator would say that his hospital has the best quality; the administrator of the latter would say, in fear of losing market share, that the numbers were wrong and misleading. In fact, these differences could be due purely to random variation alone.

HCFA could use Deming's three standard deviation cut-off points and only question those hospitals whose mortality exceeded this cut-off on the high mortality end of the distribution. Out of 5000 hospitals, one would expect that by chance alone, about 25 hospitals would be high mortality outliers. If HCFA in fact observes 100 such hospitals, then it would report that hospital X was an outlier, and there was a 75% chance that it had a real quality problem and a 25% chance that the figures reflected just bad luck.

There are two further implications. Everyone is already doing the best they can. This is true for a production process under control. It follows that there should be no rank ordering of worker performance, no bonus pay, and no firing. Performance differences are largely only a matter of chance.

The role of management is to change the whole production process, rather than badgering workers doing their best. Perhaps starting a unit dose system can reduce the nursing mean error rate from 5% to 2%. The role of management is to measure performance, not as a basis of reward or firing, but rather to assure production control. The persistent under-achiever should be educated or reassigned, not fired. The way to improve production is to change the production process itself.

DEMING'S 14 POINTS

Point 1 — Create constancy of purpose for improvement of product and service. Don't go for the fast buck and the quick fix. Don't just worry about the next quarterly financial report. Improving production processes takes time. Everyone should be involved in improving quality. Quality is central to the corporate culture. This implies stable management (not job hopping) and lifelong employment.

Point 2 — Adopt the new philosophy. Quality is not just an issue for top management and doctors: It is pervasive. Dr. Batalden of the Hospital Corporation of America said, "For everything you do about money in a hospital, do the same for quality." For example, if you have a senior vice president of finance, have a similar position for quality.

Are the conversations in the doctor's or nurse's lounge in a hospital about Florida condominiums, football scores, or supermarket sales; or are they about patient care? "Let me tell you about my patient . . . Do you think this might be a drug reaction . . .?" This is one measure of how thoroughly the commitment to quality has permeated the hospital.

Point 3 — Cease dependence on inspection to achieve quality. Having quality inspectors implies that quality is not everyone's job. The growth in the number of hospital quality assurance, utilization review, and risk management people could be good or bad depending on what these people do. If they inspect and punish, this would be harmful. If they document and give feedback information, this is a bit better, but not what Deming wants. He wants an organization where *every* worker is keeping his or her own performance charts. The quality assurance staff would act as consultants and helpers to every organizational member. How many hospital staff members currently keep track of their own performance in a quantitative way?'

Point 4 — Don't award business on the basis of price tag alone. Don't automatically buy from the lowest bidder. Instead, minimize cost by working with a single supplier over the long haul.

For example: Is a hospital's contract for physician emergency service coverage awarded to the lowest bidder? Cheapness is not always best. It is important to develop long-time, close links with suppliers who will know a hospital and what its need are. Is something lost by abandoning the hospital-based school of nursing? It is said that the Mayo Clinic, as it opens clinics in new locations, wants only Mayo Medical School graduates, because they know the Mayo style of care.

Point 5 — Improve constantly and forever every process for planning, production, and service. This follows from Point 1 — constancy of purpose, Point 2 — a total philosophy, and Point 10 — not setting targets. Don't just reach a target level of performance and stop. This also implies an organization constantly undergoing change in the unwavering pursuit of quality and the steady upgrading of production processes.

Point 6 — Institute training on the job. This is related to Point 5 — constant improvement, and Pont 13 — promoting education. For example: In one hospital, if you are a member of the medical staff, you can't show your face in the hospital if you have not read this week's *New England Journal of Medicine*. It's not in the job description; it is just deeply embedded in the culture. Workers need to learn how to measure their own performance and evaluate it.

Point 6 suggests the possibility of having the hospital's medical staff set for itself a plan for each member's continuing education, and possibly one for the board of trustees.

Point 7 — Institute leadership. Although this might sound like a trite and trivial injunction, Deming has a special definition of leadership. It includes (1) supporting the climate of concern for quality; (b) promoting widespread performance measurement; (c) maintaining constancy of purpose; and (d) changing production processes to improve quality.

For example, Dr. Victoria Cargill observed that resident physicians rarely promote preventive health measures (such as occult blood tests for colon cancer). They can be reminded, lectured, or cajoled, but they rarely cause more than a small percentage of appropriate patients to receive this test. Therefore, she changed the production process by having nurse practitioners do the testing. This resulted in a thirteen-fold increase in the number of tests returned. (Cargill, unpublished) That's what Deming means by leadership.

Point 8 — Drive out fear. Don't fire people; educate them, counsel them, test their eyesight, redesign the job, transfer the worker to a more appropriate position, but almost never fire anyone. Make sure all workers feel comfortable questioning and suggesting in a climate where quality is central. Quality circles will only work in such a climate. This is required for a high level of participation. The prospect of life-long employment can help reduce the fear of job loss. This is related to Deming's high cut-off point for defining poor quality outliers (3 standard deviations): He wants to give workers the benefit of the doubt in order to reduce fear.

For example, in one hospital the nurses frequently observed problems with the outcomes of orthopedic surgery, but in this hospital no nurse dares to question a physician, so the problem continues.

For another example, one might hear from middle management in a certain hospital, "Don't ever stick your neck out or be proactive, you will get killed. It's much safer to react to problems as they come along." That's fear.

Point 9 — Break down barriers between staff areas. Communication is not promoted in a climate of fear. Each worker can be seen as having suppliers and customers who receive their work. The x-ray, laboratory, and pharmacy departments all provide information to clinical "customers." A good working relationship requires communication.

For instance, have all the key department heads and service chiefs in a hospital met each other? How long does it take a new department head to meet the other key staff members?

Point 10 — Eliminate slogans, exhortation and targets for the work force. People are doing the best they can when the production process is under control. Slogans like "work harder" are not necessary if there is a strong total corporate commitment to quality at all levels.

If one hears slogans only from top management and reads about them in the employee newsletter, but never hears them from anyone else who works in the organization, its a bad sign. For example, the CEO might say, "Hospital Y is a great place to work." But a nurse at that hospital might say, "It's a job." When you hear such slogans over and over from the workers themselves, then it's part of the culture.

Point 11 — Eliminate numerical quotas for the work force and numerical goals for management. If performance differences are largely due to chance, don't set targets. Workers are doing their best when there is a climate of constant quality improvement.

Numerical targets can be manipulated and will be manipulated in a climate of fear and in a culture that does not care about quality. A strong culture is developed by long term relationships, and constancy of purpose.

An example of this might be the old Soviet joke about the factory whose plan called for the production of 10,000 pounds of paper clips: It fulfilled its production quota by producing one 10,000 pound paper clip.

Linking performance to rewards is not useful. If performance differences are due to chance, then rewarding these differences is arbitrary and does not promote team spirit and open communication. Here is an example of such bad thinking: If a trustee misses three consecutive board meetings she/he is automatically dismissed. Neighborhood health center doctors are required to see four outpatients an hour.

Point 12—Remove barriers that rob people of pride of workmanship. Eliminate the annual rating and merit system. Pride is necessary for a constant commitment to high quality. Merit awards are not appropriate when everyone is doing their best. Emphasize group effort rather than an individual effort. A barrier to pride can be seen in an overworked resident house staff, short of sleep, who may take on the "get rid of the patients" syndrome described by Mizrahi: (1986).

Point 13—Institute a vigorous program of education and self-improvement for everyone. Most junior hospital administrators have a clear agenda for self-improvement and skill development as they look forward to their career. If workers were randomly chosen in a hospital and asked, "What is your plan for education for yourself this year?" what answers would we get?

Point 14—Put everyone in the company to work to accomplish the transformation. This recapitulates the prior 13 points. One might ask, "If I were to read the minutes of your board of trustee meetings for the last year, would quality be discussed at all? Would it be discussed as much as money is?"

Deming's view implies that a superb quality product will be easy to sell and financial solvency will follow.

SUMMARY

Deming starts with a statistical theory of random variation and builds on this to create an entire theory of management. Some theories of human behavior start by assuming everyone is bad; Deming assumes everyone is good. Working in a corporate culture with singleness of purpose, participation, freedom from fear, job stability, and high expectations, makes Deming's hopeful behavioral assumption possible. When compared to many other types of organizations in our society, hospitals and health care organizations do well in many of these dimensions. Perhaps that's why American medicine can be the best in the world. However, Deming would say, there is a lot more to accomplish in the never-ending quest for higher quality of care.

REFERENCES

Cargill, V. et al. University Hospitals of Cleveland. Unpublished study.

Deming, Edwards. 1982. *Out of the crisis*. Cambridge Massachusetts: Center for Advanced Engineering Study, Massachusetts Institute of Technology.

Mizrahi, T. 1986. *Getting rid of patients*. New Brunswick, NJ: Rutgers University Press.

III

Organizational Design

To understand how the Professional Bureaucracy functions in its operating core, it is helpful to think of it as a repertoire of standard programs — in effect, the set of skills the professionals stand ready to use — which are applied to predetermined situations, called contingencies, [which are] also standardized.

— Mintzberg

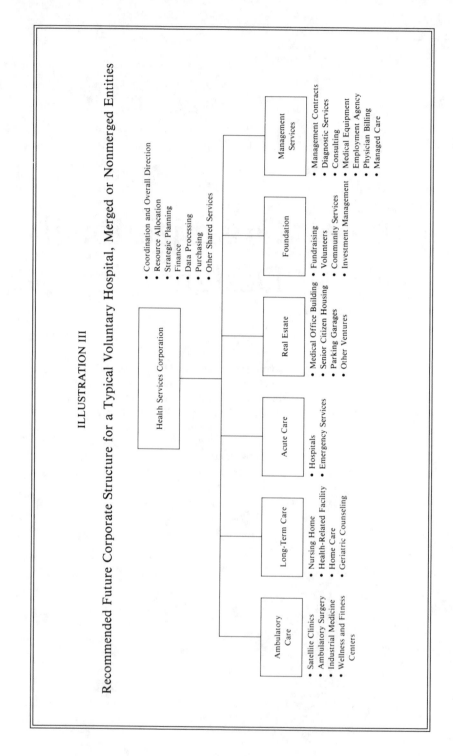

ILLUSTRATION III

Recommended Future Corporate Structure for a Typical Voluntary Hospital, Merged or Nonmerged Entities

Commentary

Anthony R. Kovner
Duncan Neuhauser

After the organizational leadership has decided what the organization will produce (i.e., what businesses it is in), they must designate the tasks, personnel, and equipment needed to achieve this production efficiently. These resources (people and equipment) are grouped together for the purpose of coordination; the way they are grouped is called the organizational design.

There are many different ways to organize work, and some ways work better than others. Strictly causal relationships between technology and organizational design, or between environment and design, have not yet been proven. Mintzberg has suggested five basic types of organizational design or structure: simple, machine bureaucracy, professional bureaucracy, divisionalized firm, and "adhocracy" (Mintzberg's term for a mutually adjusting structure).

The basic parts of Mintzberg's organizations are the strategic apex or top managers, middle management, the technological structure (such as planners and industrial engineers), support staff (such as personnel and security), and the operating core (or workers). Each of the five types of organization has a different configuration of these five parts. For example, the simple organization (e.g., a doctor's office) has managers, support staff, and an operating core but little or no technological structure or middle management.

The key means of coordination varies according to the type of organization. In a simple organization, direct supervision is the key means of coordination. In a machine bureaucracy, such as a large outpatient department for the poor, work standardization is the key means of coordination. In a professional bureaucracy, such as a community hospital, standardization of professional skills is a key means of coordinating the work. In a divisionalized firm, such as a multihospital corporation, the key means of coordination is the standardization of outputs, such as profits or market share. Finally, in an adhocracy, such as a rehabilitation unit, work is coordinated as the clinicians adjust to working with one another.

Work is sometimes organized according to the available physical facilities and may be influenced by an organization's history and the initial design of its founders. For example, most doctors still are not employees of hospitals because most physician care traditionally was provided in the homes of the patients. Organizational design also can be culturally determined. For example, most American hospitals have sizeable accounting and finance departments because of the fragmented nature of payment for medical care and the lack of national health insurance. Such departments are smaller in hospitals in other developed countries, all of which have some form of national health insurance.

According to Mintzberg, work in the operating core can be organized in one of three ways: by process or occupation (e.g., all nurses report to the director of nursing, all physicians to their department chiefs); by purpose or division, cutting across occupational specialties (e.g., all nurses and physicians report to the local clinical leadership, which may be surgery, women's health, or emergency services); or, by both process and purpose, in a matrix organization. Under this matrix method of organization, all nurses report to the clinical leadership of the division for some activities and to the director of nursing for others. Matrix organization solves certain coordination problems by process and by purpose but adds another layer to management, thereby increasing coordination costs.

Managers must decide when to use which form of organization and whether the benefits, if any, outweigh the costs. Generally speaking, process organization is favored in simpler organizations. Purpose organization is necessary in larger organizations, particularly where more occupations have to be coordinated and where there are more separate facilities. Sophistication of management favors matrix organization.

Regardless of the type of organization, a great deal of planning is needed to change the organizational design. It is not enough to say that a hospital built today would be organized differently than a previously existing hospital or nursing home. Changes in organization are costly, not only because of special pilot units and overlapping internal structures, but also because employees must care for patients while at the same time dealing with the uncertainties and frustrations of an extensive transition phase.

Many large hospitals are considering product line management. Product lines are divisions of a hospital that can be operated independently of the rest of the organization (organizing work by purpose). Examples of health products are cancer care, heart care, women's health care, emergency services, physical medicine, and rehabilitation. This type of organization encourages a greater focus on a particular product, with correspondingly more energy directed toward achieving market share or profit objectives, and with accountability for results and resources invested or removed from a product depending upon its present and predicted performance. Evidence that the benefits from such reorganization outweigh the costs and risks has not yet been gathered.

Advantages of multi-unit organizations (the divisionalized firm) include a focus on measurable outputs (thereby enhancing accountability), more specialization of function (made possible by high volumes), and more flexibility to close or open services in response to customer demand.

PERFORMANCE REQUIREMENTS

The four performance requirements are discussed below in terms of their importance for organizational design. Table III.1 shows how each of the authors of the readings in this section addresses these requirements.

TABLE III.1

Perspectives on Performance and Organizational Design

Readings	Goal Attainment	System Maintenance	Adaptive Capability	Values Integration
Griffith	Rational model, closed system			Hierarchy, collateral organization
Clement		Redefinitions for effective management	Strategies of vertical integration & diversification	
Heyssel et al.	Patient care, teaching, research	Hospital as a holding company, cost control	Decentralization	Participation by clinical chiefs in a teaching hospital
Shukla	Maximize patient care time by nurses	Technical support systems	Decentralization	Importance of good nursing care

GOAL ATTAINMENT

The appropriateness of a given combination of resources, tasks, incentives, and information systems in a health services organization is defined by its effect on the degree of goal attainment. Hospitals must try to meet many goals, and these goals differ greatly among different types of hospitals. Appropriateness in an army hospital may be defined very differently than in an investor-owned hospital.

At this level, the two overriding measures of goal attainment are efficiency, in terms of costs per unit of output, and quality of care, which is the benefit to the patient from the care received.

SYSTEM MAINTENANCE

At an implicit level, most of the readings in this section are concerned with developing organizational characteristics that are generally stable, self-adjusting, and permanent. It is perhaps natural to overemphasize change and to forget that the largest part of a manager's work is simply maintaining the organization and opposing the forces of entropy. Employees who leave must be replaced by new employees, who must be trained. Equipment and facilities must be maintained, repaired, and replaced. This information is considered obvious and, therefore, is seldom made explicit in the literature.

ADAPTIVE CAPABILITY

As goals, technology, size, personnel, and services change, structure also may need to change. Some structures are easier to change than others. For example, a centralized, hierarchically controlled organization may be changed easily by top management. If change is expected to come from professionals in the organization (as in a research laboratory), then decentralization and professional autonomy may be more appropriate characteristics in the organizational structure. Some changes are easier to implement than others. For example, it may be easy for a hospital to add a new piece of medical equipment but difficult to start a group practice.

A highly formalized organization, with a well-developed structure, task definition, and coordination, may be very efficient under stable conditions. If this organization has been, but no longer is, particularly successful, its long-established patterns may be difficult to change.

VALUES INTEGRATION

Clinician values such as independence, special expertise, and commitment to altruistic goals must be brought into organizations where managers set limits on behavior, supervise performance, and maintain economic viability. The attempt to integrate roles and values raises the need for clarification of clinician and managerial interests. To what extent are clinicians economic entrepreneurs or technical experts? Is there a sufficient degree of similarity of interest between clinicians and organizations?

THE READINGS

Griffith organizes the hospital into the following parts: governance, finance, clinical care, support services, and plant. He views the hospital organization as having three dimensions: a formal hierarchy, the informal organization, and the collateral organization, which is a network of committees and work groups providing cross-communication and linking middle managers at several different levels. He then discusses establishing the organizational design, defining responsibility centers, and the various forms of middle management.

Clement develops definitions of vertical integration and diversification. The focus of vertical integration is on the relationships among components of the production process. Diversification focuses on the relationships among final, consumable outputs. Clement points out that diversification requires skills and assets to manage businesses ranging from health promotion to selling data-processing services.

Heyssel and his colleagues describe the decentralization of Johns Hopkins Hospital, which seems directly analogous to decentralization in industrial firms. Decentralization may not be a new concept for industry, but it is new among hospitals and it raises new issues. How should a decentralized profit center like internal medicine relate to radiology and pathology? If routine laboratory tests or housekeeping services can be purchased at lower costs outside the hospital, should the purchase be allowed? How should nursing and physicians relate to each other? Should the nursing budget be folded into the profit center responsibility? If so, what will nurses think about this?

Shukla compares the distribution of supplies and working relationships for nursing in four different hospitals and shows how they relate to the amount of time registered nurses spend on direct patient care. The technical component includes distribution of supplies, medicines, and communication. The structural working relationships are between teams of primary nursing care. Shukla finds that the technical and structural systems are interactive and that a primary nursing system combined with a decentralized technical support system results in the highest amount of direct patient care.

ADDITIONAL TOPICS OF INTEREST

Architectural design also influences the way in which work is organized in health care organizations. Much thought has gone into restructuring organizations in order to shelter money, reduce taxation, and generate revenues from non-patient-care activities. These are important concerns for physicians, group practices, nursing homes, and hospitals. Readers may be interested in issues such as the way the organization of a multi-institutional system affects structuring and restructuring. How does the hospital component of a larger commercial or government organization fit into the system as a whole? How can some such organizations comprise both for-profit and nonprofit components? There are numerous variations in organizational design among health maintenance organizations (including independent practice associations) and among neighborhood health centers, preferred provider organizations, nursing homes, and other health organizations. The selected bibliography below offers suggestions for further readings on organizational design. Readers should also refer to the annotated bibliography at the end of the book.

SELECTED BIBLIOGRAPHY

Brown, Lawrence D. *Politics and Health Care Organizations: HMO's as Federal Policy*. Part I, 3–194. Washington, DC: Brookings Institution, 1983.

Clibbon, Sheila, and Marvin L. Sachs. "Like-Spaces versus Bailiwick Approaches to the Design of Health Care Facilities." *Health Services Research* 5 (Fall 1970): 172–85.

Cowan, Dale H. *Preferred Provider Organizations Planning, Structure and Operation*. Rockville, MD: Aspen, 1984.

Fetter, Robert B., and J.L. Freeman. "Diagnosis Related Groups: Product Line Management within Hospitals." *Academy of Management Review* 11, no. 1 (1986): 41–54.

Folger, James C., and E. Preston Gee. *Product Management for Hospitals*. Chicago: American Hospital Publishing, 1987.

Harris, Jeffrey E. "The Internal Organization of Hospitals: Some Economic Implications." *The Bell Journal of Economics* 8 (Autumn 1977): 476–82.

Leatt, Peggy, Stephen M. Shortell, and John A. Kimberly. "Organization Design." In *Health Care Management*, 2d ed., edited by Stephen M. Shortell and Arnold D. Kaluzny, 307–43. New York: Wiley, 1988.

Luft, Harold. *Health Maintenance Organizations: Dimensions of Performance*. New York: Wiley, 1981.

Munson, Fred C. "What Kind of Unit Management?" In *SUM: An Organizational Approach to Improved Patient Care*, edited by Richard Jelinek, Fred

Munson, and Robert L. Smith, 31–56. Battle Creek, MI: W.K. Kellogg Foundation.

Neuhauser, Duncan. "The Hospital as a Matrix Organization." *Hospital Administration* 17 (Fall 1972): 8–25.

Rosenberg, Charles. *The Care of Strangers*. New York: Basic Books, 1987.

Shortell, Stephen M. "High-Performing Healthcare Organizations: Guidelines for the Pursuit of Excellence." *Hospital & Health Services Administration* 30 (July-August 1985): 8–25.

____. "The Medical Staff of the Future: Replanting the Garden." *Frontiers of Health Services Management* 1 (February 1985): 3–48.

Shortell, Stephen M., and M. Brown, eds. *Organizational Research in Hospitals*. Chicago: Blue Cross Association, 1976.

Smith, Harvey L. "Two Lines of Authority Are One Too Many." *Modern Hospitals* 84 (March 1955): 59–64.

Starkweather, David B. *Hospital Mergers in the Making*. Ann Arbor, MI: Health Administration Press, 1981.

____. "The Rationale for Decentralization in Larger Hospitals." *Hospital Administration* 15 (Spring 1970): 27–45.

12 | Foundations of the Hospital Organization

John R. Griffith

ORGANIZATION STRUCTURE

One implication of the ethical values common to well-managed hospitals is dedication to the importance of clinical activities. Well-managed hospitals have improved and extended these services at good levels of quality for many years. As open systems theory would predict, they have been rewarded for it by substantial increases in the resources available to them. With the growth in resources has come a growth in complexity. Activities that were once the part-time tasks of a single individual now require entire sections of a much larger organization.

By the 1980s, the process of stimulus and response to exchange opportunities had resulted in the five major systems, which are subdivided into 50 or more specialized work units in even moderate-sized hospitals. A review of these parts and their approximate date of origin shows not only what the modern hospital is, but reveals much about how it came to be.

GOVERNANCE

The following are governance functions:

1. *Trustee or governing board*—The board is an old and essential part of hospitals, whose role has evolved toward boundary spanning, identification of exchange opportunities, and strate-

---

An excerpt from the chapter in John R. Griffith, *The Well-Managed Community Hospital* (Ann Arbor: Health Administration Press, 1987), 109–36, with permission, John R. Griffith.

gic planning of the organization's response. Emphasis has moved away from direct financial contribution and the contribution of specialized skills, although many examples of these still occur.

2. *Executive* — This function has emerged gradually since 1930. The title "president and chief executive officer" became relatively common in the 1970s. The number and kinds of executive personnel grew with the prominence of the office. Several dozen people now work in the executive office of well-managed hospitals, supporting the needs of the governance system.

3. *Medical staff organization* — Although the functions of the medical staff are clinical, the nature of the contract between medical staff members and the organization as a whole is a critical governance activity. It began to emerge as such when the open staffs of the early twentieth century gave way to the closed staff of the 1930s and the privileged staff of the 1970s and the 1980s. Quality reviews enforced by the JCAH were made increasingly rigorous through the postwar decades. Utilization review, that is, peer concern over the quantity of service ordered, was first mentioned in the late 1950s, became widespread in the early 1970s, and increased strikingly in importance in the 1980s. The complexity of medical staff organization grew steadily with these trends. Staff leadership was almost exclusively volunteer in community hospitals until the 1970s, when employed staff leadership became more popular.

4. *Planning and marketing* — Well-managed hospitals began rudimentary planning in the 1950s, but the concepts were not widespread until the 1970s, when planning was stimulated by federal legislation resulting from concerns over cost and equitable access to health care. Marketing, a concept that subsumes planning and extends beyond it, received great impetus in the 1980s, as pressures for cost control caused revenues to be threatened. Well-managed hospitals use the concept of marketing to assess, evaluate, influence, and respond to exchange opportunities. A more aggressive strategic planning stance developed with the marketing concept and will continue in the foreseeable future.

5. *Public relations and fund raising* — Formal efforts emerged around 1940 and grew slowly but steadily. Many hospitals paid more attention to the function around 1980. Promotion, an activity that is part of marketing, includes both advertising and public relations. The broadest concept of these activities, involving all considerations of the way the institution is perceived by

its exchange partners, is just beginning to be understood and
implemented.

6. *Information management* — Information arises from the activities of three major systems, finance, clinical, and governance.
   Contributions from these three sources developed at unequal
   rates, but by the 1980s well-managed hospitals had perceived the
   importance and interrelation of the three. Although few hospitals have formally identified information management as a governance rather than a finance function, the nature of their needs
   suggests that they will.

FINANCE

The use of private insurance and fee-for-service payment for hospital
care has led to a greatly enlarged finance system, compared to those in
other advanced nations. The spread of private health insurance (paying
either cost or charges, depending on location and kind of insurance) and
government health insurance (paying costs) stimulated first an increased
accounting capability and later a vastly improved financial analysis capability. Computer technology expanded with increased demand from the
payment sources, encouraging the strong growth of the finance function.
Fund accounting, emphasizing the proper use of donated money, was
dominant until the 1960s. Financial accounting, emphasizing accurate
identification of costs, charges, and revenue, became central with the
growth of outside payment. Last to be added was an emphasis on financial planning. This arose with the use of borrowed funds, which grew
throughout the 1970s and early 1980s in response to the stimulus of
widespread and generous insurance.

The following are controllership or accounting functions:

1. *Patient accounting* — Patient charges, or bills, generate much of
   the hospital's revenue. Patient accounting has been present
   throughout the century, grew rapidly from 1945 to 1970, and
   has continued steady growth since.
2. *Internal and external financial audit* — Audits are concerned
   with protecting owners' assets. Very little attention was paid to
   auditing until after the passage of Medicare, which demanded
   external auditing as a basic protection of public funds. Internal
   audits arose from the need to meet external standards and may
   be expected to continue to expand in the new environment of
   cost control.
3. *Payroll and accounts payable* — These routine business accounts
   have been present throughout the century, but the increase in

value of items purchased and the increases in both wages and nonsalary benefits prompted substantial growth, particularly between 1970 and 1980. Newer systems emphasize cost control by providing more specific and timely data.

4. *Cost accounting*—Efforts to determine accurate costs of treatment provided started with the use of costs to determine revenue at the close of World War II, but they remained simplistic until 1967, when Medicare adopted a cost-based reimbursement system. Cost accounting is expected to become even more important in the coming decades.

The following are functions of financial analysis:

1. *Management of capital sources*—Long-term debt became an important source of capital for hospitals in the 1970s; it was supported by extended insurance coverage and the availability of tax-exempt bonds. In the 1980s, joint ventures and for-profit capital subsidiaries introduced the use of equity finance, and the development of multihospital organizations expanded the financial management obligations.

2. *Budgeting and capital budgeting*—Careful projections of expenditures did not become routine in hospitals until the 1970s. Well-managed hospitals began to use budgets derived from careful assessment of the economic exchange environment, the hospital's long-range plan, and its long-range fiscal plan in the early 1980s. These budgets establish mutually agreed-upon expectations for future expenditures at the level of the responsibility center. Relatively short term capital budgets are used similarly, to set priorities for new programs and capital equipment. These two activities are essential elements of cost control and can be expected to grow in importance and sophistication throughout the 1980s.

3. *Financial planning*—Sophisticated financial planning controls the use of borrowed and equity capital as well as the growth of expenditures and pricing strategies. Financial planning became more elaborate as the payment mechanisms of insurers became more complex, borrowing and equity sources became more widely used, and the exchange environment became more demanding. It is a major component of strategic planning, lending reality to what would otherwise be mainly wishes and dreams.

CLINICAL CARE

Exponential growth in medical specialties, nursing specialties, other clinical professions, treatments, and diagnostic procedures can be traced throughout the century. Three major groups of clinical activity have emerged: medical staff, those making the central treatment decisions and undertaking surgery; nursing, and clinical support services.

MEDICAL CARE

The medical encounter, which occurs when a patient contacts a doctor or one of a few similar practitioners, is the central event in the health care process. In the encounter, the doctor identifies a series of patient needs for diagnosis and treatment. These needs, translated into order for services, stimulate most hospital activities. Almost all demand for inpatient or outpatient hospital services results from them.

The issues of quality and economy involve the encounter, the orders, and their fulfillment. The major outcomes of care are determined by three elements of the encounter:

1. How valid the set of needs identified is
2. How well those needs are carried out, including both professional and patient perceptions of validity
3. How satisfied the patient is with the elements of the encounter and the resulting services

Any hospital that aspires to be well managed must assure that medical encounters for its patients are done well across all three of these dimensions. Yet medical encounters are often highly individualized, intimate, and anxiety producing. Society gives physicians significant and unique prerogatives to carry these encounters out. The privacy and flexibility they demand prohibits the normal organizational approach to quality control, which emphasizes uniformity and direct oversight.

This dilemma gives rise to unique contracts between the physician and the organization that supports her or him. The one that is most common in hospitals involves the granting of annually renewed **privileges**, rights to perform certain kinds of care in the hospital. The extent of privileges is determined by professional peers, based upon the doctor's education and past performance. (Other organizations, such as HMOs or clinics, which employ or contract with physicians, develop similar structures.)

The medical staff organization conducts peer review, evaluating the credentials of applicants and annually reviewing the performance of physicians with privileges. It also fulfills several other functions supporting the quality of care. The number and importance of these functions have been growing for several decades. Representation of doctors' needs is an old but continuing function. Management of privileges has grown steadily more complex in the last 50 years; in fact, annual review of privileges was begun only recently. Recruitment of physicians as a coordinated activity is also recent. The development of consensus on methods of care, expressed as protocols that guide economy and quality, appears likely to become a fourth critical contribution of the medical staff. In addition to these four functions relating to the patient encounter, medical staffs provide education to their members and to other health professions.

The system of peer review normally stops short of direct supervision or direct observation of the medical encounter. It relies upon self-supervision by each physician with privileges. In order to assure the quality of the medical encounter, the well-managed hospital must attract doctors who are both well trained and well motivated, that is, who can be trusted to complete medical encounters well. This, in turn, requires the successful completion of all the medical staff functions.

The most common financial arrangement for medical staff members is a fee-for-service contract between the doctor and the patient, without direct involvement of the hospital. However, the form of association between the doctor and the hospital has been changing steadily. At present, about 25 percent of doctors are employed in hospitals, excluding doctors in training. The balance are independent practitioners who are paid directly by patients or their insurers; these doctors are increasingly entering into financial arrangements with the hospital or with the hospital and a third party. It is likely that multiple and hybrid forms will continue. The growth of HMOs and prospective payment contracts will stimulate more complex financial arrangements at the expense of traditional fee-for-service payment. This book assumes a model called the **conjoint medical staff**, a flexible and pluralistic relationship between doctors and the hospital that assumes increasingly close ties.

CLINICAL SUPPORT SERVICES

The services which physicians and others order as a result of medical encounters are provided by numerous health care professions, including several medical specialties. Many of these have employment relationships with the community hospital. Nursing, the oldest and largest of the clinical services, was often the source of the first members of the newer professions. The others were once called *ancillary services* but now fill too important a role in diagnosis and treatment for that label. They provide the components of health care, the intermediate products that collectively support the physician's plan for diagnosis and treatment.

Each of the clinical support services has a set of specific functions arising from its unique technology or skills, but there are several generic functions as well. All must control the processes and outcomes of their intermediate product. Quality of service, including the physician's perception of quality, is essential. In addition, the support services are responsible for several management functions, including patient scheduling, personnel logistics, planning, budget development, and cost control for the intermediate product.

NURSING

The nurse's contribution to patient care rivals the physician's in both inpatient and outpatient settings. It is defined by the concept of homeostasis, helping the patient to achieve a maximally effective interchange with his or her environment. This concept encompasses not only the traditional nursing activities, but a broad range of preventive and educational services as well. The nursing care plan arising from the concept of homeostasis is also important in lowering the final product cost.

Nursing emphasizes the development and maintenance of the comprehensive care plan in addition to functions that resemble those of the other clinical support services. Nursing is responsible for its own quality and monitors the quality of several other services in order to ensure patient and physician satisfaction. It must manage its own work force, the largest in the hospital, support a variety of logistical services for the patient, and assist the governance system with planning advice.

HUMAN RESOURCES

Several factors have spurred the growth of the human resources function beyond what is necessary to support other activities. The number of hospital employees has grown to about three per occupied bed, from fewer than two 30 years ago. In addition, hospitals employ more professionally skilled individuals, who tend to be recruited from regional or national rather than local markets. The number of such skills has increased as well. Unionization has become important in some regions. Both federal and state work force regulations have become more complex, and hospital exemptions have been removed. The human resources function includes the following activities:

1. *Recruitment and work force planning*—National markets, recurring shortages, increased labor costs, and federal equal opportunity provisions changed recruitment from a casual, local event to a regional or national one. Advanced planning of per-

sonnel needs was accelerated in the 1980s by concern over the cost of additional personnel and the need for humane policies of work force reduction.

2. *Work force support*—Large, expensive, specialized work forces demand certain maintenance activities, such as training and orientation, counselling, and promotion and termination interviewing. These have been centralized slowly in hospitals, but they now take place largely in human resources departments rather than the clinical units.

3. *Compensation*—Improved financing for hospital care, competition for employees, regulation of wages and hours, and collective bargaining have improved the once notoriously low salaries of hospital workers. Employment benefits also expanded and now constitute about 10 percent of hospital expenditures. These benefits—vacations, sick leave, health insurance, retirement pensions, and life insurance constitute a minimum package—all require administration. Federal employment law governing wages and hours, overtime, working conditions, affirmative action for disadvantaged groups, and collective bargaining rights apply to hospitals receiving payment under Medicare. State laws deal with many of the same subjects but also cover unemployment compensation and workers' compensation. Finally, many hospitals in the Northeast and some in other parts of the country have union contracts. The American Federation of State, County, and Municipal Employees and the 1199 Union of Hospital and Health Care Workers are numerically important. Some hospitals negotiate with up to six different unions, some of them representing house officers and nurses.

PLANT

Historically, each section of the hospital managed its own environmental needs, with the exception of such simple common areas as roof, corridors, and lawn. In medieval hospitals, housekeeping, food, and laundry were done on individual wards. Centralization of these activities began in the nineteenth century, when low-cost electricity and steam power became available. The combination made it cost-effective to operate plumbing and heating systems, and later kitchens, laundries, and sterilization services. The following are elements of the plant, supplies, and maintenance function:

1. *Operation of buildings, utilities, and equipment*—In the 1950s, the use of general air conditioning and devices posing radiation

hazards expanded greatly. Infection control and energy conservation became routine. Automobile parking became an essential service. Each development added to the complexity of the environmental systems. The result is that the power supply of the modern hospital is a sophisticated technical achievement in itself. Communications and computing equipment began major developments in the 1970s which appear likely to continue for some years. The proliferation of complex equipment forced specialization among repair services, with the most complex technical tasks frequently contracted to outside companies. All of this growth made careful planning and control of the use of space essential.

2. *Housekeeping and environmental safety* — Housekeeping became increasingly mechanized as wage increases justified substituting capital for labor. It is an important element in infection control. Patients, employees, and guests must be protected from environmental hazards by a routine surveillance function.

3. *Work force, patient, and visitor support services* — Hospitals provide food, various amenities, and communication services to members, patients, and guests. All but the smallest hospitals have trained security forces, and some inner-city institutions have what amounts to a small police force protecting property, patients, and personnel.

4. *Materials management* — Centralized materials management functions are relatively recent in hospital organizations. Many aspects of obtaining supplies were left to the using unit even in the 1980s, but standardization, competitive bid solicitation, and collective purchasing had grown steadily. Cost concerns accelerated their growth in the 1980s.

THE PROCESS OF ORGANIZATION DESIGN

The environment of U.S. hospitals changed radically between 1980 and 1985, but the impact of that change on organization structure is not yet known. The most successful hospitals will be those that can identify and implement the changes most satisfactorily to the American people. It is likely that hospital organization in the next decade will face as much change as it did at the peak of the post-Medicare years. Well-run hospitals therefore will be those that can manage a high rate of organizational change effectively.

THE CRITERION FOR ORGANIZATION DESIGN

Success for hospitals requires both correct assessment of community desires and effective response to them. Pressures from the outside environment affect much of the hospital organization, and a successful organization is one that responds effectively to those pressures. Some tasks are assigned by licensure laws and others by educational programs. For example, the roles of many professionals in hospitals are determined by professional practice acts. Educational programs are constructed to follow the acts; thus, even if a hospital wanted to reassign certain tasks, its personnel would not know how to carry out their new duties. Organization design is also influenced by the marketplace, including reimbursement mechanisms. A hospital operating in an affluent community or under generous reimbursement may have a different organization than one in a poorer environment. Design also depends upon technology. the growth of laboratory medicine caused the creation of a new organizational unit, the clinical laboratory, which in 100 years has grown to be the second largest department in the hospital. Computers are expected to have an important effect on organization.

To respond correctly, the hospital must coordinate the efforts of several hundred or thousand people. This begins by assigning every member of the organization to either a work group or a supervisory position. The work groups and their arrangement under various levels of supervisors creates what is called a **bureaucratic organization**. The term was coined by researchers to describe a form of human endeavor where groups of individuals bring different skills to bear on a single objective in accordance with a formal structure of authority and responsibility. The formal structure generates the familiar pyramidal shape of organization charts. Most of the economic activity of modern society is carried out by means of bureaucratic organizations (as is most religious, artistic, and social activity: the Catholic Church, the New York Philharmonic Orchestra, and the Boy Scouts of America are bureaucratic organizations). All hospitals are bureaucratic organizations.[1]

Bureaucratic organizations permit individuals to contribute to an overall objective that is larger than the sum of their individual efforts. They use specialization to enhance the individual's contribution and coordination to make the whole responsive. Coordination begins with small groups and continues with the supervisory structure. The purpose of bureaucratic structure is to facilitate responsiveness, and the two keys to responsiveness are supporting the small groups and building coordination. No hospital is ever totally successful at the effort; the well-managed hospital is more responsive, and its responsiveness underpins its success.

COMPONENTS OF ORGANIZATION

Although many people think of the pyramidal chart as describing an organization, reality is substantially more complicated. To have an effective understanding of a hospital organization, one must recognize that it has at least three broad dimensions: a formal hierarchy, represented by the pyramid; a set of formal collateral activities, or boundary spanning;[2] and informal networks, which are generated by members of the organization acting as individuals rather than through their formal authority.

The Hierarchy of Accountability

The bureaucratic organization of hospitals identifies the roles and tasks that must be accomplished, assigns them to individuals and groups, and establishes a network of communications. The network is based upon the concept of **accountability**, the notion that the organization can rely upon the individual to fulfill a specific, prearranged expectation. Just as every worker is assigned to a work group, every member of the organization should have a clear position in the accountability hierarchy.

Mintzberg notes that, in addition to the accountability hierarchy, the parts of the pyramid all have boundary-spanning activities with each other and often with the external environment. In addition, he notes that some of the accountability hierarchies serve the central purpose of the organization and are traditionally called line units, while others serve technical and support activities, sometimes called staff units, and still others constitute the strategic apex.[3] Mintzberg's models fit manufacturing better than hospitals, but it might be said that the finance group is a technical activity, and certainly the human resources and plant management groups are support activities.

Even though a work group is in a support section or is dedicated to boundary spanning, it is still in the accountability hierarchy and reports to the chief executive. Like every other work group in the well-run hospital, it has specific and often quantitative expectations for each of the closed system parameters. Assignment of accountability includes mutual understanding of the expectation, assignment and acceptance of the authority necessary to carry it out, and designation of a communication route for reporting both difficulties and performance.

The accountability hierarchy creates a form of contract between superior and subordinate components of the organization and to a large extent between the two individuals which implement it. This contract holding both parties responsible for prearranged expectations is the essence of the formal hierarchical organization. The relationship is enforced by the traditions of bureaucratic organization; by the information flows which report performance on the closed system parameters; by the authorities over expectations, appointment of individuals, and distribution of rewards; and finally, but perhaps most important, by the ability of the superior to meet the work place needs of the subordinate.

Informal Organizations

All groups of people working together develop informal organizations. They consist of the network of communications the members establish for their own desires. The informal organizations of hospitals are exceptionally important. Hospitals must give great latitude to doctors and nurses dealing directly with patients because patients' needs vary. The three-shift operation is another factor encouraging informal organization. The night crew is almost certain to encounter situations in which it must devise its own answers. Although it is usually impossible to describe the informal structure in detail, the best formal organizations not only recognize their informal shadows, but are designed to exploit their strengths and to overcome their weaknesses. One useful perspective is that the formal organization strengthens the informal one and does what the informal one cannot.

The Collateral Organization

In addition to a formal hierarchical structure, hospitals make heavy use of collaborative communications and clearances among units in different hierarchies. Such devices are used to accomplish daily work and to understand and communicate perceptions about the outside environment. These activities comprise the **collateral organization**. The collateral organization can be understood as a network of committees and work groups providing cross-communication and linking middle managers at several different levels. Members shift collateral relationships much more often than hierarchical ones, and collateral activities rarely have direct authority. The well-managed hospital uses collateral organization to build consensus about exchange opportunities and to coordinate expectations. Committee work can be time-consuming for middle managers, however, and in extreme cases may impair the hospital's function. The well-designed hospital attempts to move the consensus as quickly as possible into the formal accountability hierarchy, where quantitative expectations can be negotiated to encourage efficient responses.

The *code team*, a multidisciplinary group assisting in cases of cardiac arrest, is a dramatic example of a collateral organization. The discharge planning committee, which coordinates the efforts of nursing, medicine, and social service, is another. The oldest is the surgical team, with members from nursing, surgery, and anesthesia. The principal function of these activities internally is to integrate members of different accountability hierarchies.

Collateral activities addressing exchange issues from the external environment are frequently longer lasting and more complex. Many planning and expectation-setting activities demand the collaboration of several work groups. Attaining appropriate levels of patient care quality and satisfaction requires both in-depth technical knowledge and an understanding of customer needs. Competing opportunities for exchanges must frequently be evaluated jointly, in light of overall external needs. Well-run hospitals meet this broader need through collateral units such as the planning committee and the joint medical staff–board conference committee at the governance level. At lower levels, structures such as the pharmacy committee and the medical records committee pool technological knowledge from several areas and make decisions affecting productivity and quality.

It is impossible to dispense with the collateral organization. The dynamic nature of the environment and the variability of patient needs call for collateral activities. Control of the collateral organization can be a problem, however. Performance is improved if the collateral organization has specific expectations about its functions and reporting. Thus a well-managed collateral organization is kept relatively small, given explicit charges, supported with adequate data, monitored closely, and expected to reach conclusions on explicit schedules.

DECISIONS ESTABLISHING THE
ORGANIZATION DESIGN

The hospital organization is designed through three interrelated actions:

1. Specifying the tasks and the accountability for each small work group
2. Establishing the reporting and supervisory responsibilities of middle management, which constitutes the accountability hierarchy
3. Building collateral relationships between hierarchies, thereby allowing them to coordinate and integrate their expectations toward a common goal

The process of coordination and integration depends upon the participation of individuals and groups. One of the proven ways to gain participation is to seek it habitually in all important organizational decisions. Since the design of the organization is one important decision, it is not surprising that much of the design of the accountability hierarchy is determined by the collateral organization. The executive office stimulates and guides the participation of a variety of people in an ongoing process of designing and amending both the accountability hierarchy and the collateral organization itself.

ORGANIZATION DESIGN AS A PROCESS OF COLLABORATION

The responsibility for successful organization design falls more heavily on the executive office than on any other unit of the organization. The governing board is rarely involved in the design process, although it sometimes approves the final plan. The executive office controls the design process and its outcome.

Good executives encourage broad participation from others in the organization. Design decisions require much detailed information that the executive office is not likely to possess. On the other hand, breadth of vision and an understanding of relationships among hospital activities are important to successful organization design. It is unlikely that individuals in the clinical, financial, human resources, or plant systems will have sufficient perspective to make wise design decisions unaided. Because of the importance of the task and the value of experience, organization design is a frequent activity for the chief operating officer and his or her immediate deputies. A critical part of that activity is deciding who else will participate in the design decision at hand.

A second critical function of the executive is control of the rate of change. There are always some arguments for fixing the organization. Too much change is confusing, expensive, and fails to take advantage of learning and experience to improve performance. Too little, however, leads to insularity of viewpoint and unresolved adjustments to technological and economic changes. Identifying the correct pace of change for the organization is the responsibility of the executive.

Good practice requires that the members of the organization participate in the design of the parts that relate to their own functions. Doctors should participate in the design of the medical staff and its reporting hierarchy, food service managers, the food service, and so on. Design begins conceptually with identification of all the tasks and activities that must be performed. These are then grouped around common factors, usually equipment, training, time, or geography. Much of the success of the well-managed hospital arises from the close fit that emerges from years of effort in specifying these groupings and the resulting interfaces. The process of organization design specifies in advance the nature of this growth by structuring the flow of information. Deliberate efforts must be made to identify, discuss, and resolve conflicts and omissions of responsibilities that arise in the design process. It is the job of the executive office to assemble all the various viewpoints, hear their views, and establish formal hierarchies that will improve integration among groups.

DEFINING RESPONSIBILITY CENTERS

A responsibility center (RC) is a small group of workers and one first-level manager. A nursing station crew with its head nurse or a housekeeping crew with its foreman are typical examples. The managers are the primary monitors from the closed system model and are called **responsibility center managers** (RCMs). Even a modest hospital will have upwards of 50 RCs, with several RCs in each large department. Very large hospitals have over 100.

Criteria for Design

The design criteria for each responsibility center are:

1. *To assign every necessary task to a single RC*—Tasks assigned to more than one RC or to no RC are not accountable.
2. *To assign related tasks to the same RC*—If related tasks are assigned to different RCs, problems of continuity and coordination may arise.
3. *To assign tasks requiring similar skills to the same RC*—A work group and a manager with a common background can communicate with each other more easily.
4. *To limit each RC to a reasonable span of control*—The RCM must be able to maintain control of the activity by direct observation, to carry out the principle of no surprises (see chapter 3). Direct observation imposes geographic, temporal, and size limits on RCs.

Dealing with Conflicting Criteria

Typically hospitals have an RC for each nursing floor, or unit. They divide a large department in a single geographic location into RCs on the basis of technical function (for example, the laboratory is divided into chemistry, hematology, bacteriology, and histology RCs). They may organize a 24-hour service, such as security, into shifts. They divide a dispersed activity like housekeeping geographically in order to maintain a reasonable span of control. Laundries and operating rooms are organized around equipment—wash wheels and irons, heart pumps and lasers.

For a great many important hospital activities, the criteria for design are in conflict, and their parameters (tasks, relationships, skills, and span) cannot all be optimized at once. There are frequently two geographic units with similar functions, or two functions in the same geographic area, or two skills required for the same function. Many large hospitals have several laboratories. Emergency rooms require almost every clinical profession, plus housekeeping and other plant services. Nursing, medicine, and social service contribute to the function of discharge planning. Even the task assignment of the nursing unit RC is slightly ambiguous, because housekeeping, dietary, several diagnostic and treatment services, and medical staff are all important to the function of the nursing unit.

In every case where these conflicts arise, trade-offs must be selected to resolve them. As a result, there is no perfect list of RCs for a hospital, and, because conditions change, there is no permanent solution. Rather, well-run hospitals consider the next two steps of organization design— setting the reporting hierarchy of middle management and building collateral communications—as ways of overcoming the weaknesses of a specific set of RCs. When the RC design process is properly done, it generates three results:

1. It specifies the RCs and the RCMs.
2. It identifies the trade-offs, or departures from criteria, arising from that particular solution.
3. It suggests hierarchical relationships and collateral relationships that will optimize these trade-offs.

Another way to say this is that there are always three avenues to organizational improvement—changing the RCs, revising the middle management structure, and strengthening collateral relationships.

Responsibility Centers for the Medical Staff

Traditionally, medical practice has been left to the authority and responsibility of the individual physicians who are privileged to practice. In effect, each doctor is his or her own RC and RCM, but the closed system parameters have been only partially and ambiguously specified. More or less formal allegiances based on medical specialty have grouped doctors, but the mechanisms for accountability have also remained limited and ambiguous. The result is that an accountability hierarchy is only beginning to emerge in the very best hospitals. There are important arguments for allowing the attending physician freedom to exercise professional judgment on the patient's behalf. If done badly, specification of the activities of professionals can be more damaging than total freedom. The issues underlying the medical decision process . . . are complex, and successful medical designs will continue to recognize the importance of the individual practitioner's on-the-scene judgment.

Despite the importance of individual judgment, the trend has been toward organizing physicians into work groups and increasingly specifying closed system parameters. Several developments have eroded the tradition of completely individualized medical practice. . . . A new model of medical staff organization, the conjoint staff has emerged. Under the concept of the conjoint staff, work groups of physicians who share similar patient and disease populations are likely. These work groups have leaders, who increasingly take on responsibility for quality and appropriateness of medical care. As they do, their parallels to the traditional responsibility center and RCM become clearer. Competition for groups of patients that pay on a capitation basis is the strongest force among several supporting this trend. The emergence of explicit and annual expectations for specialty groups under HMO practice may come quite quickly in large well-run hospitals.

The absence of a well-understood hierarchy for physicians throws all communication with doctors into the collateral organization, contributing to the burdens of a relatively weak part of the organization.

ISSUES IN MIDDLE MANAGEMENT DESIGN

In the formal accountability hierarchy, each responsibility center manager reports to a supercontroller. The levels of supercontrollers between the RC and the executive constitute middle management. The sole function of middle management is to facilitate the effective performance of the RCs. Middle managers are accountable upward for adherence to agreed-upon expectations and downward for resolving issues their subordinates cannot. (That is to say, middle managers have an explicit obligation to respond to their subordinates as well as to their superiors.) They communicate expectations downward and subordinates' views upward. They must ensure that each of their RCs receives the resources it needs and meets the demands for service anticipated in the expectations.

Middle managers also constitute much of the collateral organization. The questions referred to them by the RCs are such that they must communicate across reporting hierarchies as well as within them. Meeting the expectations for the RCs reporting to them will usually be a matter of improving the fit of inputs, outputs, and demands with those of other units. Hospital managers are usually professionally trained people with unique insights into the trends of specific technology. Thus, their views are also important to issues of environmental assessment.

The nature of the responsibility center design suggests the difficulty of the middle manager's role. If each small work unit were ideally designed, with all related tasks within it, no other RC performing similar duties, and no patients presenting unusual problems, middle management would be a small cadre of experts working on planning, budgeting, and recruitment for occasional RCM vacancies. In reality, middle management is a group numbering from a few dozen to a few hundred people attacking the problems arising daily from the RCs. In poorly designed hospitals they are so consumed by these issues that they have no time for planning, budgeting, or recruitment. There is a Catch-22 involved: middle managers are overworked, so there is a temptation to add more middle managers; but the reason middle managers are overworked is that they have many problems of communication and coordination. Adding more middle managers increases the size and complexity of the collateral organization. It simply intensifies the communication problem without necessarily improving productivity or quality.

Effective design of the collateral organization is an ongoing problem. Well-run hospitals have been improving the collateral organization by establishing timetables of repetitive activities, formally reiterating certain common themes and objectives, and specifying the charges and procedures of collateral activities. Well-managed hospitals now commonly rely upon:

- Formal mission statements amplified in sufficient detail to provide guidelines on major interests or directions.
- Long-range plans for services, personnel, and capital requirements amplifying the mission statement and establishing timelines for specific events.
- An annual and multiannual cycle of environmental assessment and revision of the mission and plan.
- Grouping and annual review of specific proposals for capital expenditures and new program requests.
- An annual review of the closed system parameter expectations for each responsibility center (although this review began as a cost-oriented budget, it is spreading to demand, output, efficiency, quality, and resource conservation as a comprehensive and integrated set).

—Recruitment protocols guiding the selection of key individuals.

The current initiative among leading hospitals appears to be strengthening the planning, scheduling, and coordinating of clinical matters by improving the accountability hierarchy within the medical staff. This will transfer much activity from the collateral to the hierarchical organization, over a period of several years. As progress is made, the burdens of the collateral organization can be minimized by such tactics as the following:

- —Developing precise and complete expectations within the accountability hierarchy to clarify coordination needs.
- —Encouraging a variety of specific ad hoc collateral communications, including formal and informal, grouped and individual.
- —Strengthening the medical staff organization and recognizing the interdependence of medicine, nursing, and clinical support services.
- —Supplying information systems and capable staff support to middle management to encourage full analysis of facts and to clarify requirements for collateral discussions.
- —Increasing outcomes-oriented incentives to stimulate flexibility and acceptance of innovative solutions.
- —Using the executive group to focus, coordinate, and set priorities for agendas.

FORMS OF MIDDLE MANAGEMENT STRUCTURE

Middle management structure includes both an accountability hierarchy and a collateral organization, although, because of the complexity, the collateral organization is almost never shown on organization charts. Charts also tend to show single lines of accountability when actually there are more. Three major approaches to the accountability hierarchy have been used: conventional pyramidal organization, matrix organization, and functional organization. Most hospitals are a blend of the three, with the conventional form dominating. Well-run hospitals appear to succeed not so much because they have picked a specific structure as because they identify and correct problems as they arise from the structure they have selected.

The executive office is the only place in the organization that can resolve the problems of middle management design. It has three basic options. First, it may reconsider RC activities. Second, it may devise variations of conventional, matrix, and functional middle management structures. Third, it may develop the system of collateral communication to overcome apparent weaknesses. Sensitivity to these options is a critical part of the executive role. The third option, yet another committee, is too often pursued when the first or the second should be.

Conventional Organization

Hospitals have traditionally emphasized similar skills or professional knowledge in establishing the hierarchy of middle management. The result is an organization like that shown in Figure 12.1.

For many years it was common to indicate the medical staff as a separate and distinct organization. A variety of reporting relationships was used, many of them deliberately ambiguous about how the medical staff, executive office, and governing board shared responsibilities.[4] There was also a tendency to treat the medical staff organization as a parliamentary body representing the wishes of the staff majority rather than responding to the exchange needs of the organization. As noted above, thinking has moved steadily away from this view, and apparently will continue to do so. Although many persons are concerned with the need to protect the physician's independent authority in patient care, there is room for well-planned collective action without endangering, and possibly enhancing, the independent physician's contribution. . . . Figure 12.1 shows a medical staff hierarchy reporting to the administrator directly but otherwise similar to that of nursing or finance. This reflects the modern environment. It is noteworthy that many doctors are now employed as RCMs and middle managers in clinical support organizations. Their obligations in these roles are no different from others'. Issues of quality and appropriateness of care involving the medical staff organization might best be addressed by a variant of the conventional organization, one emphasizing intermediate and final products, as discussed below.

The conventional organization has one great strength and a number of annoying but not disabling weaknesses. Its strength is that many of the hierarchical chains—all of nursing and the clinical support services and financial system, for example—have strong professional content. This allows them to use the professional knowledge, skills, and socialization of personnel to define activities and maintain control over them. Research, education, and innovation tend to follow the same organizational lines. As a result, a new practice can be adopted quickly unless it crosses hierarchical lines. Laws of licensure and standards of practice used in malpractice trials dictate the roles of certain professionals and certain traditional hierarchies.

Conversely, the conventional organization makes each hierarchy responsive to a separate professional organization. Competition some-

FIGURE 12.1

Functional Organization Design

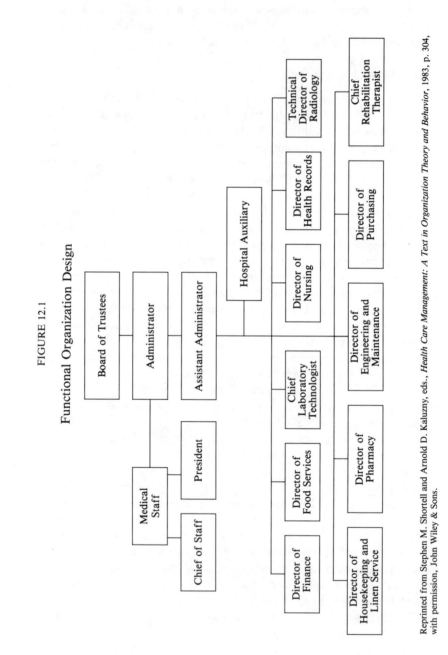

Reprinted from Stephen M. Shortell and Arnold D. Kaluzny, eds., *Health Care Management: A Text in Organization Theory and Behavior*, 1983, p. 304, with permission, John Wiley & Sons.

times develops among professions, and all of them, not just medicine, have a tendency to concern themselves with professional objectives rather than hospital objectives or exchange needs. They all pressure the hospital to give them equal recognition regardless of their relative contributions. This results in many short hierarchies, such as physical therapy or medical records, and a few long and complex ones, such as nursing or laboratory. As a result, some RCMs report directly to the executive office, while others are insulated by several layers of middle management. More important, middle managers on the same level have vastly different hierarchies reporting to them. The tendency of the professions to proliferate, driven by the increasing specialization of science, has increased the weaknesses of the conventional organization. There are more professions, more hierarchies, and more concerns about the weakness of the conventional organization in 1980 than there were in 1960.

Under the conventional model, the hierarchical organization does not enhance collateral communication among the professions. The executive group must continually stimulate the collateral organization. Informal communications among individuals treating the same patient (for example, among a doctor, nurse, pharmacist, and social worker about the care of one patient) tend to die out as the organization becomes larger. Deliberate efforts to support the informal organization often become necessary. The 1980s version of the conventional organization is supplemented by a great variety of collateral committees, task forces, work groups, networks, and affiliations, all aimed at integrating the various hierarchies effectively. Examples include discharge planning committees, ethics committees, operating room committees, planning teams and task forces, budget committees, and recruitment committees. There are usually a number of ad hoc committees and work groups as well.

Extending Accountability to the Medical Staff

In recent years, as the need for quality, economy, and appropriateness of care has increased, a variant on the conventional organization has emerged. This establishes a medical staff hierarchy divided into scientifically oriented specialties as responsibility centers. Each specialty is responsible for the cost and quality of the final product or episode of care. The specialty's accountability lies predominantly in what component services, or intermediate product services, are selected to provide diagnosis and treatment. In effect, the members of the specialty buy the units—tests, drugs, days of care—but have no control over the costs of producing the intermediate services. The intermediate producers, on the other hand, have little or no control over the quantities of services ordered, but can be held responsible for the cost and quality of each unit produced. This approach to organization design tends to continue the traditional separation of medicine from other professions. Difficulties that remain to be dealt with include:

— Defining the final product requires identifying ways in which patients can be meaningfully grouped. Some consensus pattern of care, or patient group protocol . . ., must be developed for each important group.
— Nursing, the largest intermediate service, has substantial control over both costs and quality of the final product. It is unclear how to incorporate the nursing view into patient group protocol.
— The other large, intermediate producers also affect quantities and costs, although to a lesser extent.
— Not all patients fit the scientific structure of medical specialization. Important groups of cancer and heart disease patients are treated by both surgical and nonsurgical specialists, for example.

The scheme also requires sophisticated information processing to measure both intermediate and final product parameters. It has the great virtue of assigning responsibility for cost and quality to medical responsibility centers.

The Matrix Organization

One alternative to the conventional organization is the matrix organization, so called because many RCMs and middle managers have explicit, permanent, dual reporting responsibilities.[5] Figure 12.2 shows such an organization. The matrix organization is difficult to draw in detail because the dual reporting relationships are so complex. From the perspective of the RCM, the existence of the dual responsibility is clear, although its implementation may be obscure. The housekeeping supervisor in the surgical suite, for instance, would report to both the head of the housekeeping department and the supervisor of operating room nurses. The head nurse in intensive care would report both to the supervisor for surgical nursing and to the doctor in charge of intensive care. Matrix organizations around final product protocols have been suggested, presumably with the dominant medical specialty being accountable in some part.[6]

The practical effect of the matrix organization is to emphasize the most important of the collateral relationships by making them permanent and adding them to the conventional reporting relationships. It has intuitive appeal as a description of hospital organization because many

FIGURE 12.2

Matrix Organization Design

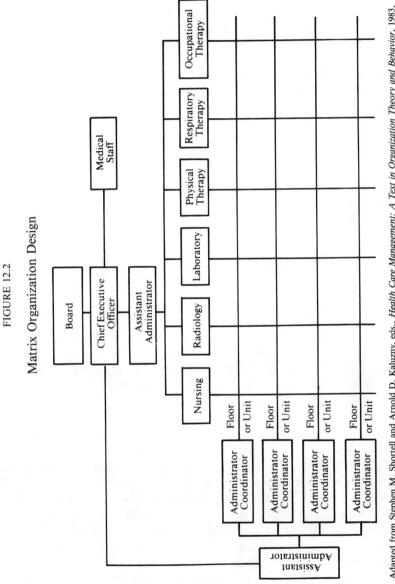

Adapted from Stephen M. Shortell and Arnold D. Kaluzny, eds., *Health Care Management: A Text in Organization Theory and Behavior*, 1983, p. 307, with permission, John Wiley & Sons.

RCMs have a subordinate relationship to another profession in addition to their hierarchical one. As the examples in the preceding paragraph suggest, these relationships are frequently with a clinical organization such as nursing or medicine as well as with the administrative organization shown in the accountability hierarchy. Under the conventional organization, such obligations can be overlooked, even though the result impairs quality of care. Matrix organization makes the most important obligation outside the RCM's own profession or trade explicit.

Despite its initial appeal, the matrix organization has not had widespread success,[7] for two reasons. First, although the communications difficulties of the conventional organization frequently involve several professions or hierarchies, it is impractical to consider more than a dual reporting matrix. Thus, many of the problems of the conventional organization remain. Second, and more serious, the dual reporting structure can easily deteriorate into a competitive relationship among three people, the RCM and his or her two supercontrollers. Three-person relationships are notoriously unstable in general, and those in hospital matrix organizations are exacerbated by conflicts in professional and status relationships (for example, among a head nurse specializing in intensive care, a doctor with the same specialty, and a nursing supervisor whose specialty is surgical nursing).[8]

Functional Organization

Hospitals frequently create separate conventional organizations for various functions, the most common being for all or part of the outpatient service. (Under functional organization, for example, the director of inpatient nursing would have no direct relationship to or responsibility for outpatient nursing.) Functional organization is also useful for geographically separate or largely self-contained units. Among inpatient activities, pediatric, obstetric, psychiatric, and long-term care units are most often considered for functional organization.

The functionally organized unit is frequently organized conventionally within itself. Some such units border on being totally separate organizations, but more commonly, they are partially self-sufficient and rely on collateral communications to receive services from conventionally organized departments. For example, the long-term care unit may have full nursing, housekeeping, and dietary services but rely on the larger organization for all other clinical and plant services.

The main problem of small, functionally organized units is ensuring effective response from their conventionally organized support services. When the functionally organized unit is geographically remote or an infrequent user of the support service, the problem is aggravated. The best known solution is to place the relationship on a quasi-external basis. In the classic case of prewar General Motors, the parts suppliers and car brands were functional divisions that "sold" to each other on an imputed price basis, with each division accountable for a profit from sales.[9] So far, hospitals have not adopted an organization in which component units can "buy" services from each other. The model holds promise, however, as the medical staff hierarchy is strengthened and the final product-intermediate product concept is implemented.

The most common variant of functional organization now in place is the multihospital system. Under for-profit versions of the system, individual hospitals or other provider units tend to be self-contained except for their planning, strategic governance, and finance functions. Not-for-profit multihospital systems have tended to decentralize even the governance function, centralizing only some elements of strategic planning and finance.[10] At present, multihospital systems are best understood as several separate hospital organizations with certain limited functions centralized; however, the trend is clearly toward more centralization.

A new variant of the functional organization has emerged from The Johns Hopkins Hospital, which assigns complete management authority and responsibility to physician chiefs who also chair departments in the medical school [see chapter 14]. This explicitly establishes the hierarchy for medical staff organization on the basis of medical specialty. The prewar General Motors conditions have been reasonably well met: in particular, doctors are responsible for resources — cost, efficiency, and revenue — as well as quality of care. In the constrained revenue situation that exists at Hopkins, they must seek efficiencies and profits to support technological advances and expansions of care. The management team of the hospital argues that their organization has done so more successfully than a conventional organization would have.[11]

The functional organization seems to hold promise for the distant future in community hospitals. There is much to be said for organizing accountability around identifiable groups of patient care needs, but this model, like its predecessors, has inherent difficulties. It is noticeably easier to apply to a medical school hospital, where the hierarchical organization of medicine by specialty already exists, than it would be for a typical community hospital. It requires full-time medical managers, a situation that is outside the tradition of most hospitals and politically demanding. Very few doctors are trained for such a role, either by education or experience. The model also requires a sophisticated cost-finding system to calculate the necessary imputed prices.

MULTIHOSPITAL SYSTEMS

The affiliation of individual hospitals into groups and superorganizations, sometimes called **horizontal integration**, began only 15 years ago, but it has evolved rapidly. It is estimated that 40 percent of all community hospitals had such an affiliation in 1985. The nature of the affiliation ranges from simple contracts for services to elaborate ownership structures involving several corporate layers combining both for-profit and not-for-profit charters. The impact is similarly diverse, but in general, hospitals that are part of even the most centralized system still look much like their independent competitors. They have better resources in governance, finance, training, information systems, and recruitment which they are still learning to exploit but which have already given them significant advantages. The greatest contributions of the multihospital system seem to be in resources rather than in structure.

In general, well-run hospitals and multihospital systems recognize that there are legal, financial, marketing, and organizational dimensions to integration and that it is desirable to address each one separately. Some may be centralized while others are not. Under this philosophy, the organizational questions are driven by management needs rather than by theories.

The most obvious organizational influences of multihospital systems are in the governance function. For-profit hospitals have a trustee or director function, but it is likely to be at the corporate office rather than in the local community. Not-for-profit organizations use their corporate offices to guide local boards; they provide expanded environmental assessment, enhanced financial planning information, and suggestions for procedural questions. Increasingly, they are reserving certain decisions for themselves: final approval of long-range plans, annual budgets, and the selection and compensation of the chief executive officer are often centralized.

The future is likely to bring more centralization: services that can be purchased from the parent company more effectively than they can be provided by the local unit will disappear from local sites. These are likely to be such easily transported services as finance, information systems, human resources, plant maintenance, and laundry. Laboratory service is the obvious candidate among clinical services.

In addition to the integration of hospitals into multihospital systems, outreach to new kinds of services, particularly supporting the aged and the mentally ill, is common, and hospitals are making new, more formal affiliations with their physicians. These expansions, often called **vertical integration**, are supported by joint ventures, partnerships, subsidiary corporate structures, and holding companies, as are the multihospital systems. (Several multihospital systems are involved in both horizontal and vertical integration.) Vertically integrated units are obvious candidates for functional organization.

Many common communication and accountability tasks must be performed in health care delivery. As a result, most health care institutions look like hospitals organizationally. The names of the components often differ more than the functions, and the profile of services offered is far more distinctive than the nature of the hierarchical and collateral structures. This is likely to remain true in more integrated horizontal organizations in the future. There may be many labels and much expedient variation but similar underlying structures. All operating health care units must have a medical staff, a laboratory, and a laundry; even if the function is geographically remote, it must fill local needs for the unit to thrive. In fact, geographic remoteness becomes less and less important with advanced technology. It is organizational remoteness, even in the simplest, smallest health care provider, that is fatal: it signals the failure of accountability for quality, productivity, and patient service. . . .

NOTES

1. George F. Wieland, *Improving Health Care Management: Organization Development and Organization Change* (Ann Arbor, MI: Health Administration Press, 1981); Stephen M. Shortell and Arnold D. Kaluzny, *Health Care Management: A Text in Organization Theory and Behavior* (New York: Wiley, 1983).

2. J.D. Thompson, *Organizations in Action* (New York: McGraw-Hill, 1967).

3. Henry Mintzberg, *The Structuring of Organizations*, (Englewood Cliffs, NJ: Prentice-Hall, 1979), 18–34.

4. E. Johnson, "Revisiting the Wobbly Three-Legged Stool," *Health Care Management Review 4* (Summer 1979): 15–22.

5. Duncan Neuhauser, "The Hospital as a Matrix Organization," *Hospital Administration* 17 (Fall 1972): 8–25.

6. L.F. McMahon, Jr., et al., "Hospital Matrix Management in DRG-Based Prospective Payment," *Hospital & Health Services Administration* 31 (January-February 1986): 62–74.

7. L.R. Burns, Matrix Management in Hospitals: Patterns and Developments, unpublished.

8. L.F. McMahon, Jr., et al., "Hospital Matrix."

9. Alfred P. Sloan, Jr., *My Life With General Motors* (New York: Doubleday, 1972).

10. Sisters of Mercy Health Corporation, *Integrated Governance and Management Process, Conceptual Design* (Farmington Hills, MI: SMHC, 1980).

11. Robert M. Heyssel, et al., "Decentralized Management in a Teaching Hospital," *New England Journal of Medicine* 310 (1984): 1477–80.

| 13 | Vertical Integration and Diversification of Acute Care Hospitals: Conceptual Definitions |

Jan P. Clement

As the reimbursement system and the competitive environment for hospitals have changed, so have the business strategies employed by hospital managers. While horizontal integration was a dominant strategy in the seventies, strategic changes in the service and product mixes of hospitals have recently become dominant. Hospitals are branching out by developing sports medicine clinics, management consulting businesses, freestanding urgent care centers, insurance products, and more. The terms vertical integration and diversification have been used interchangeably to describe these same changes. The confusion in terminology arises because, until recently, these terms have been used in reference to manufacturing firms. It is only lately that they have been applied to service firms.

To facilitate a discussion of the effective management of new investment strategies, the definitions of vertical integration and diversification for hospitals must be clarified. This article will define these terms specifically for nonuniversity acute care hospitals that produce secondary and tertiary care services.[1] Therefore, the definitions presented below differ from those in casual use today. Hospital managers need precise defini-

Reprinted from *Hospital & Health Services Administration* 33 (Spring 1988): 99–110, with permission, Health Administration Press.

tions of vertical integration and diversification to formulate realistic expectations regarding the potential benefits of these strategies and to allocate and manage resources effectively.

VERTICAL INTEGRATION

A vertically integrated firm links the stages of production and distribution of its product into a chain spanning all or part of the distance from ownership and procurement of raw materials to the distribution channels that get the goods or services to the consumer. An outline of the production-distribution chains of vertically integrated housing and automobile manufacturing firms is presented in Figure 13.1.

Harrigan (1985) proposes four dimensions that refine the definition of vertical integration: stages, breadth, degree, and form. "Stages" refers to the number of production stages in which the firm participates. The firms depicted in Figure 13.1 each participate in four stages. Firms integrate backward, or upstream, when they produce raw materials or intermediate products that would otherwise have been purchased from independent suppliers. Forward, or downstream, integration occurs when firms add another stage that moves further toward finishing and distributing products to consumers. "Breadth" describes the number of production processes performed at any stage. For example, the automobile firm

FIGURE 13.1

Examples of Vertically Integrated Firms

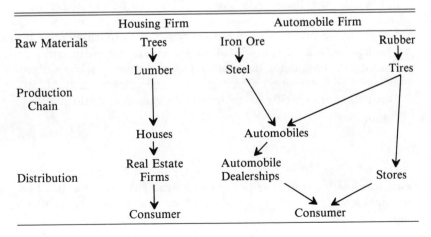

has two processes at the second stage in Figure 13.1 — production of both steel and tires. The "degree" of vertical integration is the proportion of total input or output of required resources transferred to a later in-house production stage.

If, for example, half of the tires needed by the automobile firm are purchased from outside suppliers, the degree of vertical integration at stage 3 in Figure 13.1 is 50 percent. Finally, "form" refers to ownership. It is not necessary for a firm to own each stage of production to be vertically integrated. Both shared ownership and contractual arrangements allow firms to control the production and distribution stages, and consequently, to reap the rewards and incur the losses associated with vertical integration.

The most common definition of vertical integration for acute care hospitals concentrates on the stages dimension. Vertical integration is defined as owning more than one link in a linear chain extending from insurance through ambulatory care, secondary inpatient care, and tertiary care to home health or nursing home services. The pitfalls inherent in this definition of vertical integration will be shown as a more precise definition is presented.

The framework for developing this definition requires answers to the following four questions: (1) who is the ultimate consumer of the hospital's final output, (2) what does the hospital produce, (3) how is the final output produced, and (4) how is the final output distributed to consumers? In the following discussion, each question is examined and its importance in defining vertical integration is shown.

THE CONSUMER

In any market exchange relationship, there must be a producer and a consumer. Hospital outputs are ultimately consumed by patients. Although this seems obvious, the consumer is not explicitly defined in the vertical integration chain listed above. His or her participation in purchasing and consuming the hospital's output is never acknowledged. In the alternative definition of vertical integration developed in this article, the patient is explicitly recognized as the consumer of the hospital's final output.

OUTPUT

The definition of vertical integration requires a reference point with respect to which a firm is vertically integrated. That reference is a final consumable output such as an automobile. The acute care hospital's main businesses, inpatient and outpatient care, are considered to be its final consumable output here. Each consists of a package of services produced when a patient visits the hospital. Since services cannot be held in inventory, each patient, in essence, places a special order for specially tailored services.

Although the patient's demand for the hospital's services is derived from his or her demand for health, the actual output for consumption is the package of services. To assume that hospitals produce health as a final product or even a predictably altered human body is to ignore the critical significance of both the nonstandardized input and the uncertainty inherent in medical care. Heredity, previous morbidities, and comorbidities are among the reasons that the same production process applied to two patients may not produce the same results, or that restoration to health may be impossible. Vertical integration is defined by the hospital's linkage of services into a package, not by its production of health. It is by focusing on the linkages that managers may realize benefits from vertical integration.

PRODUCTION

Previous use of vertical integration with regard to production by acute care hospitals has concentrated on the stages of production (for example, levels of care), and ignored the breadth, degree, and form dimensions. Closer examination of the stages and of Harrigan's other three dimensions, however, clarifies important aspects of vertical integration for acute care hospitals.

Even though the stages of vertical integration have been the focus of previous definitions, there have been two important oversights. First, acute care services are mistakenly pictured in a linear sequential order, and second, some services that actually are arranged linearily, namely ancillary services, are forgotten.

Patient consumption of acute care hospital services is more realistically depicted in Figure 13.2. Three characteristics of that consumption are especially important. First, secondary, tertiary, nursing home, and home care services may either be final stages of production or intermediate links in a sequence of consumption during an episode of illness. In addition, even though a patient may consume all of the hospital's services during his or her lifetime, the time gap between, for instance, secondary care and nursing home care is usually so long that the previous stage is irrelevant for the next. Information collected on the patient's physical characteristics and, perhaps, medical technology, will have changed so much that none of the previously collected information can be forwarded for use in later care. The stages consumed earlier in the lifetime consti-

FIGURE 13.2

Vertical Integration of Hospital Services

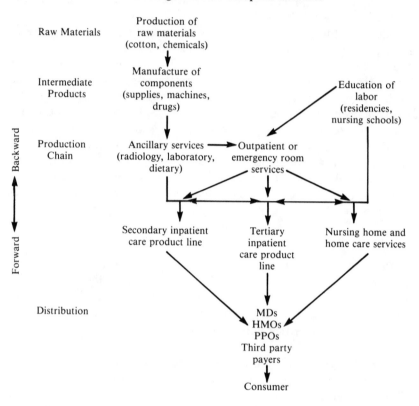

tute final consumption products, not intermediate links in a sequential production chain. Thus, an episode of illness and care is a critical element in defining vertical integration; it is more useful than a lifetime, which is implicitly the time period of reference for the definition noted above.

A second important feature detailed in Figure 13.2 is that patients may return to previous "stages" during an episode of illness. There is no necessary linear procession toward a common final production process. Secondary care may follow tertiary care rather than the other way around.

The third especially noteworthy characteristic depicted in Figure 13.2 is that the patient may skip stages. In a linear sequence, processing at the third stage implies that processing at the first and second stages has also been completed. Although provision of secondary and tertiary services does imply that ancillary and outpatient services have been, or are concurrently being, provided, the same cannot be said with regard to services later in the chain. For example, nursing home care does not imply that secondary services have been provided.

Harrigan's second dimension of vertical integration, breadth, is also useful for defining vertical integration of acute care hospitals. Breadth refers to the number of activities at any stage of production. The number of secondary inpatient care services, such as obstetrics, ophthalmology, and medical-surgical, or the number of different laboratory tests available quantifies the breadth of vertical integration of acute care hospitals.

Harrigan's third dimension is degree, the proportion of total input or output of required resources transferred in house. Information about patients is the critical resource to be transferred when ancillary services are provided or patients consume more than one level of the hospital's services. Since patients do not always follow a linear pattern in their consumption of services progressing to the same stage, degree is an important addition to the definition of vertical integration for acute care hospitals. Potential measures of degree include the proportion of ancillary services purchased from other hospitals or firms and the proportion of patient transfers into the hospital's tertiary care, nursing home, and home health care units from other hospital units. The higher the number of services or patients coming from other organizations, the lower the degree of vertical integration of the hospital.

Finally, ownership need not be complete for a hospital to be vertically integrated. Vertical relationships may exist when the hospital has only partial ownership in a joint venture. In addition, according to Harrigan, vertical control may be exercised through contracts, for example, when several nursing home beds are reserved for the hospital's patients.

DISTRIBUTION

The final weakness of the previous definition of vertical integration for hospitals is that the process of distribution of the hospital's services to consumers is ignored. Exchange between hospitals and patients is intermediated by both physicians and third party payers (Figure 13.2).

Physicians distribute the hospital's services to patients through their determination of testing, and length of hospitalization, among other variables. Hospitals have been called doctors' workshops because, although most are usually not directly employed by hospitals, doctors are influential in a number of managerial investment and production decisions.

Distribution of the hospital's services and products is also performed by third party payers that sell contingent claims contracts to potential consumers. They lower the out-of-pocket cost to consumers for the use of hospital services, making more consumers able to order services. Contracts with health maintenance organizations (HMOs) and preferred provider organizations (PPOs) are more specific; they are means of ensuring that the patients will choose that particular hospital's services.

MANAGEMENT PERSPECTIVE

The definition of vertical integration presented above may assist managers of acute care hospitals in realizing the benefits of vertical integration. Because an extensive discussion is beyond the scope of this article, the illustrations are brief and limited to cost-minimization benefits. The costs minimized may take the form of production or transaction costs, such as the costs of gathering information, contract negotiation, and contract enforcement (Williamson 1975). Such costs should be lowered when the number of stages of production is high, and the degree is high.

As the number of stages of production controlled by the hospital increases, production and transaction costs during an episode of illness can be expected to decline. When the hospital is able to satisfy all of the patient's consumption needs during an episode of illness, market transactions between successive stages of that patient's consumption of services are eliminated. For example, when a patient is transferred from secondary to nursing home services in house, referral contracts with nursing homes do not have to be written or monitored. In addition, information needed to produce patient care does not have to be regathered, nor do diagnostic tests have to be repeated. Managers, however, must not assume that simply adding stages will necessarily minimize costs. Both production and transaction costs should be lower when the time interval between consumption of various services is short, as in the episode of illness model of vertical integration. The actual length of the production chain depends upon the flow of patients during episodes of care rather than the list of all possible hospital services.

Cost savings are also more likely when most of the input to later production stages comes directly from earlier stages controlled by the hospital. That degree may be important for cost reduction can be seen with both ancillary service and nursing home examples. As more ancillary services are provided to patients in house, the hospital's costs should fall because there are no transportation or contracting costs incurred in transferring the results from an external supplier. When most of the patients for the hospital's nursing home unit are transferred from its other service units, contract negotiation, marketing, and information-gathering costs are lowered. This is not true when most of them are admitted from an external hospital or clinic. Therefore, it is important to identify the degree of vertical integration as well as the number of stages.

As is shown by these brief examples, conclusions concerning the cost-minimization effects of vertical integration drawn only from examination of the purported linear production stages of medical care may be inaccurate. To realize cost-minimization benefits from vertical integration, managers must evaluate the actual production chain and the degree of vertical integration.

DIVERSIFICATION

The focus of vertical integration is on relationships among components of the production process for a particular final consumable output of the hospital. In contrast, diversification refers to the relationship among two or more final consumable outputs. Specifically, diversification refers to producing outputs that cannot be substituted for each other at any stage of production, unlike a visit to an emergency room that may be substituted for a visit to a physician's office. Nor are the outputs part of the package of inpatient or outpatient care services; they are not complements for a part of the package. Thus, when a hospital adds another inpatient care service, it expands the breadth of production or lengthens the production chain of one product but does not diversify.

When a firm does diversify, it must acquire new assets and develop new skills to deal with one or more of three important types of diversity: production technology, consumer group, and consumer function.[2] The latter two can occur when new markets are entered. For example, if an automobile firm diversifies into housing production, the firm must develop or manage a different production technology and market the additional final output to different consumer groups for a different function. Although diversification in production technology is frequently recognized, the two types of market diversification are often ignored.

It is quite clear that some recently adopted hospital services differ in technology from those services we typically associate with inpatient hospital care. For example, wellness centers, health clubs, and some occupational health services promote health rather than diagnose and treat illness. In contrast, managing the production technology of data processing services sold to other businesses should not require new production skills or assets. Although these services are used in house to support the production of patient care services, when sold to other businesses they are final consumable outputs distinct from patient care services.

Personnel of diversifying hospitals may also have to develop competence in different skills or acquire assets to serve new consumer groups. Consumers of health promotion services have different needs, payment mechanisms, and decision criteria than do patients. Similarly, businesses in the market for data processing services constitute a new consumer group. It is important to recognize that these consumer groups may have to be courted more than patients because there is usually more market competition among providers of these other services.

Finally, managers have to expand their expertise to deal with new consumer functions. Hospital managers familiar with managing inpatient medical care may not be as knowledgeable about consumer demands, assets, or operational cash flows needed for health promotion services or real estate operations. Likewise, when a customer for data processing services requests support for in-service education programs, a new consumer function is served that requires new skills and assets.

These three types of diversity introduced by corporate diversification provide a convenient and meaningful means of identifying related and unrelated diversification. A firm's diversification is related when its new products employ production technologies similar to those already used, or the firm serves markets similar to those already served. As a result, assets and skills may be transferred from managing the firm's current products and markets to the diversifying products and markets. Unrelated diversification, on the other hand, involves use of dissimilar assets and skills because of dissimilar production technologies, consumer groups, or consumer functions.

When one or two, but not all three, types of diversity are introduced, the diversification can be related, because firms can draw upon some of their existing production or market-specific management skills in managing the diversification. However, when all three types of diversity are present, far less knowledge and fewer skills and assets are directly transferable to the new situation. Only the most general skills are transferable; thus, diversification is unrelated.

A classification of several hospital products according to whether they diversify the hospital and whether that diversification is related or unrelated is presented in Table 13.1. The acute care hospital's initial product consists of outpatient and secondary or tertiary medical care services provided to ill people seeking care. These customers are usually covered by a third party payer.

Simply offering new secondary or tertiary medical care services does not constitute diversification. In addition to not being a separate prod-

TABLE 13.1

Related and Unrelated Diversification of Acute Care Hospitals

Service or Product	Production Technology	Consumer Groups	Consumer Functions	
Burn center				
CCU				
Nursing home				Not diversification
Birthing center				
Sports medicine				
Hospice				
Mental health	X			
Home health care	X			
Services sold to other businesses:				
Laundry		X		Related diversification
Management		X	#	
Data processing		X	#	
Dietary		X		
School health		X	#	
Occupational health		X	#	
Stress management	X	X	X	
Wellness	X	X	X	Unrelated diversification
Real estate management	X	X	X	
Education materials development	X	X	X	

X = Source of diversity.
# = Potential source of diversity.

uct, the production technology required is only incrementally different from the technology required to provide most secondary or tertiary inpatient care; consumer groups and functions remain the same.

Mental health services, on the other hand, require a unique technology (Table 13.1). Although patients are diagnosed and treated, as are other inpatients and outpatients, the treatment is significantly different than the treatment provided to medical or surgical patients. But the consumer group is composed of ill people, many of whom are covered by third party payers. Because some production skills can be transferred, this diversification is said to be related.

Services that are already performed in house to support inpatient care services, such as laundry, dietary, data processing, and management services, may be sold to other businesses. Although the technology to provide these services is already in place, the hospital is diversified because it produces a different final product serving a new customer group — other businesses. These services may also serve a different consumer function.

Finally, some services incorporate each of the three types of diversity. Educational materials development is characterized by a different production technology and a new customer group (other hospitals or educational institutions) and serves a different consumer function (education) than inpatient care services. To offer stress management and wellness programs, hospital personnel must acquire the skills and assets to use new production technologies, attract new consumer groups, and serve new consumer functions. Although they may be able to transfer some general skills in managing these services, because of the distinctive characteristics of the services, managers must develop substantially new skills. Thus, this type of diversification is unrelated.

MANAGEMENT PERSPECTIVE

As with vertical integration, precise definition of diversification is especially useful to managers for minimizing costs. Costs may be minimized if inputs can be shared in the production of two or more products. Such sharing is more likely with related than unrelated diversification. The three types of diversity help managers to identify the production and marketing resources that can be shared.

Another potential motive for unrelated diversification may be to avoid business cycles. Since related businesses or products rely on the same consumer groups, or consumer functions, downturns of demand for one output are likely to be correlated with downturns for those that are market related. Such corresponding cycles are less likely for unrelated diversified firms.

A more precise definition of diversification can help managers choose the investment projects that are appropriate for their goals. Moreover, after the initial investment decision has been made, managers may be more cognizant of the special management needs of the projects.

Conclusion

The definitions of vertical integration and diversification developed in this article for acute care hospitals concentrate on the distinguishing features of these types of investment. An important distinction between vertical integration and diversification is focus. While the focus of vertical integration is on the relationships among components of the production process, the focus of diversification is on the relationships among final consumable outputs. Diversification requires different skills and assets to manage the diversity of production technologies, consumer groups, or consumer functions as required by several different final outputs.

Careful definition of vertical integration and diversification is a necessary precursor not only to clear communication, but also to sound management. Examples of how these definitions may be useful for managers have been presented. Ultimately though, empirical research is crucial for determining the usefulness of these definitions and, indeed, of these investment strategies.

ACKNOWLEDGMENTS

Valuable comments on an earlier draft were received from Thomas D'Aunno, John R.C. Wheeler, James Suver, Vivian Valdmanis, and Doug Conrad. Any remaining omissions or errors are the responsibility of the author.

NOTES

1.   University hospitals are excluded because they produce research in addition to inpatient medical care services.

2.   Abell uses these descriptors in a different context. See Abell, D.F., *Defining the Business: The Starting Point of Strategic Planning*. Englewood Cliffs, NJ: Prentice-Hall, Inc., 1980.

REFERENCES

Harrigan, K.R. "Vertical Integration and Corporate Strategy." *Academy of Management Journal* 28 (June 1985): 397–425.

Williamson, O.E. *Markets and Hierarchies: Analysis and Antitrust Implications.* New York: The Free Press, 1975.

14 | Decentralized Management in a Teaching Hospital

Robert M. Heyssel
J. Richard Gainter
Irvin W. Kues
Ann A. Jones
Steven H. Lipstein

For more than a decade American hospitals have been asked to contain costs. The most recent program is the Medicare prospective payment system, which reimburses hospitals a fixed price per case based on diagnosis-related groupings (DRGs). If this approach proves successful, it may be adopted by other payers and perhaps extended to the reimbursement of physicians through prospective professional fees.

Hospital reaction to the new payment scheme varies. Some look for cost controls and more efficient management techniques to reduce expenses; others carefully analyze their mix of DRGs to measure which are profitable and which involve unusual and expensive services. The less-profitable services are typically provided by teaching hospitals — institutions that are already a subject of concern because of their high costs and dependence on shrinking public dollars.[1-4]

To survive, teaching hospitals must look to innovative approaches in both medical care and management practice. Medical practices must aim at reducing lengths of hospitalization by performing a higher proportion of the necessary diagnostic tests and therapeutic procedures in outpatient settings. Changes in management practices should encourage physician involvement; most of the costs associated with hospital care result from

Reprinted from *The New England Journal of Medicine* 310, no. 22 (1984): 1477–80, with permission, Massachusetts Medical Society.

physician decisions. Given the traditional hospital organizational structure, with central supervision of costs but little control over decisions that affect them, a new management approach is in order. For ten years Johns Hopkins Hospital has operated with a management structure designed to control expenditures by placing responsibility for costs in the hands of physicians. In this article we briefly summarize that experience.

THE JOHNS HOPKINS EXPERIENCE

BACKGROUND

Johns Hopkins Hospital opened in 1889 with 330 beds, 25 physicians, 200 employees, and an annual operating budget of about $85,000. The central administration was small. Services related to medicine, nursing, and support functions were each headed by an administrative director.

Over the years the hospital grew in size and complexity. By 1972 Hopkins had 1000 beds, 1300 physicians, 4100 employees, and an annual operating budget of $58 million. The size and titles of the administrative staff had changed, but its organization was basically unaltered. Medical services still reported to a vice-president for medical affairs, nursing and support services to a vice president for administration, and accounting and budgeting to the treasurer. Although clinical departments controlled staff appointments, beds, and diagnostic and therapeutic services, they had minimal involvement in budget preparation and limited accountability for financial performance. Expenses originated in the units but were the responsibility of central administration.

To address problems of cost control and accountability, Hopkins adopted a decentralized management system frequently used in industry.[5] This system required more extensive financial and management information and, for the first time, involved physicians in management decisions.

DECENTRALIZED MANAGEMENT

With the introduction of decentralized management in 1973, Hopkins shifted operating responsibilities and financial accountability to the clinical departments. Under this structure the larger hospital in effect became a holding company for a series of specialty hospitals referred to as functional units. The organizational design shown in Figure 14.1 reflects the status of each department as an operating unit reporting to the president of the hospital. Although the direct reporting line of the functional-unit directors to the president is unambiguous, the structure allows most

FIGURE 14.1

Organizational Design at Johns Hopkins Hospital

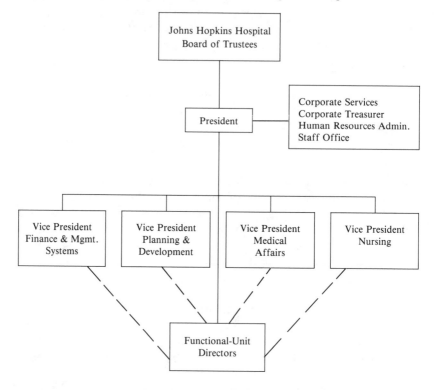

The functional units include anesthesiology and critical-care medicine, gynecology and obstetrics, laboratory medicine, medicine, neurology, oncology, ophthalmology, pathology, pediatrics, psychiatry, radiology, and surgical sciences.

decisions to be made at the level of the functional-unit director and vice presidents, or vice presidents in their areas. Regular meetings occur between the corporate officers and functional-unit directors to ensure a broad understanding of policies and decisions and to provide a routine forum for discussion.

As structured, each functional unit is headed by a physician chief who is also the chairman of that department in the school of medicine. Reporting directly to each chief are a nursing director and an administrator. These three function as a management team and are accountable for all direct costs associated with the operation of the unit, including services acquired from other departments, such as laboratory medicine and radiology. Costs that pertain to the operation of the institution as a whole—e.g., central personnel administration, security, accounting, billing, and insurance—are allocated to the functional unit. Each unit may use services such as housekeeping, dietary, and maintenance from central hospital departments, but the unit may also switch to other providers if services of equal quality can be purchased at a lower price. Although outside-purchase options are seldom exercised, competitive pressure requires the hospital to provide good, affordable central services.

Each functional unit must operate within the general policies of the hospital relating to overall institutional goals, capital-resource allocation, personnel policies, and rate setting. Capital allocation is reviewed by a joint committee of central and functional-unit management. Salary guidelines are established centrally to ensure uniformity and parity within the institution. Financial data and data on use of services are maintained in central files and made available to units for budgeting and volume projections. As the units have gained more experience, they have developed individual data sets pertaining to their own use of services and patterns of physician practice. These data are invaluable in the analysis of use and planning for new services.

Ten years of decentralized management at Johns Hopkins have had two major sets of consequences. The first is measured by financial performance. The second is less objective and pertains to the role of physicians who double as managers of institutional resources.

FINANCIAL CONSEQUENCES

Before 1972, more than 80 per cent of the hospital's costs were allocated by central administration. By fiscal year 1983 the allocation pattern was reversed. Clinical departments directly controlled 51 per cent of their expenses, with departmental use (or purchase) of ancillary services such as laboratory tests and radiology accounting for an additional 20 per cent. Overhead expenses and institutional costs amounted to 22 per cent and 7 per cent, respectively.

Trends in unit costs have been used to measure the impact of physician management. Allowing several years for implementation of the decentralized system, the eight-year period from fiscal year 1976 through 1983 shows that the compound growth rate of unit costs at Hopkins was 10.5 per cent—slightly less than the 11 per cent growth rate for all Maryland hospitals and considerably less than the national growth rate of 14.1 per cent. The 10.5 per cent rate represents stable costs if inflation and patient-care volume are held constant. Furthermore, within the rate-setting guidelines of the Maryland Health Services Cost Review Commission, the hospital has been able to retain a positive operating balance in each of the years since 1976. This includes the past seven years, in which there have been the added capital expenses of a complete rebuilding program.

While holding unit-cost increases below state and national averages, Hopkins has continued to grow in terms of overall budget and the ability to support new programs, technologic advances, and new buildings, including a regional oncology center. Table 14.1 shows the eight-year cost trends. Base-year costs are adjusted each year for inflation, changes in patient care volume, depreciation, interest on new buildings, cost improvement (productivity increases), new programs, and operating requirements. The new-programs/operational-requirements line shows that an average of 3.9 per cent of base-year dollars are used annually to support new applications of medical science and technology. These include noninvasive diagnostic procedures, advanced radiographic-imaging techniques, automated laboratory testing, and additional patient-care and family-care services.

MANAGEMENT FACTORS

Decentralized management is not easily implemented in an environment that has traditionally been centralized. The key factors essential to successful implementation are the willingness of corporate officers to delegate decision-making authority to functional-unit management; the assumption of responsibility by the functional-unit directors (physicians who are chiefs of services) for their units; the acceptance and support of the professional nursing staff; the development of management and financial information systems to support decentralization; and the development of effective communication between the central administration and the decentralized functional units and within central and functional areas.

The transfer of responsibility must be accompanied by the authority to make decisions. Hopkins' management and trustees were willing to delegate the necessary authority to decentralized management even though the chiefs of services were generally considered to have primary commitments to the academic pursuits of teaching and research. The intent was to strengthen the chiefs' management skills, as well as to make departmental administration a primary activity. Physician involvement in management decisions, policy direction, day-to-day operations, and hospital economics became the norm rather than the exception. In transferring responsibility, the central administration had to redefine its own

TABLE 14.1

Eight-Year Cost Trends (Actual) at the Johns Hopkins Hospital, Fiscal Years 1976–1983*

	1976		1977		1978		1979		1980		1981		1982		1983	
	$	%	$	%	$	%	$	%	$	%	$	%	$	%	$	%
Base costs in previous years	73,238	—	84,730	—	93,933	—	101,915	—	110,937	—	125,920	—	136,025	—	154,960	—
Inflation-factor cost	5,559	7.6	5,151	6.1	6,363	6.8	6,802	6.7	9,696	8.7	10,908	8.7	12,075	8.9	10,281	6.6
Volume (internal)	1,353	1.8	(27)	(0.0)	78	0.1	980	1.0	1,186	1.1	(2,019)	(1.6)	(634)	(0.5)	3,719	2.4
New programs/ buildings	172	0.2	458	0.5	2,221	2.4	748	0.7	2,874	2.6	156	0.1	835	0.6	1,427	0.9
New programs/ operational requirements	4,911	6.7	5,610	6.6	1,455	1.5	1,302	1.3	3,020	1.3	3,030	2.4	7,644	5.6	7,094	4.6
Cost improvements†	(503)	(0.7)	(1,989)	(2.3)	(2,135)	(2.3)	(810)	(0.8)	(1,793)	(1.6)	(1,970)	(1.6)	(981)	(0.7)	(1,244)	(0.8)
Total costs	84,730	—	93,933	—	101,915	—	110,937	—	125,920	—	136,025	—	154,964	—	176,241	—
Net new programs/ cost improvement†	4,408	6.0	3,621	4.3	(680)	(0.7)	492	0.5	1,227	1.1	1,060	0.8	6,663	4.9	5,850	3.8

*For actual dollar values, add three zeroes to each amount.
†Parentheses indicate negative values.

role. The new role focused on policy development and monitoring functional-unit performance rather than on control through administrators reporting directly to the central administration.

The second key factor is the assumption of responsibility by the unit directors. Although physicians frequently think that hospital administrators are not responsive to their needs and that decisions are not made in a timely manner, they shy away from direct involvement. Although involvement of physicians in management could clarify and expedite the decision-making process, the necessary commitment of time would be in addition to the time required by the traditional responsibilities of the academic physician. To provide needed management support, nonphysician administrators were added to the unit management teams. Nursing directors also assumed increased departmental responsibilities for staffing and budgeting. In addition, each functional unit now has a financial manager and support staff. This team provides financial expertise for both the hospital and the school of medicine, alleviating the need for large central departments.

The effect of this kind of management can be seen in the department of surgery, where the surgeon-in-chief, the administrator, and the unit director of nursing jointly manage what is in effect a 250-bed hospital with an annual operating budget in excess of $20 million. When responsibility for the school of medicine's budget is added, the total operating budget approaches $40 million, with supervisory responsibility for 1,000 employees. The team concept has made it possible to assume this kind of responsibility and has resulted in a management organization that is more accessible than a central bureaucracy.

The third major issue, decentralization of nursing, is potentially the most difficult. Some of the opponents of decentralizing management in large hospitals have been nurses in local and national leadership positions. They may have mistaken perceptions of what decentralization both implies and accomplishes for nursing. Organized nursing seems to believe that it must have absolute control of a centralized budget to protect the position of nursing in the hospital hierarchy and to maintain the professional identity of nurses. Concern has also been expressed about the idea of nurses working for and reporting to physicians.

The professional role of nurses at Hopkins is in fact strengthened under decentralization. The role of nurses in patient care is no more changed in the sense of nursing functions than the role of physicians is changed in terms of direct medical care of patients. The focus is on strengthening nursing management at all levels within the organization. As strong managers placed in a collegial forum among administrators and physician chiefs of services, nursing directors are better positioned to promote the professional practice of nursing. To those who argue that nurses cannot be professionally accountable to physicians since doctors know little about professional nursing, the Hopkins experience is most revealing. The decentralized system has attracted competent nurse-managers who can advocate the role of nursing to administrators and functional-unit directors. They are capable of managing large numbers of people, budgeting resources appropriately, developing strong head-nurse leaders, and evaluating the capability of nurses for promotion. The outcome has been joint decision making in the best interest of the entire functional unit.

Recruitment of directors of nursing is carried out by the vice-president for nursing. The chief of service and the administrator in the functional unit make the final selection from among the group of candidates recommended by central nursing. The major functions of the vice-president for nursing include setting nursing-care standards, reviewing nursing practice, directing the total nurse-recruitment program, and along with other senior central-management officials, reviewing and approving the budgets and plans of the units. The vice-president is also responsible for overseeing the management of in-service and continuing-education programs. Finally, and most important, the vice president for nursing provides institutional leadership for professional nursing by participating in all key central decision making and by setting the tone for nursing practice throughout the hospital.

The fourth issue concerns the provision of meaningful management information to facilitate operational decisions at the level of the functional unit. Information systems in hospitals have traditionally been focused on cost finding to meet the reporting requirements of Medicare, Medicaid, and Blue Cross. Although necessary for effective management, systems to monitor performance have not been widely developed. Through decentralization Hopkins has developed a series of reports that recognize each functional unit as an independent operation. Units receive detailed statements of direct income and expense and reports on resource use, including productive nursing hours and ancillary consumption. On a quarterly basis, units are given case-mix data with indicators of performance, such as total charges and length of stay by DRG. A fully allocated profit-and-loss statement is prepared to determine how each service performs as an independent financial and operating entity. Building these information systems has been time-consuming and expensive and has required a major commitment from central management. However, the information generated is critical to the success of the decentralized approach.

The final issue is communication. At Hopkins communication

revolves around a highly structured planning, budgeting, and monitoring process. Each fall central administration circulates budgeting guidelines and timetables, asking each functional unit to develop goals for the next year within the constraints of the economic climate. The units then prepare their budgets for a subsequent detailed review, based on projections of occupancy, use of services, staffing, and cost inflation. Units are also asked to prepare five-year plans (updated annually) and to review any proposed new programs, other additions to their expense base, and plans for cost reduction. Budget meetings between representatives from central management and the functional-unit management team result in an annual operating plan, presented to the board of trustees each May. The units receive monthly and quarterly reports of operations, based on performance measures against the operating plan. These reports are discussed with the units and in the professional groups of the hospital, such as the medical board. The meetings of the board of trustees are open to all functional-unit directors, allowing them to interact directly with the trustees and central management.

The development of management-information systems has lessened but not eliminated the problems in communication between central administration and the functional units. Gaps in understanding result from a lack of coordinated effort among corporate officers (e.g., officers of finance, planning, and medical affairs) and between central and functional-unit managers. Regular communications, as well as ad hoc problem-solving meetings, are essential.

DISCUSSION

The decentralized management system at Hopkins has been effective in involving physicians in budgeting and budget management. The process is now moving forward to allow decentralization of both revenue and expense budgeting. The intent is to have the process evolve in a manner conducive to budgeting both revenues and expenses by case or DRG. Positive operating results achieved through control of expenses, case-mix adjustments, and reduced levels of unnecessary care will then be translated into support for clinical programs, new technologic procedures, and higher-quality patient care.

This approach recognizes that decisions to bring patients into the hospital, to prescribe courses of diagnosis and treatment, and to discharge patients generate the majority of hospital expenses. Decentralized management gives the institutional responsibility for these decisions to those who make them — the physicians. Management strategies aimed at reducing lengths of stay and controlling the use of ancillary services are then more likely to be successful because they are directed by physician-managers who can influence the behavior of their colleagues.

REFERENCES

1.   Rogers DE, Blendon RJ. The academic medical center: a stressed American institution. N Engl J Med 1979; 298: 940–50.

2.   Lewis IJ, Sheps CG. The sick citadel: the American academic medical center and the public interest. Cambridge, Mass.: Oelgeschlager, Gunn & Hain, 1983.

3.   Goldsmith J. The health care market: can hospitals survive? Harv Bus Rev 1980; 58(5): 100–12.

4.   Relman AS. The new medical-industrial complex. N Engl J Med 1980; 303: 963–70.

5.   Drucker PW. Management tasks, responsibilities, and practices. New York: Harper and Row, 1973.

15

Technical and Structural Support Systems and Nurse Utilization: Systems Model

Ramesh K. Shukla

Nurse utilization, the percentage of nurses' time devoted to direct patient care, has been the subject of research since the 1940s, when there was an acute shortage of nurses. In the last two decades, hospital administrators have adopted a variety of strategies to improve utilization of registered nurses. For example, some administrators have implemented a unit dose medication distribution system to reduce nurses' involvement in medication procurement and distribution. Material supplies and linen distribution systems have been improved to reduce nurses' time performing indirect care tasks. Implementation of unit management systems has reduced nurses' time performing clerical and managerial duties. The design and construction of hospitals and/or nursing units has reduced time walking and performing nonproductive tasks. Computerized communication systems have facilitated tracing and using information. The recently devised primary nursing care system has reduced registered nurses' time coordinating care compared with the time required by a team of nursing personnel.

These strategies were expected to increase the efficiency of nurses' time for providing more professional and direct care. The results of one controlled study, however, indicate that changing the structure of nursing

Reprinted from *Inquiry* 20 (Winter 1983): 381–89, with permission, Blue Cross and Blue Shield Association.

care from a team to an all-RN model of primary nursing in fact reduces the efficient utilization of nurses.[1] Another study of an all-RN model of primary nursing indicates an improvement in the utilization of nurses for direct patient care of about 6%.[2] Improving distribution and communication systems also has been shown to increase the amount of time registered nurses spend providing direct care to patients, from 12% to 35% of their time.[3]

Inconsistencies in the evaluation of primary nursing care and large variations in the results of improving distribution and communication systems can be systematically explored by analyzing the relationships between the structural and the technical dimensions of nursing support systems. A framework for such an analysis is presented herein. Four controlled nurse utilization studies are analyzed to show that reduced utilization of primary nurses in one hospital was primarily the result of inefficiencies in the distribution and communication systems.

It is strongly suggested that hospitals that are considering implementation of an all-RN model of primary nursing should ensure that their support systems will maximize the utilization and effectiveness of their RNs. When distribution and communication systems cannot be improved because of economic or physical constraints, it is suggested that modified forms of primary nursing that utilize aides or LPNs to perform routine tasks can buffer RNs from the inefficiencies of distribution, transportation, and communication functions.

NURSING SUPPORT SYSTEMS

Nursing support systems can be conceptualized as having two major subsystems: technical and structural. The definitions of the technical and the structural support systems, and their impact on nurse utilization, are reviewed next.

TECHNICAL SUPPORT SYSTEMS

Technical support systems (TSSs) are the physical subsystems designed to facilitate nurses' ability to deliver direct patient care. The higher the efficiency of the TSS, the less time nurses must spend performing indirect care and nonprofessional tasks. There are several factors that affect the degree of support nurses receive from the TSS. These factors can be grouped into two subsystems: 1) the distribution system and 2) the communication system.

Distribution System

Distribution systems on nursing units ensure the appropriate distribution of medications from pharmacy to patients, linen from laundry to patient rooms, and supplies from central supply to patients and staff on the units. Many studies have reported on the implementation of various types of improved distribution and storage systems. One of the most common medication distribution systems implemented is the unit dose system.[4] Several studies have determined that registered nurses' time per patient is saved with this system.[5]

A more comprehensive approach to distribution systems was developed in the early 1960s by a hospital architectural consultant, Gordon Friesen. Specializing in hospital design, Friesen developed many innovative storage, distribution, and communication systems with the goal of increasing efficiency and decreasing costs of operation through automation[6] and innovation in hospital design.[7] Friesen argued that different distribution systems (medication, linen, and supplies) within a hospital must be consistent in method and procedure to increase simplicity and rationality, which in turn will provide maximum distribution effectiveness.

The Friesen nursing unit differed from the conventional unit in a number of ways. The storage of general supplies, medications, and patient charts were decentralized and placed within the patients' immediate environment by the use of a "nurserver." The nurserver is a structural innovation consisting of a pass-through double-door cabinet that allows access from both inside and outside the patient's room. Supply technicians are responsible for the processing and distribution of supplies to the individual nurservers on the unit. The Friesen distribution system was comparatively evaluated with a traditional distribution system in a hospital.[8] It was shown that the time nurses spent in patients' rooms increased by 12% to 19% under the Friesen system. Since then researchers have done similar studies and have found significant increases in the utilization of nurses with the Friesen distribution system.[9]

The underlying premise of the Friesen system and its modified forms is that the indirect care activities of obtaining medications and supplies can be performed by nonnursing personnel to increase the direct patient care functions of registered nurses. That is, the indirect care functions become relatively independent of the direct-care functions under Friesen-type distribution systems with the delegation of indirect-care functions to nonnursing personnel.

Distribution systems can be conceptualized on a continuum between centralized systems and decentralized systems. In centralized systems medications, linen, and supplies are kept in a centrally located place on the nursing unit and the nurses obtain them when needed, whereas in decentralized systems medications, linen, and supplies are distributed directly to patient rooms by nonnursing personnel for use by nurses in given direct care. Most systems today fall in between the two extremes of the continuum. Some hospitals have partially decentralized the unit dose medication distribution system and the centralized material supply system. From the previously cited studies,[10] one can make the proposition that the greater the decentralization of distribution support functions, the greater will be the delegation of indirect care tasks to nonnursing personnel and thus the greater will be the utilization of registered nurses in providing direct care to patients.

Communication Systems

Communication systems can be viewed as having an intraunit function and an interdepartmental function. Friesen argued that patient charts, which represent a source of communication among the care providers within a unit, should be kept in patient rooms rather than centrally at a nursing station. Under decentralized communication systems, charts are kept in patient rooms and there is no traditional nursing station. Information on a patient—his or her assessments, plan of care, and nursing notes—are available to nurses in the patient's rooms, and communication among hospital personnel occurs closer to the source of the information.

In the Friesen-type design, the efficiency of communication and nurse utilization is improved by replacing the traditional nursing station with an administrative communication center (ACC). The ACC is staffed with nonnursing personnel who coordinate both intra- and interunit communications. Paging systems, nurse finders, and computer-assisted communication centers improve the communication efficiency on these nursing units. More recently, the use of computers for interdepartmental communication within a hospital has also shown promise in improving the utilization of nursing staff.[11]

It should be noted that decentralizing patient charts to patient rooms is an effective method of improving intraunit professional communication only if this decentralization is supported by a highly technical and centralized ACC. The link between the ACC and the charts is the physicians and nurses who make the flow of information feasible. With advancements in communication and computer technology, it may one day be economically feasible to have decentralized computer terminals in patient rooms.

For the purpose of this paper, a communication system is considered decentralized when charts are kept in patients' rooms and communication between nurses and the ACC is feasible through a nurse-finder system or a wireless radio receiver system. A communication system is considered centralized when there is a nursing station with charts and an interdepartmental communication system. The interdepartmental communication system generally consists of telephones and a pneumatic tube system or a manual messenger service system.

STRUCTURAL SUPPORT SYSTEMS

The function of structural support systems on nursing units is to organize the activities of nursing care into a systematic, workable assignment pattern for the staff. Nursing delivery structures have evolved greatly since the advent of the case method and the functional assignment method that were prevalent in the early 20th century. In the last 30 years, team nursing and, more recently, primary nursing care structures have improved the utilization of nurses.

Team Nursing

In the early 1950s team nursing was suggested as a way to fully utilize the various skill levels of nursing personnel, in response to the increased complexity of medical care and the shortage of professional nurses. With the proliferation of various therapists, dietitians, and other health personnel, the professional nurse took on the role of coordinator of this group of care providers. Team nursing would allow a variety of professionals and nonprofessionals to contribute to patient care and would maximize the use of nursing staff skills to provide cost effective nursing care.[12] The literature cites the advantages of team nursing over functional nursing, including the increased availability of professional nursing staff skills to a larger number of patients,[13] greater continuity of care,[14] continuous supervision of care provided by other team members,[15] greater interaction between nurses and patients,[16] maximum use of skill levels,[17] and reduction in time spent by professional staff performing nonprofessional tasks.[18]

A typical team nursing unit consisted of two RNs, an LPN, and an aide, who provided care to a group of 20–25 patients. The role of the team leader included the participative planning of nursing care, delegation of specific tasks to team members, provision of professional care, and the supervision, coordination, and evaluation of care provided by the team members.

Primary Nursing

Primary nursing is a relatively recent phenomenon in nursing in which a specific nurse, called a primary nurse, is assigned to each patient on the unit. The primary nurse is given full responsibility and accountability for the assessment, planning, delivery, and evaluation of nursing care given to her or his patients. The primary nurse remains the patient's nurse throughout the patient's hospitalization on a 24-hour basis. Primary nursing is clearly an emulation of the medical model. Responsibility for care is sometimes delegated to an associate primary nurse, who carries out the primary nurse's patient care plan during the primary nurse's off times. Essential to primary nursing is the acceptance of nursing as a profession and the recognition of the professional nurse as a care giver accountable for her or his actions. In an ideal primary nursing system, the primary nurse is responsible for all the direct and indirect care of about six patients.

Primary nursing is thus seen as an organizational innovation to 1) reduce coordination requirements, 2) improve accountability of care, 3) improve continuity of care, 4) improve nurse utilization, and 5) improve nurse autonomy in providing care.

Studies that have compared primary and team nursing report that primary nursing results in higher patient satisfaction and quality of nursing care.[19] It has also been reported to be less expensive than team nursing.[20] The findings of these studies were challenged by the results of two quasi-experimental controlled research studies. One study concluded that the competency of nurses rather than the structure of primary nursing was responsible for the higher quality of care.[21] The study also pointed out that the previous studies had not controlled or accounted for the differences in the competency of the registered nurses. The second study showed that when the competency of nurses is the same on a team unit and a primary unit, the primary unit does not provide better quality of care and is more expensive because of the higher proportion of registered nurses on the staff.[22]

There have been few studies to date on the impact of nursing care structures on nurse utilization. One study reported a decrease in the utilization of registered nurses in an all-RN model of primary nursing,[23] whereas another showed a positive impact.[24] That study suggested that the contradictory results of nurse utilization could be explained by the efficiency of distribution and communication systems. The lower nurse utilization in the former study was more the result of deficient support systems rather than the primary nursing structure.

In the remainder of this paper, four studies undertaken within the framework of a systems approach are analyzed to show the interrelationships between technical support systems and structural support systems on nursing units.

SYSTEMS FRAMEWORK

Nurse utilization, the percentage of nurses' time attributed to direct patient care activities, depends on the efficiency of nursing support systems. The higher the efficiency of the nursing support system, the higher the nurse utilization. There are two components of the nursing support system: the technical support system (TSS) and the structural support system (SSS); see Figure 15.1. If the TSS and SSS were not interrelated, one could adopt strategies to improve the SSS from team to primary nursing irrespective of the nature of the TSS. It will be shown, however, that the TSS and the SSS are interrelated and that the choice of a team or a primary SSS would depend on the nature of the TSS.[25]

The TSS can be classified as either centralized or decentralized. The TSSs in most hospitals fall between the two extremes of the centralized/

FIGURE 15.1

A Framework of Nursing Support Systems

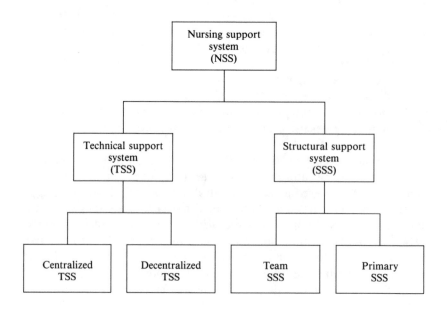

decentralized continuum. For the sake of simplicity, I shall classify TSSs into two discrete — centralized and decentralized — systems. Similarly, the SSS can be classified as either team nursing or primary nursing.

CHANGE STRATEGIES

A hospital can attempt to improve nurse utilization by changing the nature of its technical support system from a centralized to a decentralized system (*A* to *B* or *C* to *D* in Figure 15.2), by changing its structural support system from team to primary (*A* to *C* or *B* to *D*), or both (*A* to *D*), which would require simultaneous change to primary nursing and to decentralized distribution and communication systems.

Which of these strategies will provide greater improvement in nurse utilization? And, is there an interaction between the two basic strategies — changing the TSS and the SSS — that will improve nurse utilization? The theses of this paper are:

1. Changing the TSS from a centralized to a decentralized system will improve the utilization of nurses, irrespective of the nature of the SSS.
2. Changing the SSS from a team to an all-RN model of primary

FIGURE 15.2

Strategies for Improving Nurse Utilization

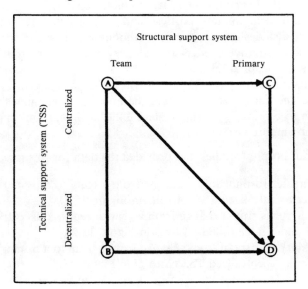

nursing in a decentralized TSS will improve the utilization of nurses.

3. Changing the SSS from a team to an all-RN model of primary nursing in a centralized TSS will reduce the utilization of nurses.

If the above propositions can be supported, one can argue that the optimal strategy to improve nurse utilization would be to improve the TSS first and then implement a primary nursing system. Implementation of the all-RN model of primary nursing in a hospital with an inefficient TSS will reduce the utilization of nurses, because a higher proportion of professional nurses' time will be devoted to non-professional and indirect care tasks, which are performed by aides and LPNs on a team unit.

DATA BASE

To test the above theses, we identified four hospitals that had adopted one of the three strategies described in the foregoing to improve their nursing support system. We chose to study the experiences of these four hospitals for the following reasons:

- Each of the hospitals had implemented and evaluated one of the three change strategies with respect to nurse utilization.
- Each hospital had used the work-sampling technique to study its nurse utilization; the data were thus comparable.
- Each of the hospital studies had evaluated changes in nurse utilization by using pretest, posttest, and control group designs. The use of such designs has proven methodologically sound for comparing alternative change strategies, even with data from more than one hospital setting.
- Each of the hospitals had a similar unit management system, which permitted us to compare the impact of changing from a team to a primary nursing system under a similar unit management support system.

The four hospital studies that provided the data for this research are:

- Riverside Hospital study: change from a team to a primary SSS under a centralized TSS (*A* to *C* in Figure 15.2).
- Chi Systems study: change from a centralized to a decentralized TSS under a team SSS (*A* to *B* in Figure 15.2).
- St. Mary's Hospital study: change from a team to a primary SSS under a decentralized TSS (*B* to *D* in Figure 15.2).
- Wausau Hospital study: change from a team SSS and a central-

ized SSS to a primary SSS and a decentralized TSS (*A* to *D* in Figure 15.2).

An appropriate study could not be identified that evaluated the strategy of changing from *C* to *D* and that met the four criteria for inclusion in this study. There were several hospitals that changed from *C* to *D*, but no data were collected to evaluate the change.

In all four studies data were collected using the work-sampling technique. This technique of studying nurse utilization is well accepted in the field and is described elsewhere.[26] Briefly, the technique is based on the statistical principle that when observations are taken at random, activities that utilize more nursing time are more likely to be observed. If large enough random observations are made, an activity that takes twice as much time, for example, will be observed twice as frequently.

RESULTS

Results from the four nurse utilization studies are presented in Figure 15.3. The percentage figures indicate the differences in nurse utilization before and after the implementation of the change strategies.

RIVERSIDE HOSPITAL STUDY (*A* TO *C*)

Nurse utilization within the team as well as the primary nursing structure was examined at Riverside Hospital, Newport News, Virginia.[27] The two 48-bed units studied had comparable centralized TSS levels; utilization was computed based on the proportion of the nurses' time spent in direct care and professional care activities. The study was undertaken only after assurances were given that the registered nurses on both the team and the primary units were compatible in terms of educational background, age, experience, and nursing competencies on the Slater scale.[28] The sample size for the work-sampling study was 3,000 observations, which provided a sampling error of ±2.5%.

Results of the study indicated that the RNs on the team unit spent more of their time performing direct-care activities (41.5%) than did the RNs on the primary nursing unit (37.5%); that is, the utilization of registered nurses was reduced by 4% as a result of changing the SSS from team to primary nursing. We used the *z* distribution to test the statistical differences in the mean proportion of time for direct care. The 4% difference in nurse utilization between team and primary nursing was statistically significant at the $p < .05$ level. It was also shown that the time needed for coordinating care on the primary nursing unit (22.6%) was significantly less than the time needed on the team unit (30.2%).

FIGURE 15.3

The Percentage Increase in Nurse Utilization Following
the Changeover from a Team to a Primary Nursing
Structural Support System and from a Centralized
to a Decentralized Technical Support System

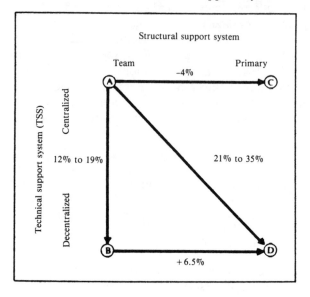

However, the time saved in coordination of care under primary nursing
did not translate into increased direct care. It is suggested that in the
absence of aides on the primary unit, the registered nurses spent a greater
amount of time in supportive activities.

CHI SYSTEMS STUDY (*A* TO *B*)

The Friesen concept was evaluated by Chi Systems, Inc., at the Scarborough Centenary Hospital in Toronto, Canada.[29] The data were collected on four Friesen units during a total of 2,500 observations. The
time spent in direct care in patient rooms was computed for each of the
skill levels: head nurse, registered nurse, licensed practical nurse, and
aide. The data were compared with those from an AHA nursing study of
55 hospitals and those from a Community Systems Foundation (CSF)
study of 15 hospitals.[30]

The staffing hours per patient day in the Friesen, AHA, and CSF studies were 3.49, 4.44, and 4.21, respectively, which indicate that the decentralized distribution and communication systems (i.e., the Scarborough Hospital) required less staffing time than did the centralized support systems in the 70 AHA and CSF hospitals. The Friesen system is essentially a comprehensive approach to improving and decentralizing the TSS. When the Chi Systems study compared the Friesen approach with another conventional, centralized nursing unit at Scarborough Hospital, the Friesen nursing unit was found to permit RNs to spend 19% and LPNs to spend 12% more time with patients. This study shows that nurse utilization can be substantially improved by improving the TSS, even within the team nursing framework.

ST. MARY'S HOSPITAL STUDY (*B* TO *D*)

This study compared direct and indirect patient care times on a primary nursing unit and a team nursing unit, each having a decentralized TSS.[31] The data were collected using the work-sampling technique; 600 observations were made on each of the units. Ratios of direct to indirect care time of 1.57:1 on the primary unit and 1.21:1 on the team unit were observed. Because the same amount of money was budgeted for the two units and because the primary nursing unit was staffed with only registered nurses, there were fewer nursing personnel and fewer hours of care per patient per day on the primary nursing care unit. However, the registered nurses were better utilized on the primary unit than on the team unit, as indicated by the ratio of direct to indirect care time. In percentage terms, the registered nurses spent 54.6% of their time on the direct care of patients in the team unit and 61.1% in the primary unit, or a difference of 6.5%.

WAUSAU HOSPITAL STUDY (*A* TO *D*)

Researchers at Wausau Hospital conducted a work-sampling study to evaluate the effects of simultaneously changing both the TSS and the SSS.[32] The experimental unit was operating with a centralized TSS and team SSS before the change. Approximately 10 months after the implementation of a modified Friesen design and primary nursing concept, the unit was sampled again, using the same elements and observers. Work sampling was also done on a control unit. On each of the units, 500 observations were made at each sampling. The results clearly demonstrate an increase in utilization (direct care) of 35% for RNs and 21% for aides and LPNs after the changeover to a decentralized TSS and primary SSS.

CONCLUSION

In this era of cost containment and nurse shortages, the utilization of nurses is a major concern of hospital and nursing administrators. The utilization of nurses is also very important from another perspective — that of nurses seeking job satisfaction. Many studies have indicated that nurses want hospitals to provide support systems so that they can fully utilize their professional skills and concentrate on direct care functions. During the last two decades administrators have supported several innovations to improve the utilization of nurses in hospitals. Some of these innovations have included changing the nursing care structure from functional to team, and now to primary, as well as improving the efficiency of distribution and communication systems. There is no study, however, that examines the interrelationship between the technical support (distribution and communication) system and the structural support (team or primary) system.

This paper reviews four studies and suggests that the interaction between the TSS and the SSS in the nursing framework is significant. In fact, the contradictory findings of nurse utilization in the primary setting can be explained by the interrelationships between the structural support system of primary nursing and the technical support system. The decision to adopt primary nursing should not be made independent of the nature of the technical support system. The results presented here support the use of a primary nursing system coupled with a decentralized technical support system to maximize RN utilization. Likewise, the results also indicate that an all-RN model of primary nursing should not be adopted if a centralized technical support system remains in place. If RNs do not have adequate support for routine and nonprofessional activities, they will have to perform most of the indirect and nonprofessional tasks themselves before they can attend to professional and direct-care responsibilities. The optimal utilization of professional nurses would thus occur within the primary nursing structural support system that utilizes a decentralized technical support system.

In those hospitals where the technical support system cannot be changed because of physical or economic constraints, the use of LPNs or aides is necessary to buffer the registered nurses from the inefficiencies of the system. Modular nursing and modified primary nursing models are alternative structures that are generally used to maximize the patient care time of registered nurses in such settings. Modular nursing combines the features of team and primary nursing to reduce the involvement of registered nurses in activities that diminish the amount of time they can spend in direct patient care.[33]

NOTES AND REFERENCES

1. R. K. Shukla, "Nursing Care Structures and Productivity," *Hospital & Health Services Administration* 27 (December 1982): 45-58.

2. Mohan Kirtane, "Pilot Study on 7 Orange," unpublished report (Milwaukee, WI: St. Mary's Hospital, March 1978).

3. *Nurse Utilization: A Patient Care Systems Project: Final Report* (Madison, WI: Wisconsin Regional Medical Program, Inc., August 1972), p. 32; "New Patient Care Method," unpublished project report (Wausau, WI: Wausau Hospital, May 1975).

4. J. Black and W. W. Tester, "Decentralized Pharmacy Operations Utilizing the Unit Dose Concept," *American Journal of Hospital Pharmacy* 24 (March 1967): 120-129.

5. See Eugene Lane, "Nurse and Patient Benefit From Unit Dose," *Hospital Management* 104 (November 1967): 58 passim; E. M. Price, "A Nurse Looks at Hospital Drug Distribution Systems," *American Journal of Hospital Pharmacy* 24 (1967): 104-109; D. M. Reynolds, M. H. Johnson, and R. L. Longe, "Medication Delivery Time Requirements in Centralized and Decentralized Unit Dose Drug Distribution Systems," *American Journal of Hospital Pharmacy* 35, no. 8 (1978): 941-943; and P. F. Parker, "Unit-Dose System Reduces Error, Increases Efficiency," *Hospitals* 42 (December 1968): 65-69.

6. Gordon A. Friesen, "Integrated Communication Through Construction," *Hospital Progress* 41 (August 1960: 64-67, and "A Mechanized Supply System Provides Supplies Where Needed," *Hospitals, J.A.H.A.* 40 (May 1, 1966): 109-112.

7. Gordon A. Friesen, "Why Not Build a Patient Room as a Special Care Unit?" *Modern Hospital* 110 (March 1968): 92-93.

8. *The Friesen No-Nursing Station Concept: Its Effects on Nurse Staffing* (Ann Arbor, MI: Chi Systems Inc., 1970).

9. See note 3.

10. Ibid.

11. H. H. Schmidts, *Hospital Information Systems* (Germantown, MD: Aspen Systems Corp., 1979), chap. 6.

12. See E. A. Brooks, "Team Nursing—1961," *American Journal of Nursing* 61 (April 1967): 87-91; L. M. Douglass and E. O. Bevis, *Team Leadership in Action: Principles and Application to Staff Nursing Situations* (St. Louis; C. V. Mosby Co., 1970); Thora Kron, *Nursing Team Leadership*, 2d ed. (Philadelphia: W. B. Saunders Co., 1966); E. C. Lambertsen, *Nursing Team Organization and Functioning* (New York: Columbia University Teachers College, Bureau of Publications, 1953); M. A. Williams, "The Myths and Assumptions About Team Nursing," *Nurses Forum* 3, no. 4 (1964): 61-73.

13. G. G. Peterson, *Working with Others for Patient Care*. 2d ed. (Dubuque, IA: William C. Brown, 1973).

14. G. G. Peterson, *The Management of Patient Care: Putting Leadership Skill to Work*, 4th ed. (Philadelphia: W. B. Saunders Co., 1976).

15. Williams (see note 12).

16. E. L. Clark, "A Model for Nurse Staffing for Effective Patient Care," *Journal of Nursing Administration* 8 (February 1977): 24.

17. M. G. Auld, "Team Nursing in a Maternity Hospital," *International Journal of Nurses Study* 7 (June 1970): 57–66.

18. See note 1.

19. See Reidun J. Daeffler, "Patients' Perception of Care Under Team and Primary Nursing," *Journal of Nursing Administration* 6 (March–April 1975): 20–26; G. Felton, "Increasing the Quality of Nursing Care by Introducing the Concept of Primary Nursing: A Model Project," *Nursing Research* 24 (January–February 1975): 27–32.

20. Gwen Marram, "The Comparative Costs of Operating a Team and Primary Nursing Unit," *Journal of Nursing Administration* 6 (May 1976): 21–24.

21. Ramesh K. Shukla, "Structure vs. People in Primary Nursing: An Inquiry," *Nursing Research* 30 (July–August 1981): 236–241.

22. R. K. Shukla, "All-RN Model of Nursing Care Delivery: A Cost-Benefit Evaluation," *Inquiry* 20 (Summer 1983): 173–184.

23. See note 1.

24. See note 2.

25. R. K. Shukla, "Primary or Team Nursing? Choice Depends Upon Two Factors," *Journal of Nursing Administration*, November 1982, pp. 12–15.

26. Faye G. Abdellah and Eugene Levine, "Work Sampling Applied to the Study of Nursing Personnel," *Nursing Research* 3 (June 1954): 11–16.

27. See note 1.

28. Mabel Wandelt and Doris Stewart, *Slater Nursing Competencies Rating Scale* (New York: Appleton-Century-Crofts, 1975).

29. See note 8.

30. Stanley E. Jacobs, Naomi Patchin, and Glenn Anderson, *AHA Nursing Activities Study: Project Report* (Chicago: AHA, 1968).

31. See note 2.

32. See note 8.

33. See note 1.

IV

Professional Integration

... in the United States, the physician is not so much part of the hospital as the hospital is part (and only one part) of the physician's practice.

— Freidson

ILLUSTRATION IV

Predicted Dimensions of Hospital Medical Staff Organization Structure

Dimension	Measures	Mean or Percent	Standard Deviation
Resource Capability	Percent of Active Staff Board Certified	41.0%	27.0
	Percent of Active Staff Pathologists and Radiologists	14.0%	14.0
	Number of Active Staff Members per Bed	.34	.37
	Existence of a Director of Medical Education	20.0%	40.0
	Percent of Active Staff Funded for Research	5.0%	21.3
	Number of Services and Benefits Provided to Active Medical Staff—e.g., In-Hospital Clinical Office Space, Bookkeeping Services, etc.	1.87	2.63
	Number of Interns and Residents per Bed	0.18	0.06
	Hospital Bed Size	167	171
Formalization	Number of Staff Requirements—e.g., Board Certification, County Medical Society Membership, etc.	1.2	0.8
	Whether or not the Proportion of Maximum or Minimum Medical Staff Members Appointed to Board is Specified	12.0%	32.1
	Percent of Committees with a Quorum Requirement	45.0%	45.1
Centralization	Percent of Departmental Chiefs Appointed instead of Elected	49.7%	46.1
	Percent of Committees for which Members are Appointed instead of Elected	58.0%	40.0
	Physicians are Elected to the Governing Board by the Medical Staff rather than Appointed	5.9%	23.5
Commitment to Hospital	Percent Nonactive Staff Physicians	36.0%	27.0
	Percent of Active Staff on Contract	20.0%	22.0
	Percent of Contract Staff on Salary	23.0%	35.0
	President of Medical Staff on Contract	4.0%	20.0
	Percent of Department Chiefs on Contract	28.2%	31.6
	Percent of Contract Active Staff Holding Committee Assignments*	49.0%	0.49
	Percent of Noncontract Physicians with Major Professional Activity in Your Hospital	83.0%	28.0
Communication/ Control	Number of Committees per Logarithm of Bed Size	4.3	1.8
	Number of Meetings per Committee	11.1	5.1
	Number of Members per Committee	6.5	3.8
Participation in Decision Making	Medical Director Votes on Governing Board	3.0%	17.2
	Director of Medical Education Votes on Governing Board	0.5%	7.3
	President of Medical Staff is on Governing Board	39.2%	48.8
	Other Medical Staff Officers are on Governing Board	19.0%	39.0
	Active Staff are on Governing Board	42.0%	49.0
	Physicians are on Executive Committee of Governing Board	25.7%	43.7
	Percent of Medical Staff Committees with Nonphysician Voting	37.0%	31.0
Primary Care Orientation	Ratio of Outpatient Visits per Bed	145	186
	Percent of Active Staff in Generalist Care (FP, GP, Pediatricians)†	38.0%	27.0
	Percent of Generalist Care Physicians on Contract	5.0%	18.6
	Number of Activities Involved in Cooperation with Outside HMOs—e.g., Emergency Care, Education, Peer Review, etc.	0.68	1.21

* The Percent of Contract Active Staff Holding Committee Assignments rather than all staff was used due to data problems in the latter measure.

† The term "generalist care" is used rather than "primary care" because there is as yet no widely accepted common definition of primary care, nor is it known how much primary care is actually delivered by family practitioners, general practitioners, and pediatricians. Internists and obstetrician-gynecologists were excluded in order to arrive at what was felt to be a closer approximation to generalist as opposed to specialist care.

Reprinted from Stephen M. Shortell and Thomas E. Getzen, "Measuring Hospital Medical Staff Organizational Structure," *Health Services Research* 14 (Summer 1979): 100–101, with permission, the Hospital Research and Educational Trust.

Commentary

Anthony R. Kovner
Duncan Neuhauser

The integration of professional and organizational goals is one of the key problems facing managers in health services organizations. Increasing attention is being paid to the need for clinician managers to link professional objectives to organizational objectives.

Some divergence between organizational and professional objectives is functional. Physicians and nurses are concerned with the best possible care for their patients. Managers are concerned with the best possible care for all patients and potential patients. This divergence is functional to the extent that claims for resources on behalf of both objectives can be effectively represented and adjudicated in the organizational decision-making process. If there is no divergence, the result may be a lack of sufficient organizational or professional response on behalf of their different constituents. If the divergence is too great, the result may be suboptimization, as professional objectives are achieved at the expense of organizational objectives or vice versa.

Managers are few and professionals are numerous. Can managers achieve organizational objectives when these conflict with the priorities of professionals? Some opportunities for managers result from the following characteristics of health services organizations:

— Key interest groups in the organization have different objectives. For example, professionals may oppose and a governing board may favor increased hospital emphasis upon chronic and ambulatory care.
— Physicians and nurses often compete for scarce organizational resources. For example, surgeons and surgical nurses may favor acquisition of expensive equipment, while internists and medical nurses urge increased investment in highly skilled professional nursing staff.
— There is often goal divergence among physicians and nurses in

the same clinical areas. Full-time surgeons are probably more interested in research than are surgeons in private practice. Hospital outpatient nurses believe outreach services are more important than do nurses who work for fee-for-service group practices.

Physicians and hospitals can be viewed as partners joining their skills and resources to create new programs in a rapidly changing competitive environment. In such joint ventures, both may provide capital and commitment. These ventures may be carried out by new corporate entities that are for-profit and jointly owned. "Intrapreneurs" are entrepreneurs within an existing organization who are encouraged to create and develop new programs and products. Encouraging hospital-associated physicians to develop new programs is one form of this "intrapreneurship." Describing these activities with new words like "joint ventures" and "intrapreneurs" reflects the greater attention now being paid to them.

Professionals respond differently to the changing environment for health services organizations. Some will wish to respond in the direction of the change, others to resist changes that seem to be fads or ill-advised responses. Professionals differ in their responses to new medical care programs such as hospices, urgent care centers, or milieu therapy, as well as in their responses to new management initiatives such as matrix management, performance budgeting, and product line planning. Professionals favor, are indifferent to, or oppose some or all of these programs and initiatives, some of which are more suited to certain organizations and services than to others. Managers must test the external and internal environments of their organizations and adapt to inevitable change. They must differentiate between the inevitable and the uncertain, and to choose programs and directions after the pioneers have worked out the bugs but before the latecomers have jumped on the bandwagon.

THE READINGS

Delbecq and Gill propose that the hospital professions have fundamentally different concerns, working styles, and values. Working together does not require homogenizing the views of these groups; however, it does require a fair process by which decisions can be made. This process should be based on a definition of justice and should include due process and the opportunity to be heard through representative problem-solving groups.

Kovner and Chin also examine the decision-making process in hospitals, giving particular attention to the role of physician leaders. They describe the context that determines appropriate models for decision making.

Although nursing goes through periodic shortages, some argue that the current shortage of nurses is the most severe. However, these shortages bring about a renewal of interest in making life tolerable for hospital nurses and creating a work environment where nurses can fulfill their professional aspirations. Mottaz reports that autonomy, participation, salary, and the nature of supervision are factors that contribute to work satisfaction among nurses.

Shortell contrasts the advantages and disadvantages of three innovative models of medical staff organization. He evaluates the models according to (1) their recognition of differences in professional socialization and training, and (2) their ability to maximize effective problem solving and communication, generation of useful alternatives, effective implementation of solutions, and professional and organizational training.

PERFORMANCE REQUIREMENTS

The four performance requirements are discussed below in terms of the readings in Section IV. In addition, Table IV.1 summarizes the authors' approaches to professional integration.

GOAL ATTAINMENT

Each of the articles in this section is concerned with commitment and the satisfaction of health care professionals. The authors all recognize that these two factors are essential for organizational goal attainment.

SYSTEM MAINTENANCE

Particularly in health care organizations, members value the technical knowledge and shared culture provided by the organization. As turnover increases, this shared knowledge is lost. Thus a shared knowledge of the organization's development and a limit on turnover are essential components to system maintenance.

ADAPTIVE CAPABILITY

The process of decision making is at the core of adaptive capability. According to Delbecq and Gill, and Kovner and Chin, the appropriate process for decision making depends on the circumstances. As Mottaz

TABLE IV.1

Perspectives on Performance Requirements
and Professional Integration

Readings	Goal Attainment	System Maintenance	Adaptive Capability	Values Integration
Delbecq & Gill	Success	Integration, teamwork, cohesion	Decision rules	Due process & justice
Kovner & Chin	Physician leaders	Physician-hospital relations	Strategic decision making	
Mottaz		Turnover	Participation	Work values & satisfaction
Shortell		Independent corporate model maintains system	Parallel model encourages adoption	Division model encourages values integration

suggests, the degree of participation in decision making is an important component of nursing satisfaction.

Shortell's parallel model involves the creation of a separate organization for purposes of conducting certain activities, such as adaptation, which are not handled well by the formal organization. According to Shortell, the parallel model has particular advantages in enhancing communication, generating alternatives, and implementing new programs across organization boundaries.

VALUES INTEGRATION

Belief that the organization is just and that it will seek out opinions can be a central value among organization members. Delbecq and Gill suggest that values need not be uniform, but that there must be acceptance of diverse values and ways to bring these values into the decision process.

Shortell's divisional model promotes integration of values across occupational lines, as each division has the necessary functional support services to do its tasks and is responsible for the management of those functions. Shortell observes that the nursing staff may be upset because they are required to report through a physician clinical staff chief in each division rather than through their own administrative hierarchy. Physicians would be similarly upset if the divisional clinical chief were a nurse.

ADDITIONAL TOPICS OF INTEREST

The readings in this section focus on the organization of professionals in hospitals. Readers may also be interested in studying topics such as the way clinician managers integrate professional preferences with organizational objectives, the integration of professionals other than physicians and nurses, and professional integration in organizations other than hospitals. The selected bibliography gives suggestions for further reading on professional integration. Readers should also refer to the annotated bibliography at the end of the book.

SELECTED BIBLIOGRAPHY

Aiken, Linda, and Connie F. Mullinix. "Special Report: The Nurse Shortage: Myth or Reality." *The New England Journal of Medicine* 317, no. 10 (1985): 641-51.

Beauchamp, George R. "Occasional Notes: Superstar Opthalmology: A Modern Parable." *The New England Journal of Medicine* 319, no. 17 (1987): 1159-61.

Begun, James. "Managing with Professionals in a Changing Health Care Environment." *Medical Care Review* 41 (Spring 1985): 3-10.

Brown, Lawrence D. "Organization Building: The HMO as a System of Contributions." In *Politics and Health Care Organization*, 31-74. Washington, DC: Brookings Institution, 1983.

Broyles, Robert W., and Bernard J. Reilly. "Physicians, Patients and Administrators: A Realignment of Relationships." *Hospital & Health Services Administration* 33 (Spring 1988): 5-14.

Bucher, Rae, and Joan Stelling. "Characteristics of Professional Organizations." *Journal of Health & Social Behavior* 10 (March 1969): 3-15.

Dear, Margaret, Carol S. Weisman, and Sharon O'Keefe. "Evaluation of a Contract Model for Professional Nursing Practice." *Health Care Management Review* 10 (Spring 1985): 65-77.

Felch, William C., and Abraham L. Halpern. "Coping with Physician Incompetence." *New York State Journal of Medicine* 79 (November 1979): 1921-24.

Flood, Ann B., and W. Richard Scott. *Hospital Structure and Performance.* Baltimore: Johns Hopkins University Press, 1987.

Freidson, Eliot. "The Medical Profession in Transition." In *Applications of Social Science to Clinical Medicine and Health Policy*, edited by Linda H.

Aiken and David Mechanic, 63–79. New Brunswick: Rutgers University Press, 1986.

Fuller, Gerald, and Eugene M. Beaupre. "Physicians and Administrators Can Work Together." *Hospital Financial Management* 9 (October 1979): 14–23.

Gill, Sandra L., Eric W. Springer, and Andre L. Delbecq. "Commitment and Discipline in Hospitals: Leadership Protocols and Legal Precedents." *Health Care Management Review* 12, no. 3 (1987): 75–82.

Glandon, Gerald L., and Michael A. Morrisey. "Redefining the Hospital-Physician Relationship under Prospective Payment." *Inquiry* 23 (Summer 1986): 166–75.

Gordon, Paul. "Top Management Triangle in Voluntary Hospitals." *Journal of Academic Management* 36 (December 1961): 205–14; (April 1962): 66–75.

Luft H.S., J.P. Bunker, and A.C. Enthoven. "Should Operations Be Regionalized? The Empirical Relation Between Surgical Volume and Mortality." *New England Journal of Medicine* 301, no. 25 (1979): 1364–69.

Mechanic, David, ed. *Handbook of Health, Health Care and the Health Professions. Part 4: The Health Occupations*, 407–538. New York: Free Press, 1983.

Pauly, M.V. "Medical Staff Characteristics and Hospital Costs." *Journal of Human Resources* 13 (1978 Supp.): 77.

Pelligrino, E.D. "The Changing Matrix of Clinical Decision Making in the Hospital." In *Organization Research in Health Institutions*, edited by Basil Georgopoulos, 301–29. Ann Arbor, MI: Institute for Social Research, The University of Michigan, 1972.

Redisch, Michael A. "Physician Involvement in Hospital Decision Making." In *Hospital Cost Containment*, edited by Michael Zubkoff, Ira E. Raskin, and Ruth Hanft, 217–43. New York: Prodist, 1978.

Roemer, Milton I., and Jay W. Friedman. *Doctors in Hospitals*. Baltimore: Johns Hopkins University Press, 1971.

Schenke, Roger. *The Physician in Management*. Tampa, FL: American Academy of Medical Directors, 1980.

Shortell Stephen M. "Physician Involvement in Hospital Decisionmaking." In *The New Health Care for Profit*, edited by Bradford H. Gray, 73–102. Washington, DC: National Academy Press, 1983.

Shortell, Stephen M., Thomas M. Wickizer, and John R.C. Wheeler. *Hospital-Physician Joint Ventures*. Ann Arbor, MI: Health Administration Press, 1984.

Sigmond, Robert M. "Changing Hospital Goals." *Journal of the Albert Einstein Medical Center* 17 (Spring 1969): 7–16.

Smith, Harvey L. "Two Lines of Authority Are One Too Many." *Modern Hospital* 84 (March 1955): 59–64.

Stevens, Barbara J. *The Nurse as Executive*. Rockville, MD: Aspen, 1980.

Stone, Deborah A. "The Nature, Sources and Limits of Physicians' Power." In *The Limits of Professional Power*, 1–18. Chicago: University of Chicago Press, 1980.

Thompson, Richard E. *Physicians and Hospitals: Easing Adversary Relationships*. Chicago: Pluribus Press, 1984.

Weisman, Carol S., Cheryl S. Alexander, and Laura Morlock. "Hospital Decision-Making: What Is Nursing's Role?" *The Journal of Nursing Administration* 11 (September 1981): 31–36.

Young, David, and Richard Saltman. *The Hospital Power Equilibrium: Physician Behavior and Cost Control*. Baltimore: Johns Hopkins University Press, 1985.

16 | Justice as a Prelude to Teamwork in Medical Centers

André L. Delbecq
Sandra L. Gill

The need for integration and teamwork in health care organizations seems obvious as the struggle continues to reduce the cost of conflict and inefficiency. Yet recent accounts of teamwork and collaboration efforts in hospitals and medical centers have been noticeably ineffective.[1-3] Since conventional rationales for teambuilding are unlikely motivators in health care settings, it seems prudent to explore the potential of structured decision processes as an alternative route toward cohesive problem solving and organizational justice.

THE TEAMWORK CONTEXT IN MEDICAL CENTERS

In considering teamwork in medical centers, it is helpful to conjure an image of teamwork in another setting: the military. It is not difficult to imagine one's self seated in an audience in which the majority wear military uniforms, or even to imagine one's self as one of the great leadership personages of all time, George Patton, standing in front of that audience. A physician who had been in the military has confessed that this was his fanciful image—that he would be a medical George Patton, with a pearl-handled stethoscope, and that he would stand up in front of the "troops" and lead them onto new and innovative beachheads in medicine.

He said the difference between the Patton image and the reality of his medical leadership could be exemplified by a typical meeting in which:

Reprinted from *Health Care Management Review*, Vol. 10, No. 1, pp. 45–51, with permission of Aspen Publishers, Inc., © Winter 1985.

(1) three of the people critical to the meeting and whom he counted on to provide support would arrive late; (2) two other key physicians would argue vigorously against the concept that he was proposing; (3) several other physicians indicated that they would not be at all interested in participating in the program; and (4) one physician would indicate that unless he was authorized to expend more money on specialized equipment for traditional programs he would not participate in any new efforts by the organization (but would be willing to head a committee to organize the purchase of the equipment). This limited leadership appears to be a much more realistic image of teambuilding in medical organizations than the command power of Patton.

PHYSICIAN DECISION STYLES

The senior author participated in the Physician-in-Management Seminars (PIMS) funded for the American Academy of Medical Directors (AAMD) by The Robert Wood Johnson Foundation.[4] Kurtz collected data on these physicians.[5] There were 800 physicians in the sample from PIMS. Of these, 94 percent were male; ages ranged from 30 to 60. Instrumentation in the data gathering effort included Fundamental Interpersonal Relations Orientation—Behavior (FIRO-B), Life Orientations Survey (LIFO) and Hall's Style of Leadership Survey. FIRO-B was designed to assess individuals' behavior preferences regarding the expression and reception of inclusion, control and affection in general interpersonal interactions.[6,7] LIFO assesses behaviors the individual uses under conditions of stress or conflict, and can be used to identify behavioral reactions to conflict situations.[8] In this way, individuals can assess the circumstances in which their behavior is most productive—or counterproductive, i.e., the "fit" of their behavior with stressful circumstances.

What can be said about these medical leaders with respect to their team interactions? With respect to their attitudes toward interpersonal interaction, these physicians would prefer not to be interactive. The majority would prefer solo activity and like to remain detached and distant. This means that a realistic image of teambuilding with physicians has to begin with the realization that many of the key actors will not give it rave reviews.

NEEDS AND VALUES

Kurtz's data suggest that physicians represent a high "need for control" population. They have a very high need for influence, a very high need for dominance and a very high need to be the focal point in decision structures. Under conditions of stress or conflict, i.e., when disagreement occurs (and when other populations of managers would move toward group consensus as a problem-solving strategy), these physicians tend to withdraw support from the group, assert authority, stubbornly fight for suboptimal points of view, and define success as winning and failure as losing, as opposed to defining success as a mutually acceptable compromise. In short, under stress they prefer to impose their point of view on colleagues.

This tendency was manifested over and over in group exercises and case analyses in seminars focusing on problem-solving and negotiation situations in the PIMS series. Graduate students who worked with the senior author described the physicians as "non-collegial" and "primitive battlers."

The anomaly, in light of these personality or behavioral tendencies, is that 84 percent of the physicians do not value authoritarianism. It is a paradoxical situation. Their behavior under conditions of stress reverts to authoritarian behavior, but their expressed value is that authoritarianism is undesirable. Their value preference may reflect what they would prefer from others, but their behavior may reflect (perhaps at a somewhat subconscious level) an action orientation contrary to their value orientation.

DIFFERENCES BY SPECIALTY AND REGION

Of course, there are individual and subgroup differences in the data; what are cited here are central tendencies. For example, psychiatrists have lower control needs than physicians in other subspecialties. Internists are much more tolerant of conflict and tend to be more collaborative (as long as they can exercise final control). Pathologists, of all subspecialists, are the most willing to be confronted and the most difficult with whom to deal.

To make matters more stark, all of the "non-teamwork" behaviors tend to increase with age. Managers in other industries are shown to be less affiliative as they get older. Colloquially, it can be said that interaction rates decrease as waistlines increase in most studies of managerial personnel. The right to be moderately obstinate seems to be one of the features of the mid-life evolution. The reason to point this out is that seniority often goes together with either the willingness to volunteer for or the likelihood of election to medical leadership.

There are also some differences by region. The Southeast is the most blatant in terms of need for control by physician leaders. The Northeast is in the middle, and the West is somewhat less control oriented.

STRUCTURAL BARRIERS TO COHESION

Some other barriers to teamwork should be mentioned. Medical organizations are loosely coupled systems.[9,10] That is, physicians see themselves affiliated with but not employees of the organization, so that in their minds income and productivity are often seen as somewhat independent from the administration of the organization. Their focus is on medical technology. Consequently, administration and medical leadership are seldom the "apple of the physician's eye."

There is a strong tendency to view the organization as an institutional support service, which otherwise interferes with what is good for a specialty or practice. This leads to stressing personal needs as opposed to valuing what is good for the organization as a whole. The very physical ecology of the hospital (placing subspecialties in proximity) reinforces this behavior. Physicians can interact much of the time in the medical center only with a small subset of actors within their own medical department who share the same biases.

An additional barrier is "time squeeze."[11] The managerial and organizational decisions that have to be made are processed under conditions that allow only limited time for participation. Physicians who see management as interfering with work (seeing patients) are not going to spend a long afternoon engaged in organizational problem solving. It is often difficult to capture key physicians for 30 minutes. In this respect, physicians do not have shared norms requiring participation in committee work that managers in Xerox, IBM, Intel, Rolm or any other corporation would have.

For organizational development, this reduced focus on cohesion reflects a very different situation than is seen in conventional teambuilding. Interventions focused within a subspecialty (medical department or unit) may indeed approach the preconditions of interdependency and affiliation that are the groundwork for conventional teambuilding. However, when the focus is on the organizational boundaries (between medical units) or on the strategic level of decision making (the medical center as a whole), approaching teamwork from a standpoint of affiliation as opposed to due process is likely to be doomed to failure. To put it another way, when coping with the macrostructure, due process is probably more important.

To a lesser degree, this holds true in industry as well.[12] Approaches to creating cohesion within a marketing department or within a production unit can focus on affiliation. Put production, marketing and finance representatives into a meeting to make a strategic decision, and affiliation is often not the manipulative variable. Due process becomes more important. However, this structural differentiation is reinforced in the medical setting by the unique personality tendencies of physicians. It is then heightened by the loosely coupled structure of medical centers.

JUSTICE VERSUS COHESION

What does this individualist, controlling, combative behavior imply for teamwork in medical centers? What style of leadership does it require? The first premise must be that physician leaders are obviously not individuals who are going to value cohesive harmony in their group as they work through problem solving. Nonetheless, despite these behaviors there is a key value that physicians hold that provides the central approach.

Physicians do express a very strong positive value toward due process. (This is probably the result of the incredible competition in medical school. After medical school, residencies, subspecializations and boards—between 12 and 17 years depending on the specialization—secure, mature physicians often seek an alternative to win–lose combat.) Consequently, they look within the organization for leadership that assures appropriate due process.

Furthermore, physicians believe in majority rule. They recognize that at some point individual expression of strong points of opposing views must cease and a decision must be formulated. Finally, physicians are concerned about maintaining high morale within a professional organization. In short, they are aware of the complex, competitive, individualistic environment and seek to achieve positive morale in the organization by due process and majority rule, realizing that teamwork in the sense of high affiliation is not typically part of the medical culture.

This concern with due process must be the keystone when approaching teamwork among physicians. Responding to this value also provides a positive context for decision making. An organization with key leaders, who believe in due process and majority rule and who seek to come to decisions that create high morale, has to be seen as a positive starting point, even if the interpersonal styles of physicians make achieving this end somewhat more difficult. It is also important to note that if physician leaders do not perceive due process occurring in the organization, and if they do not perceive that there has been sufficient attention to majority rule (if they do not perceive that they have been treated as involved constituents), then they either withdraw from interaction or engage in forms of political fighting that are particularly destructive. As a result, the medical leader has a viable but restricted "zone of tolerance" for leadership.

The conclusion from over 30 collective years of working with physicians is that approaches to teamwork that focus on high norms for affiliation are doomed to failure. Instead, teamwork in medical organizations must acknowledge that medical centers are made up of very independent professionals with high needs for power and control. The mechanisms for enacting leadership must include (1) clearly perceived representative structures, (2) visible processing of decisions and (3) clear decision rules. In a sense, justice is substituted for cohesion. There are prerequisite structures for each of these three necessary elements for morale in medical centers.

ELEMENTS FOR SUCCESS

CLEAR REPRESENTATIVE STRUCTURES

A representative structure is a decision group wherein all relevant factions are represented and have their position voiced by a spokesperson capable of bringing to bear the concerns and values of their particular faction to the political process.[13] In the abstract, this seems to be a viable mechanism. In the concrete, physicians in the PIMS series constantly violated the spirit of such decision groups, confusing three other structures — formal hierarchy, formal standing committee and seniority — with the representative structure.

Formal Hierarchy

The most frequent error made by physician administrators (evidenced through critical incident exercises in The Robert Wood Johnson program) was to substitute formal hierarchy for representative groups when engaged in strategic problem solving. Hierarchy is not the "sole source provider" of legitimacy in medical centers. In fact, key opinion leaders for subspecialties or units, standard settlers for professional standards and central communicators to the political networks having to support decisions in health care organizations often include individuals who do not occupy hierarchical positions.

Hierarchy may be included, but composition must be expanded beyond those who hold formal office. Later, these decisions can be ratified and responsibility for enactment turned over to hierarchy. In other words, if the approach is to make decisions only through hierarchy, many key informants will not have input, and much of the diversity of professional opinion implicit in the strong personality profiles cited earlier will be glossed over.

This implies that, in any given planning period for strategic decisions, leaders will have to form special ad hoc problem-solving groups that assemble individuals who both possess unique competencies appropriate for that decision and are representative opinion leaders. Creating representative structures for critical decisions is the manifest enactment of due process. Processing all decisions through hierarchy will inevitably be perceived as decision by power as opposed to decision by due process. To a lesser extent, tendencies to refer matters to standing committees, or to senior staff can, in the same fashion, underrepresent concerned factions who hold strong views and who will be affected by decisions.

Representative structures are not only superior to hierarchy for creating a sense of teamwork, but they are superior to global participation. If participation includes everyone (e.g., all partners in a medical center as opposed to representatives), then it is unlikely that timely decisions will ever be made. Data on multispecialty group practices show that in group practices where all partners have to approve decisions there are low rates of innovation.[14] Where all physician partners participate town meeting style, the diversity of opinion leads to stalemate. Differing points of view cancel each other out. Thus the effective middle ground between hierarchy and global participation is a representative structure composed of seven to nine representatives who bring to bear a cross section of opinion.

Criteria to consider for membership include multiple ages, varied length of service, multiple specialties, differentiated training and experience, clinical as well as research orientations, inside (from within the organization) and outside resource persons. Global participation fails because there are too many diverse opinions and too little time to process the decision. Hierarchy does not work because it is seen as the exercise of arbitrary authority.

In the absence of representative structures, political networks (made up of physicians who major in politics and minor in medicine) will emerge in the attempt to control decision making in an informal but less representative manner. Counterproposals are presented by aggressive physicians. In medical centers where political energy substitutes for reasoned debate, there will be very few who perceive due process.

In summary, it is a bad choice to process strategic decisions only through hierarchy. A second bad choice is engaging everyone in debate. A final bad choice is allowing a random, informal organization to impose politicized decisions on the organization. Thus representative structures are the desired strategy.

Formal Committees

Representative structures do not emasculate hierarchy for the majority of day-to-day decisions. Such representative structures are not proposed as a replacement for existing executive or standing committees. Rather, on key issues affecting the welfare of the organization, a representative structure can augment existing hierarchy. And they do not exclude hierarchical participation in representative structures. However, a good behavioral index of enacted due process is the appointment of two or three carefully composed representative structures in any given year inclusive of but not restricted to formal office holders. Issues such as establishment of satellite services, mergers or new services would be examples of topics appropriate for ad hoc task forces.

VISIBLE PROCESSING OF DECISIONS

Membership composition, which has been the focus of the discussion so far, does not by itself assure due process. The second requirement is that the representative group participate in an open and visible process of strategic decision making.

Decisions arrived at behind closed doors, with no early warning signals regarding the evolving thinking of the committee, and sprung on the larger constituency with the request for immediate ratification, will achieve little endorsement and create as little a sense of teamwork as a decision arrived at behind closed doors by hierarchy. What is required is a visible process in which the evolution of the final decision by the representative structure is understandable and predictable (even if not totally agreeable). How is this achieved?

Information Search

Representative groups should always seek information from a broader sample of opinion than their own ranks. The classic error of the average committee is that it does not seek external data. Rather, each person on the committee represents his or her own personal "infinite wisdom." That, of course, destroys any concept of a representative group. thus, by definition, a representative group must seek additional information at three critical stages of problem solving: (1) identifying the problem, (2) exploring elements that must be included in an adequate solution and (3) reviewing preliminary proposals.

With respect to problem identification, simple surveys, interviews, observational techniques, nominal groups,[15] etc., should be employed by the representative group to be sure that the critical dimensions of the problems are fully understood by the committee, and that relevant concerns of each critical constituency are included in the problem matrix.[16] A briefing by the committee, in a public meeting at the end of the problem-solving phase, to the larger medical center constituency allows professionals at large one last opportunity to be sure that their individual concerns are included in the deliberations of the committee.

Second, a powerful research finding is that solutions based on a committee's talking only to people inside the organization are a lower quality than solutions that include elements identified by talking to informants outside the organization.[17] A sophisticated problem-solving committee always seeks opinions from outside experts, other organizations with prior experience and professionals from other medical centers who have grappled with the problem at hand. Obviously, seeking the input of professionals within the organization but not on the committee is important as well.

The more the preliminary proposal is seen as incorporating conversations with numerous experts and informants, the more the larger constituency in the medical center will see the committee's efforts as well-founded and objective. By contrast, the more the solution is perceived as being developed only by an advocacy committee that engaged in dialogue only with itself, the less likely it will be perceived as arriving at an objective or sophisticated proposal.

Chances for Input

The second critical briefing by the committee to the larger constituency (medical center as a whole) should be in the form of an early, unrefined, loosely focused solution concept. This allows the larger constituency to again suggest modifications or solution elements that ultimately increase the acceptability of the proposal.

Only after two public briefings with relevant members of the medical center dealing with problem definition and solution elements should the representative committee refine a proposal for final vote. When the refined proposal emerges, there will be few surprises. The larger constituency will have already been briefed on the committee's perception of the problem, will have had the opportunity through such means as interview and survey to share in this definition, will have been briefed on the preliminary solution concept and will have had a chance to suggest modifications, so that the final refined proposal will be perceived as evolving through a fair and open process.

Such a process requires a certain amount of patience. The process through which such strategic proposals evolve takes a number of weeks (sometimes months). It is not something that occurs after one or two meetings. But it is important to contrast the sense of justice and due process that such a visible and open decision process creates with the alternative. A group's members talk among themselves and mysteriously arrive at a recommendation in closed meetings to which the rest of the medical staff perceives no access or ability to influence. The committee's recommendation is a surprise. Once again an informal organization typically arises to try to bring to bear alternative views that seem to have been neglected in the deliberations of the committee, and decision making gets stalemated.

To summarize, the second requirement, in addition to a representative structure, is an open and visible decision process in which problem definition and solution development encompass opinions beyond those of the formal committee, and the preliminary solution concept is openly discussed with opportunities for modification before bringing the recommendation to final decision.

CLEAR DECISION RULES

It should not be assumed that such an open and visible process creates consensus among physicians. It is simply part of the due process norm that underlies a fundamentally just approach to arriving at a difficult strategic decision around which divergent points of view have focused. If consensus is not possible, the norm of majority rule is still present. However, the question remains: which majority? Is it the majority of the hierarchical team who reviews the recommendation, the majority of the committee members themselves or the majority of the total relevant professional staff asked to vote in parliamentary style?

An important part of the mandate to any representative committee is to clarify the decision rule ahead of time. Does it make a decision or recommend a decision? If the latter is the case, to whom is the recommendation given? This can differ by character of the decision, size of the organization, time urgency and governance traditions. This final decision authority should be clear to staff as a whole and to the committee before the committee's deliberation. Likewise, the voting statistics of the final decision authority should be honestly reported, even closed votes. Minority opinions will leak out in any case, so accurate ballot reporting is necessary to create a sense of fairness and openness.

BACK TO TEAMWORK

Such a structure, process and final decision rule does relate to conventional concepts of teamwork. Simply mixing constituencies on representative structures creates overlapping networks of interaction that do not occur in the day-to-day communication patterns within the organization. Praise and pride can be lavished on responsible committees who have worked through difficult problem-solving processes. Exhortations for mutual support of fair decisions can be legitimately voiced.

Furthermore, since due process is alive and well, destructive behaviors (rude remarks and neurotic defensiveness) can be confronted and reprimanded. It costs an individual nothing to make rude remarks; the expense to the organization in terms of civility and creative problem solving is very high. Thus a core value is to reinforce rules of civilized and helpful conduct and to sanction hurtful behavior.

In this sense, many of the conventional aspects of teamwork apply and do help. However, more time than is probably warranted is spent in talking about building teamwork in medical centers. Although it is an important task, until medical center personnel become skilled at enacting justice in decision processes, cohesion is a long way off. Administrators are faced with the challenge of testing the due process model as a behavioral enactment of justice on actual issues. Attention to representative structures, open and visible decision processing and clear final decision rules allow relatively independent, non-affiliation-oriented physicians (the real colleagues) to stand at ease and accept cajoling as pleasant. After all, justice is in place in the organization. Why not join the team?

REFERENCES

1. Margulies, N., and Adams, J. *Organizational Development in Health Care Organizations.* Reading, Mass.: Addison-Wesley Publishing, 1982.

2. Lammert, M. "Power, Authority and Status in Health Systems: A Marxian-Based Conflict Analysis." *Journal of Applied Behavioral Science* 14, no. 3 (1978): 321-33.

3. Weisbord, M. "Why Organization Development Hasn't Worked (So Far) in Medical Centers." *Health Care Management Review* 3, no. 1 (Spring 1976): 17-38.

4. Schenke, R., ed. *Physician in Management.* Tampa, Fla.: American Academy of Medical Directors, 1980.

5. Kurtz, M.E. "A Behavioral Profile of Physicians in Management Roles." In *The Physician in Management*, edited by R. Schenke, pp. 33-44. Tampa, Fla.: American Academy of Medical Directors, 1980.

6. Schutz, W. *FIRO-B.* Palo Alto, Calif.: Consulting Psychologists Press, 1958.

7. Schutz. W. *FIRO: The Interpersonal Underworld.* Palo Alto, Calif.: Consulting Psychologists Press, 1966.

8. Stuart Atkins, Inc. *LIFO.* Beverly Hills, Calif.: Atkins, 1971.

9. Weick, K. *The Social Psychology of Organizing.* Reading, Mass.: Addison-Wesley Publishing Co., 1979.

10. Alderfer, C.P. "Boundary Relations and Organizational Diagnosis." In *Humanizing Organizational Behavior*, edited by L. Meltzer and F. Wickert. Springfield, Ill.: Thomas Publishers, 1976.

11. Merrill, M.J., and Moosbruker, J. "Building an Organizational Development Effort in a Teaching Hospital." In *Organizational Development in Health Care Organizations*, edited by N. Margulies and J. Adams, pp. 75-104. Reading, Mass.: Addison-Wesley Publishing, 1982.

12. Lawrence, P., and Lorsch, J. *Organization and Environment.* Homewood, Ill.: Irwin Publishers, 1967.

13. Delbecq, A. "The Management of Decision Making within the Firm: Three Strategies for Three Types of Decision Making." *Academy of Management Journal* 10, no. 4 (December 1967): 329-39.

14. Delbecq, A., and Pierce, J. "Organization Structure, Individual Attitudes and Innovation." *Academy of Management Journal* 2, no. 1 (January 1977): 27-37.

15. Van de Ven, A., and Delbecq, A. "The Effectiveness of Nominal Delphi and Interacting Group Decision Making Processes." *Academy of Management Journal* 17, no. 4 (1974): 605-21.

16. Delbecq, A. "Effective Meeting Leadership." In *The Physician in Management*, edited by R. Schenke, pp. 203-27. Tampa, Fla.: American Academy of Medical Directors, 1980.

17. Delbecq, A., Van de Ven, A., and Gustofam, D. *Group Techniques for Program Planning: A Guide to Nominal Group and Delphi Processes.* Glenview, Ill.: Scott Foresman, 1974, pp. 124-37.

Physician Leadership in Hospital Strategic Decision Making

Anthony R. Kovner
Martin J. Chin

INTRODUCTION

Hospitals are facing greater competition, and their freedom to make changes in the scope of clinical services is becoming more restricted by financial and regulatory constraints. These environmental pressures are recognized by hospital officials, but there has been little attention paid to the role of physician leaders in strategic decision making.

The changing relationship between hospitals and their physicians requires study by both parties as resources become more scarce and as competition increases. This article identifies key variables that influence hospital strategic decision making and presents three models of physician participation in hospital strategic decision making and the findings from a study of eight acute general hospitals.

DEFINITIONS

Physician leaders are those physicians who occupy formal positions of authority in the hospital organizational structure. Such positions include chiefs of clinical services, officers of the medical board, and occupants of formal administrative posts such as medical director, director of medical education, or chief of the medical staff.

Reprinted from *Hospital & Health Services Administration* 30 (November–December 1985): 64–79, with permission, Health Administration Press.

The emphasis of this article is on formal leaders who control many of the channels relating to strategic planning, channels available for interaction between managers and the medical staff. Managers ultimately must communicate with and seek out the formal physician leadership even if the informal physician leadership is very influential. Formal leaders are often informal leaders as well.

One special group excluded from the group of physician leaders are those physicians who serve as chief executive officers of hospitals. In these cases, physician CEOs are considered to be managers because they are held accountable for their managerial performance, not their performance as physicians.

Strategic decisions are choices made by hospital officials to initiate, expand, diminish, or close clinical programs and services. These decisions involve changes in hospital scope of service, usually referred to as changes in product mix.

Strategic decisions involve major changes in the commitment of resources in terms of financing, personnel, equipment, facilities, and organization. Examples of strategic decisions are discontinuance of inpatient pediatric or obstetric service due to low volume, expansion of cardiac diagnostic capabilities, establishment of a hospital-sponsored HMO, acquisition of a nursing home, participation in a multi-institutional system, and creation of a clinical/research institute.

THE LITERATURE

There has been limited research on the subject of physician participation in hospital strategic decision making. Most research has focused on how physicians affect hospital operational outputs such as costs and utilization. These articles reflect the prevalent method of study of hospital-physician relations which is to examine structural characteristics of physicians and hospitals (e.g., how many doctors, what size of hospital) and relate these to hospital cost and utilization performance.

While this research addresses the role of physicians in hospital operational, rather than strategic, decision making, there are findings from this research which apply to both forms.

Shortell and his colleagues have produced the major body of research on the characteristics of physicians and their impact on hospitals. In a paper on physician involvement in hospital decision making, Shortell argues that environmental changes are causing both for-profit and not-for-profit hospitals to move from dual and separate authority structure (where physicians and managers control different types of decisions) to shared authority in hospital decision making.[1]

Shortell and Evashwick studied characteristics of the medical staffs of 4,212 acute general hospitals.[2] They found that medical staffs could be differentiated according to the extent to which all physicians had a contractual orientation toward their hospitals and according to the level of participation of physicians on governing boards. They found that for-profit hospitals tended to have higher proportions of physicians in a formal contractual relationship than not-for-profit hospitals. Larger hospitals also tended to have greater proportions of contracted physicians. Medical staff participation on governing boards also was greater in for-profit hospitals, but there was less medical staff participation on governing boards in larger hospitals (more than 500 beds) than in medium-sized hospitals (300–499 beds).

Pauly suggested that coordination and control of hospital output (where output is defined units of service such as an inpatient day) becomes more difficult as this output is dispersed among a larger number of physicians.[3] Harris critiqued the decision-making structures of hospitals by depicting the hospital as made up of feudal territories.[4] These fiefdoms were controlled by competing chiefs of services who dominated the resource allocation process. He called for changes in the regulation and organization of hospitals in order to deal with the lack of coordinated resource allocation.

Sloan echoed this notion by noting that, "very few hospitals can afford to be managed by a loose coalition of attending physicians."[5] Sloan found that the vast majority of hospitals do not place limits on the ability of its physicians to have close relations with other hospitals, although this differs substantially between hospital-based physicians (such as pathologists and radiologists) and non–hospital-based physicians.

All of these authors allude to the increasing complexity of hospital operations and the concurrent need for more formal structures for decision making.

Sloan and Becker conclude that a more decentralized medical staff structure (more control at the departmental level) results in higher hospital costs.[6] Thus, if chiefs of clinical services have more delegated powers, they must also have strong accountabilities, otherwise the hospital will experience poorer cost and utilization performance. This study suggests that having physicians paid by hospitals is not alone sufficient, but that there must exist other structures which integrate physicians into the hospital management structures such as having more formal control systems, regular reporting relationships, and performance appraisal systems. Once again, formal structures for control and communication are cited as necessary for improved hospital performance.

In one of the few studies of the process of decision making, Heyssel *et al.* conclude that contractual relationships for physician leaders must be supported by other organizational control devices.[7] [See Chapter 14.] Costs were found to be lower where there were salaried chiefs who were accountable for their performance as managers and supported by managerial staff at the departmental as well as at the hospital level. This suggests that greater integration of management staff with physician leaders improves operating performance.

A NORMATIVE, CONCEPTUAL SCHEME

This article offers a normative, conceptual scheme for selecting an appropriate model of physician participation in hospital strategic decision making [see Figure 17.1]. The model is normative in that performance on each of the independent variables determines which model of decision making is most appropriate. The model is applied to acute general hospitals.

The dependent variable, strategic decision making, is operational in terms of three models:

- Fractionated model
- Dual domain model
- Integrated model

The four independent variables consist of:

- The competitiveness of the hospital's environment.
- The complexity of the strategic decisions facing the hospital.
- The strategic orientation of physicians in leadership positions.
- The contractual relationships of these physician leaders to the hospital.

The following five sections in this article deal with independent and dependent variables. Findings from an empirical study of eight hospitals are also presented.

INDEPENDENT VARIABLES

COMPETITIVENESS OF THE ENVIRONMENT

Health delivery organizations compete for patients, physicians, capital funds, and for the right to offer new services through the certificate-of-need process. Competitors include other hospitals, private physician groups, or alternative delivery organizations such as HMOs and free-

FIGURE 17.1

Normative Conceptual Scheme for Selecting the Most Appropriate
Model of Strategic Decision Making

Independent Variables	Recommended Model of Strategic Decision Making		
	Fractionated	*Dual Domain*	*Integrated*
Competitiveness of the environment	Low	High	High
Complexity of decisions faced by the hospital	Low	Low	High
Strategic orientation of the MD leaders	Low	Low	High
Contractual relationship of the MD leaders to the hospital	Low	Low	High
Total	Low	Medium	High

standing ambulatory care centers. A more competitive environment is characterized by a greater number of competitors over a wide scope of services.

The competitiveness of the environment is an important independent variable for selecting a decision making model because it determines how many and how quickly decisions must be made. If the environment is highly competitive, this suggests that a hospital must confront a greater number of strategic decisions which may necessitate a more sophisticated model.

COMPLEXITY OF STRATEGIC DECISIONS

Hospitals vary in the scale or impact of these decisions on their organizations. Complexity of decisions refers to the scale of decisions which a hospital must consider, relative to the size and sophistication of the hospital. The complexity of decisions is particularly great if a hospital considers a major change from the existing mission.

Decisions are more complex if they:

- Represent a major change in the hospital mission.
- Entail greater risk and uncertainty.
- Consume a larger proportion of hospital resources.
- Affect several departments or services.
- Require major organizational restructuring.

STRATEGIC ORIENTATION OF PHYSICIAN LEADERS

Physician leaders assume their positions for different reasons, and there is substantial variation in the willingness of physicians to participate in strategic decision making. Some physician leaders have more advanced management skills, greater knowledge, and an eagerness to participate; others are either unwilling or unable.

In many hospitals, there are physicians in key leadership positions who choose to be informed and who are active participants in the assessment of strategic choices and in the making of decisions about services which do not directly relate to their own personal clinical domains. In the same institutions, other physician leaders may choose to focus on the delivery of clinical care, teaching, or research and will leave the overall strategic decisions to be made by managers. They will only interact on strategic issues which directly relate to the services which they control.

The strategic orientation of physician leaders is high if there are physicians in formal leadership positions who have the following characteristics:

- Knowledge of a hospital's competitive position and willingness to communicate this to other decision makers.
- Interest in working on administrative committees, task forces, and work groups.
- Ability to distinguish between personal, departmental, and hospital-wide objectives and acknowledgement of these distinctions.

CONTRACTUAL RELATIONSHIP OF PHYSICIAN LEADERS

The literature suggests that the formal relationship of physician leaders to the hospital may be an important determinant of the ability of hospitals to effectively make decisions. Given the loose coupling of physicians to most hospitals, contracted physician leaders may serve a vital function in improving the contribution of physicians to hospital strategic decision making.

Contracted physician leaders have loyalties and biases which are favorable to medical staff-hospital relations. The contractual relationship of physician leaders is measured on a hospital-wide basis by:

- The number of physician leaders who have a formal, specified financial arrangement with the hospital.
- The number and extent of formal reporting and accountability responsibilities which physician leaders must fulfill.

DEPENDENT VARIABLE: THREE MODELS

FRACTIONATED MODEL OF DECISION MAKING

The fractionated model of decision making is characterized by the absence of formal systems for strategic decision making. These decisions are made with few data or analyses concerning the hospital's market conditions, competitive positions, or financial plans. Long-range planning is not considered to be valuable or feasible, thus the issues which are considered have a short (one-year) time frame.

Under the fractionated model, one to three key decision makers assume all responsibility for assessing the environment and evaluating alternatives. There is little awareness of and no influence over the strategic choices on the part of anyone in the hospital's management or medical staff other than the one to three key decision makers.

Hospitals able to make strategic decisions effectively under this model face environments which are noncompetitive and slowly changing. Such hospitals are geographically isolated from competing provider organizations, are in areas of short supply of inpatient facilities relative to the population needs, and serve well-insured patient populations.

Decision making tends to be of low complexity because relatively few decisions are made; these decisions involve limited choices and are made as responses to short-term crises. The longer-term, strategic problems are seen primarily in terms of short-term threats or opportunities. Thus, there is little need for a formalized system of gathering data, setting priorities, and selecting actions.

Fractionated decision making is appropriate for hospitals that face little environmental change, where physicians lack a strategic planning orientation, and where physicians do not have contractual accountability to the hospital for managerial responsibilities. This occurs in geographically isolated hospitals, hospitals which serve more affluent populations, and smaller hospitals which have defined their market niche as being that of a low-cost, low-technology institution. Fractionated decision making is also appropriate where management is nonspecialized or lacking in financial and personnel resources to conduct a formal strategic-planning program.

However, there are examples of hospitals which attempt to retain fractionated decision making even when the environment changes.

DUAL DOMAIN MODEL OF DECISION MAKING

The dual domain model is characterized by a division of responsibility and authority to make strategic decisions. Under this model, managers engage in formal strategic planning, but the scope of services that can be affected by this planning process is limited to the domain not closely guarded by physician leaders.

Hospitals which operate under the dual domain model face environments they see as becoming more competitive. Managers set the planning agenda, collect the data, and then work with selected board members and physicians to select the courses of action. Managers may seek physician input but discourage proactive participation of physician leaders because they may not want physicians to alter the managerially determined agenda. They may not completely trust the physicians, or they may not want too many parties participating in the decision making process. In the dual domain model, physicians are informed and are asked to react to strategic initiatives posed by managers.

Physician leaders in hospitals which typify the dual domain model see their primary roles as clinicians and not as managers of their departments. Most of them are elected by their peers rather than appointed or hired by the chief executive officer.

While the strategic-planning process is largely influenced by managers and trustees in dual domain hospitals, changes in scope of service and product mix do occur (as they do under the fractionated model), largely as a result of changes in the day-to-day physician practice patterns, not from any centrally planned policy.

Service changes occur as a result of new admitting practices, referral patterns or treatment preferences of individual physicians and not as the result of a strategic redirection of resources. The consequence is a divided course of action; some decisions derive directly from the formal strategic planning process, others derive from uncoordinated physician behaviors.

Dual domain hospitals are characterized by a reluctance or inability on the part of the formal strategic planning bodies to make decisions regarding acute-care services. In dual domain hospitals, rarely are decisions made which involve major changes in the mission of the hospital.

When managers and trustees attempt to make decisions in these areas, physicians often resist because they are unwilling to allow nonphysician intervention in clinical services. The motivation for the resistance may be economical or philosophical.

Because of this resistance, many managerially controlled strategic-planning efforts focus on services which fall outside of the main interests of most physicians. Many managers and trustees find it is easier to strategically plan for long-term care services, hospices, and alcoholism services because these do not directly touch on acute inpatient care.

Thus, if there is a low level of complexity of decisions, the dual domain model is recommended because decisions do not require extensive interaction between physician leaders who dominate the traditional major clinical services and managers who dominate other services.

Today, the dual domain model may be the most common form of strategic decision making used in hospitals. Many hospital managers have become comfortable only recently with the tools and techniques of strategic planning, particularly as applied to the major clinical departments. Many hospitals lack information about which services comprise separate markets, and they lack data to evaluate the hospital's market niches. However, they have pursued formal strategic planning in the hopes of improving the sophistication and influence of the process for a later use.

The dual domain model is inappropriate when the skills of the managers do not allow them to carry out a formal strategic decision-making process or when the environment is so competitive that individual physician leaders cannot make decisions which serve both the interests of key physicians in their departments and the interests of the hospital as a whole.

Some hospitals may inappropriately rely on the dual domain model because managers fail to recognize that physician participation is crucial when the environment is most competitive or because managers have not yet sufficiently developed their own staff's skills in strategic planning.

INTEGRATED MODEL OF STRATEGIC
DECISION MAKING

Under the integrated model, regular communication occurs among managers, board members, and the physician leadership. There is a regular formalized process for soliciting physician input in decisions regarding changes in service mix. Physician leaders assist in specifying which data should be gathered to study strategic options.

There is a formal process by which key physicians, board members, and managers jointly determine the courses of action. Hospitals which operate under the integrated model assume that formal strategic planning is a necessary and routine activity. They also assume that active physician leader participation is essential for the process to be effective.

Hospitals which operate under the integrated model also have the ability to consider a broader range of decisions, but they have difficulty prioritizing the choices. The process also tends to be slow and prone to miscommunication due to the larger number of people analyzing issues and contributing to the process.

The integration of physicians into strategic planning may take different forms. Physician leaders may be held directly accountable for their managerial performance by board members, other physicians, or managers. Chiefs of services may be required to take on full or part-time managerial duties and an associated salary. New physician leader positions entitled "vice-president for medical affairs" or "medical director" may be created to serve as a liaison between managers and physicians.

EMPIRICAL FINDINGS FROM EIGHT CASE STUDY HOSPITALS

We conducted structured interviews with 120 physicians in formal leadership positions, 20 trustee board members, and 40 administrators in eight not-for-profit, nongovernmental, acute general hospitals (greater than 200 beds) in the Northeast. The interviews consisted of a set of open-ended questions related to the four variables described above. Questions were asked regarding:

- Competitiveness of the environment: How many competitors and how intense was the competition? In what service areas was competition most keen?
- Complexity of decisions: What were the major strategic issues considered by the hospital during the period 1980–1982? What difficulties were encountered in the process of decision making?
- Strategic orientation of physician leaders: How were physicians involved in strategic decision making? What types of information did they receive, and what input did they provide to the process?
- Contractual relationship of physician leaders: To what extent were physician leaders contractually obligated to the hospital?

What formal accountability was required of physician leaders to hospital officials?

The interviews were conducted by a team of six researchers who worked in pairs. Interviewers were randomly assigned. Notes from each interview were transcribed and used by the interviewers to assist them in rating each hospital's performance on four independent variables.

A four-point measurement scheme was used for each of the four variables. The six researchers rated each hospital on each of the four variables. Raters relied on the interview notes and their personal experiences in the interviewing process. The highest and the lowest scores from the six raters were dropped for each variable. The mean of the remaining four scores was calculated, and this provided the final score for each variable. The scores on the four variables were added to create a total score for each hospital.

A test of agreement was conducted to investigate whether there was consistency among the ratings provided by the six researchers. Using the agreement rule of five out of six raters scoring within one point, we found agreement in 75% of the 32 scoring trials. Based purely on chance, this kind of agreement would occur only 22% of the time. Thus, there was strong evidence that the raters had agreement which was not due to chance.

Once total scores for each hospital were obtained, these were used to classify each institution in one of the three models. The categories for these total scores were:

Fractionated Model	4.0 to 6.99
Dual Domain Model	7.0 to 12.99
Integrated Model	13.0 to 16.00

The categories were constructed so that a hospital would have to score low (1 or 2) on most variables to be classified in the fractionated model. To be classified as an integrated model, a hospital would have to score high on most variables.

By design, this classification scheme has a wider range of scores for the dual domain model. Having a larger central category was preferable to uniform assignment of scores for categories to ensure that the fractionated model was truly differentiated from the integrated model.

FINDINGS

Our interviews in eight hospitals suggest there may be different levels of strategic orientation and contractual relationship of physician leaders for different types of hospitals. Figure 17.2 shows how the scores on the four variables placed each of the case study hospitals in one of the three models of strategic decision making.

DISCUSSION AND IMPLICATIONS

Physician leaders serve an important function by bridging the gap between attending physicians and the hospital trustees and managers. Their role in strategic decision making may be minimal as under the fractionated model; it may be limited to specific areas as under the dual domain model; or it may be highly proactive as under the integrated model. As changing financial, regulatory, and competitive pressures are brought to bear on physicians and hospitals, the role of the physician leader becomes increasingly complex and difficult.

The results indicated that the strategic orientation of physician leaders was low in many hospitals. Chiefs of services often had large private

FIGURE 17.2

Scores for Eight Case Study Hospitals on the Independent Variables

	Competitiveness of the Environment	Complexity of Decisions Faced by the Hospital	Strategic Orientation of the Physician Leaders	Extent of Contractual Relationship of MD Leaders	Total Score	Model
Affiliated Hospital	3.25	3.25	3.5	3.75	13.75	Integrated
Catholic Hospital	3.75	3.75	1.5	3.75	12.75	Dual
TATCH	3.5	2.5	2.25	4.0	12.0	Dual
Hope Medical Center	3.5	3.5	1.75	2.25	11.0	Dual
Borough Hospital	3.0	3.25	1.5	2.5	10.25	Dual
Inner City Hospital	1.25	2.25	2.0	3.25	8.75	Dual
Community Hospital	2.5	1.75	1.0	1.0	6.25	Fractionated
Union Hospital	2.25	1.75	1.25	1.0	6.25	Fractionated
	$\bar{x} = 2.875$	$\bar{x} = 2.75$	$\bar{x} = 1.844$	$\bar{x} = 2.689$		

practices and did not identify with the strategic concerns of hospital officials. Physician leaders in these hospitals were primarily concerned with their private practices and tended to see the interests of the hospital from the viewpoint of independent practitioners rather than as hospital clinical managers. Managers and board members may have discouraged these physician leaders from attaining a higher strategic orientation because they did not trust physicians' judgment or loyalty to the hospital.

The physician leader must balance the often conflicting responsibilities of representing colleagues versus protecting the larger interests of the hospital. He runs the risk of either being perceived by attending physicians as selling out to managerial pressures or being seen by managers and board members as guarding the parochial interests of physicians. This balancing of interests must be considered by physician leaders, although the role of the physician leaders varies under each different model of strategic decision making.

Seven out of the eight hospitals in our study were free-standing community general hospitals. These free-standing hospitals were 300–700 beds and were not part of an academic medical center. Free-standing community hospitals and their physician leaders may be in the most precarious strategic position. They are faced with many complex decisions regarding their mission and scope of services.

The hospital may lack some specialized market and planning staff which larger entities may possess. They may face more competition than smaller, more isolated, and locally dominant hospitals. They may be unable to muster the resources needed to sustain a complete research and teaching program that is found in academic medical centers.

Figure 17.3 illustrates how the strategic orientation and contractual relationship of physician leaders may vary by type of hospital. For free-standing community hospitals to make strategic decisions which are timely and sufficient, they may be forced to move toward one of the other cells depicted in Figure 17.3. Since the constraints to becoming an academic health center are increasingly formidable, most free-standing community hospitals may be forced to move, either to become part of a multi-institutional system or to become a hospital which is more limited in terms of its market served and the services offered.

There is nothing in the literature to indicate that multi-institutional systems score higher on strategic orientation or contractual relationship of physician leaders. Such multi-hospital systems do tend to have sophisticated planning and marketing capabilities to support physician leader integration.

FIGURE 17.3

Expected Physician Leader Characteristics and Hospital Setting

		Contractual Relationship of Physician Leadership with the Hospital	
		HIGH	LOW
Strategic Orientation of the Physician Leadership	HIGH	Multihospital System	Smaller, Geographically Isolated Hospital
	LOW	Academic Health Center	Free-standing Community Hospital

STRENGTHS AND LIMITATIONS

There are several strengths to this conceptualization of strategic decision making in hospitals. First, the emphasis of these models is on the role of the physician leader. Previous studies focused on the medical staff as a whole and ignored the dominant role of medical officials. By focusing on the chiefs of services and appointed medical officials, a model for exchange among managers, board members, and specifically identified physicians can be developed.

A second strength of this conceptual scheme is its reliance on a recommended model of decision making which is contingent on a hospital's performance on selected environmental and physician leader variables. The recommendations for change are conservative. Hospitals and physician leaders should not engage in sophisticated forms of strategic planning unless the conditions are largely satisfied.

A third strength of this conceptual scheme is the ability to make recommendations for different types of hospitals. The role of physician leaders can be substantially different in small community hospitals than in academic medical centers; these in turn may differ greatly for physician leaders in multi-unit hospital systems. The variables used to select strategic decision-making models are flexible enough to apply to different types of hospitals.

There are several limitations to the concepts and models proposed in this article. First, the models assume that there is homogeneity of requirements among physician leaders; that is, all chiefs of services will require similar levels of strategic orientation or similar contractual relationships. Clearly this is an oversimplification, since in any hospital there is likely to be wide variation by service as to competitive situation and complexity of decisions.

There are differences in the power of physician leaders as well. In some hospitals, only one or two physicians may be strategically oriented, yet this may be sufficient to move the hospital toward an integrated model. In other hospitals, the vast majority of physicians may be strategically oriented, but a few key physician leaders may be resistant. This could prevent the adoption of an integrated model. Interphysician variation can be important and should be considered in analyzing strategic decision making in any hospital.

The ability to assess the informal power relationships among physician leaders, board members, and managers is another limitation. The variables used for these models relate to formal and visible characteristics of managers and physician leaders. This article avoids questions of informal influence, historical relationships, and personality traits, important determinants of organizational behavior in the hospital setting. If the board members and physician leaders have strong informal or social ties to each other, this can drastically alter the selection of the most effective model of strategic decision making.

A third limitation concerns the identification of clear boundaries between the three different types of strategic decision making. This is an inherent problem for any organizational model. The determination of which model a hospital fits into can be muddied by scoring on the independent variables. As a result, we sometimes are faced with hospitals on the border of different categories. Further work on operationalizing the independent variables and separating out their effects is required to refine the classification rules.

A fourth limitation is the sample of hospitals on which observations were based and generalizations grounded. These were eight medium to large-sized, not-for-profit hospitals in the Northeast. Our models are biased to the extent that these hospitals are not representative of hospitals in other parts of the country.

We suggest further research to see if the models in specified hospitals are associated with changes in the scope of clinical services, a result of strategic decisions.

REFERENCES

1. Stephen M. Shortell, "Physician Involvement in Decision-Making," in Gray B.H. ed. *The New Health Care For Profit: Doctors and Hospitals in a Competitive Environment* (Institute of Medicine, National Academy Press, Washington, D.C., 1983).

2. Stephen M. Shortell, and C. Evashwick, "The Structural Configuration of U.S. Hospital Medical Staffs," *Medical Care* 19 (1982): 419–430.

3. M.V. Pauly, "Medical Staff Characteristics and Hospital Costs." *Journal of Human Resources* 13 (1978) Supplement: 77–111.

4. J.E. Harris, "The Internal Organization of Hospitals: Some Economic Implications," *Bell Journal of Economics* 8 (1977): 467–482.

5. F.A. Sloan, "The Internal Organization of Hospitals: A Descriptive Study," *Health Services Research* 15 (1980): 203–230.

6. F.A. Sloan and E.R. Becker, "Internal Organization of Hospitals and Hospital Costs," *Inquiry* 18 (1982): 224–239.

7. R.M. Heyssel et al. "Decentralized Management in a Teaching Hospital: Ten Years at Johns Hopkins," *New England Journal of Medicine* 310 (1984): 1477–1480.

18 | Work Satisfaction among Hospital Nurses

Clifford J. Mottaz

Over the years, the concept of work satisfaction has generated considerable interest. The tremendous amount of research conducted on the topic expresses this interest. Locke (1976) and others (Campbell et al. 1976) point out that the literature on work satisfaction contains over 3,000 studies and the number grows yearly. One of the major reasons for the keen interest in this area is the widely held view that work satisfaction influences such factors as productivity, absenteeism, and turnover, creating consequences for organizational effectiveness (Gruneberg 1979). Another important reason for the popularity of the concept is the belief that work satisfaction may have serious consequences for the well-being of the individual (Gruneberg 1979). Thus, the research results in this area have interested both administrators and workers considerably. Most of this research has been conducted on employees in business and industry. Recently, however, work satisfaction research has expanded to include other areas such as the health care field, nursing in particular. The intent of the present study is to investigate the nature and sources of work satisfaction among registered nurses.

Concern over the potential shortage of nursing personnel has centered attention on the problems of retention (Neumann 1973; Munro 1983). Several recent studies suggest that employee turnover among nurses is a very serious problem approaching epidemic proportions (Brief 1976; Wandelt 1981; Wolf 1981; Munro 1983). According to Donovan (1980), the national average turnover rate for registered nurses is between 30 and 40 percent, suggesting that three or four out of every ten nurses voluntar-

---

Reprinted from *Hospital & Health Services Administration* 33 (Spring 1988): 57–74, with permission, Health Administration Press.

ily leave their jobs each year. Price and Mueller (1981a) report that nurses have more than three times the turnover rate of teachers and one-and-a-half times the rate of social workers.

The implications of turnover for organizations are many though only a few examples will be mentioned here. The most obvious consequence is the financial cost associated with turnover. Turnover often results in costs for recruitment, selection, and training. Wolf (1981) suggests that a hospital may spend more than $2,500 to replace one registered nurse who quits the job. A more important consequence is that turnover may adversely affect the quality of care given to patients (Wolf 1981). If there is a shortage of nurses, or if the available nurses lack experience, the quality of nursing care may seriously decrease. Additionally, high turnover rates may have a demoralizing effect, resulting in both lower levels of productivity and lesser group cohesion. For a more detailed discussion of the consequences of turnover, see Mowday et al. (1982).

Research on work organizations in general and in the health care field strongly suggests that turnover is, for the most part, an outcome of work dissatisfaction (Diamond and Fox 1958; Saleh et al. 1965; McCloskey 1974; Price and Mueller 1981b; Seybolt et al. 1978; Wandelt et al. 1981; Weisman et al. 1981). In summing up this research, Wolf (1981) states "Although some nurses leave their jobs for unavoidable reasons, studies show that the primary reason is job dissatisfaction." Thus, it is not surprising that work satisfaction among nurses has been a major concern of hospital administrators and the nursing profession, alike.

One commonly used approach to the study of work satisfaction is the interactionist perspective. From this point of view, work satisfaction is an affective response resulting from an evaluation of the work situation. For instance, Locke (1969) has defined the concept as the "pleasurable emotional state resulting from the appraisal of one's job as achieving or facilitating the achievement of one's job values." It is widely accepted that work satisfaction is largely a function of work-related rewards and values (Katzell 1964; Vroom 1964; Locke 1969; Kalleberg 1977). Work rewards refer to the intrinsic and extrinsic benefits that workers receive from their jobs (Herzberg 1966). Rewards are the major determinants of work satisfaction, although they do vary in their effect on work attitude (Kalleberg 1977; Mottaz 1985). The relative importance of the various rewards for determining work satisfaction depends on the individual's work values. Work values refer to what the worker wants, desires, or seeks to attain from work (Locke 1969). The greater the perceived congruence between work rewards and work values, the greater the work satisfaction. If this argument is valid, then the present problem is to determine the way work rewards and values combine to influence work satisfaction among nurses.

Although the majority of studies on work satisfaction have been conducted in business and industry, the field of nursing does contain satisfaction research. Most of the studies done on the nursing profession have attempted to identify the correlates of work satisfaction. McCloskey (1974) for example, found that intrinsic rewards, such as achievement, were more strongly related to work satisfaction than extrinsic factors, such as pay. Everly and Falcione (1976) found that interpersonal relations followed by intrinsic rewards were the most important sources of satisfaction. Cronin-Stubbs (1977), in her study of recently graduated nurses, reported that achievement and recognition were the best predictors of satisfaction. A study by Godfrey (1978) revealed that lack of appreciation, poor communication, and conflict with superiors all contribute to dissatisfaction. Perry (1978), on the other hand, found supervisory support, responsibility, and promotion strongly related to work satisfaction. Still other studies have found autonomy to be the major source of work satisfaction (Slavitt et al. 1978; Seybolt and Walker 1980). Wandelt et al. (1981) argued that the quality of care given to patients most influences satisfaction among nurses. Munro (1983) discovered that the importance and challenge of work followed by work conditions were the most important determinants of work satisfaction. Finally, Neumann (1973) reported that social service (patient care), intrinsic job factors, and supervision were the best predictors of satisfaction.

While the existing literature contains many valuable clues regarding the nature and sources of work satisfaction among nurses, the findings tend to be inconsistent and confusing. As a result, it is not possible to draw any definite conclusions. There appear to be several reasons for this. The major weakness of these studies is that the models used are incomplete. A key research variable in one study may not even be considered in another study. This lack of comprehensiveness makes it impossible to compare the results of one study with those of another. A second shortcoming is that until recently, most studies have used bivariate, rather than multivariate analytical techniques to identify the determinants of work satisfaction. The use of bivariate procedures, however, does not allow for accurate assessment of the relative importance of the various determinants of work satisfaction when the effects of other important variables are held constant. A third problem is that many studies dealing with the work satisfaction of nurses have failed to control for the possible effects of important status variables such as age, tenure, gender, and education. Another limitation is that the majority of existing studies have not included samples of workers from other occupational settings. As a result, we have little comparison between nurses and members of other occupations in terms of levels and sources of work satisfaction. Additionally, a number of studies have been based on extremely small samples of nurses (50 respondents or less), making the results highly tentative. Finally, few studies on nurse satisfaction have been guided by a well-specified model of work satisfaction.

Considering nursing's critical importance and the serious consequences work satisfaction may have for both the organization and the individual, it is a topic warranting further investigation. The present study will attempt to overcome limitations of past research by: (1) analyzing the potential sources of work satisfaction by including work-related variables and status variables frequently reported in the literature, (2) using multivariate analytical procedures in addition to bivariate techniques, (3) comparing the nature and sources of nurse work satisfaction to the results for other occupational groups, (4) conducting the analysis on a broad sample of nurses, and (5) applying the interactionist model of work satisfaction.

METHODS

SAMPLE

The present research was part of a larger project examining the work attitudes of 1,615 employees representing eight occupational groups. The data were from several diverse organizations located in a large midwestern metropolitan area. Within each organization, simple random or stratified random sampling procedures ensured an adequate representation of workers from all major occupational groups participating in the study. The sample includes both full-time and part-time nurses representing diverse clinical areas; the 312 nonsupervisory registered nurses work in four large hospitals. The other occupational groups involved in the study are: university faculty (N = 169), organizational administrators (N = 167), elementary school teachers (N = 108), police officers (N = 440), secretaries (N = 112), factory foremen (N = 68), and factory workers (N = 249).

The questionnaire distributed to these employees contained sections on status variables, overall work satisfaction, perceptions of work rewards, and work values. The workers participating in the study were guaranteed complete anonymity. The overall response rate was 74 percent, while that for nurses was 79 percent.[1]

RESULTS

LEVEL OF WORK SATISFACTION

In order to put work satisfaction among nurses into perspective, the sample of nurses was compared with samples of workers from several other occupational groups. The mean score, standard deviation, and analysis of variance results for overall work satisfaction by occupational group are presented (Table 18.1). As might be expected, the findings indicate that work satisfaction generally increases from blue-collar to professional occupations. Moreover, the workers in the sample report moderate to moderately high levels of work satisfaction. Nurses, however, have a fairly low level of work satisfaction relative to other professional occupations. Only police officers, factory foremen, and factory workers report lower levels of satisfaction. Although the nurse's level of work satisfaction is not extremely low, the present findings should be viewed with some concern as even a modest amount of dissatisfaction may affect job performance.

DETERMINANTS OF WORK SATISFACTION

The present study proposes to identify the determinants of work satisfaction among nurses. To pursue this objective, multiple regression analysis was used to assess the effects of the intrinsic and extrinsic rewards on overall work satisfaction. Both standardized (B) and unstandardized (b) regression coefficients show the relative contribution and predictive power of each factor. Each occupational group was analyzed separately.

TABLE 18.1

Mean, Standard Deviations, and Analysis of Variance Results for
Overall Work Satisfaction by Occupation

	Occupation			
	University Faculty	*Administrative Personnel*	*Elementary School Teacher*	*Registered Nurse*
Mean	3.17	3.10	3.18	2.87
Standard deviation	.483	.524	.440	.480
N	(169)	(167)	(108)	(342)

The possible range for mean scores is between 1 and 4; the higher the score, the greater the work satisfaction.

In each case, the possible moderating effects of age, gender (where appropriate), education, total income, and marital status were held constant (Table 18.2).

These results suggest that the predictive power of the regression model is quite strong across all occupational groups. Together, the nine work rewards account for a considerable proportion of the variance in overall work satisfaction. This is indicated by the fact that the adjusted R^2 values range between .536 and .713. This finding suggests that work satisfaction in the various occupational groups is based essentially on the same set of determinants. At the same time, the effects of these determinants may vary in intensity.

Further analysis reveals that a similar hierarchy of determinants emerges within each of the occupational groups. Generally, intrinsic task rewards consistently and powerfully predict overall work satisfaction. This accounts for a greater proportion of the explained variance in most cases than both types of extrinsic rewards combined. Of the extrinsic rewards, social rewards appear to be a fairly strong predictor in each group, organizational rewards having a much smaller effect and emerging as a significant predictor in only a few occupational groups. Overall, the results suggest that the nature of the task itself primarily determines one's attitude toward work. Autonomous, meaningful, and interesting tasks appear to have a very strong positive effect on work satisfaction at all occupational levels. This finding calls into question the widely held notion that intrinsic rewards are not a major source of satisfaction among workers in lower-level occupations.

The results for nurses indicate that while the determinants of work satisfaction are similar to those found in other occupational groups, important differences exist. The data suggest that all three intrinsic task

TABLE 18.1 Continued

	Occupation				
Police Officer	Clerical Worker	Factory Foreman	Factory Worker	F	P
2.81	3.03	2.85	2.57	29.34	.000
.540	.530	.544	.580		
(440)	(102)	(68)	(249)		

rewards are significant predictors of satisfaction. At the same time, the results indicate that two extrinsic rewards, supervisory assistance and salary, also have a significant effect. The remaining extrinsic rewards appear to have virtually no impact on work satisfaction. The beta weights in Table 18.2 indicate that supervisory assistance is the most powerful determinant of satisfaction among nurses followed by task significance, task involvement, task autonomy, and salary, respectively.

INTERPRETATION OF RESULTS

The analysis to this point indicates that: (1) nurses report a moderate level of work satisfaction, (2) the level of satisfaction among nurses tends to be somewhat lower than in other professional occupations included in the study, and (3) the major determinants of work satisfaction are supervisory assistance, task significance, task involvement, task autonomy, and salary. While these results are informative and important, they do

TABLE 18.2

Multiple Regression of Work Satisfaction on Work Rewards
by Occupation

Work Reward	Occupation							
	University Faculty		Administrative Personnel		Elementary Teacher		Registered Nurse	
	B	b	B	b	B	b	B	b
Task autonomy	.224	.227*	.206	.270*	−.019	−.019	.223	.257
Task significance	.381	.377*	.190	.198*	.381	.429*	.300	.330*
Task involvement	.389	.386*	.389	.386*	.198	.208*	.209	.221*
Supervisory assistance	.118	.114	.127	.145	.156	.121	.320	.327*
Co-worker assistance	.171	.158*	.113	.131	.182	.169*	−.028	−.028
Working conditions	−.053	−.050	−.048	−.006	.095	.088	.009	.008
Salary	.006	.005	.086	.083	−.010	−.075	−.033	−.021
Promotional opportunity	.119	.114	.102	.078	.060	.045	.016	.015
Fringe benefits	−.036	−.026	.012	.012	.001	.008	.10	.074
	$\hat{R}^2 = -.713$		$\hat{R}^2 = .642$		$\hat{R}^2 = .536$		$\hat{R}^2 = .637$	
	$F = 38.92*$		$F = 28.02*$		$F = 10.09*$		$F = 13.06*$	

*Significant at the .05 level or better.

not illuminate the nature of the process underlying the attitude of work satisfaction.

According to the interactionist model presented earlier, work satisfaction is an an effective response resulting from an evaluation of the work situation. The evaluation process consists of assessing the balance between perceived work rewards and work values. Thus, from this perspective, work rewards and values are the main explanatory concepts accounting for work satisfaction.

If the above argument is valid, one would expect nurses to place greater value on the intrinsic task rewards, supervisory assistance, and salary than on any of the other work rewards. Moreover, because nurses express a moderate level of work satisfaction, they might perceive the returns on one or more of these valued rewards as somewhat low (Table 18.3).

The data reveal that the value hierarchy for nurses is quite similar to the hierarchy for other professional occupations. Nurses appear most concerned with intrinsic task rewards followed by extrinsic social and finally, extrinsic organizational rewards. More important, the findings

TABLE 18.2 Continued

Occupation							
Police Officer		Clerical Worker		Factory Foreman		Factory Worker	
B	b	B	b	B	b	B	b
.104	.127*	-.075	-.099	.283	.219*	-.057	-.069
.313	.362*	.225	.266*	.270	.256*	.346	.404*
.306	.308*	.367	.320*	.026	.025	.166	.164*
.053	.049	.185	.185*	.211	.258	.251	.259*
.097	.118*	.211	.255*	.225	.299*	.087	.100
.082	.098*	-.069	-.079	-.036	-.038	-.006	-.008
-.071	-.068	.111	.088	-.143	-.126	.108	.110*
.092	.074*	.067	.057	.177	.142	.123	.114*
.052	.044	.058	.055	.162	.130	-.085	-.082
$\hat{R}^2$ = .614		$\hat{R}^2$ = .699		$\hat{R}^2$ = .636		$\hat{R}^2$ = .543	
F = 64.59*		F = 22.33*		F = 11.66*		F = 25.55*	

indicate that task significance, task involvement, task autonomy, supervisory assistance, and salary, rank first through fifth, respectively.
Nurses also assign greater importance to supervisory assistance than do
workers in any other occupational group. These results support the interactionist argument that workers assess their jobs primarily in terms of
what they consider to be important in work.

An effort to account for the moderate level of work satisfaction found
among nurses suggests that they perceive the returns on one or more of
the highly valued rewards as relatively low. The data in Table 18.4 support this notion. Nurses report a fairly high level of task significance and
a moderate level of task involvement compared to workers in other
occupational groups. More important, however, the data indicate that
nurses perceive their jobs as providing relatively low levels of task autonomy, supervisory assistance, and salary. Only factory workers report
lower levels of task autonomy and salary, while only police officers
report a lower level of supervisory assistance. These results suggest that
task involvement plays a much smaller role than task autonomy, supervisory assistance, and salary.

Job tenure is a potentially important factor deserving consideration.
Work satisfaction among nurses may increase significantly with length of

TABLE 18.3

Means and Analysis of Variance Results for Work-Related Values
by Occupation

	Occupation			
Work Value	University Faculty (N = 169)	Administrative Personnel (N = 167)	Elementary Teacher (N = 108)	Registered Nurse (N = 312)
Task autonomy	8.32	7.36	7.23	7.02
Task significance	8.04	6.77	7.55	7.68
Task involvement	7.76	6.80	7.01	7.16
Supervisory assistance	5.11	5.52	5.79	6.37
Co-worker assistance	4.98	5.55	5.75	6.18
Working conditions	4.51	4.52	5.53	5.81
Salary	6.18	6.00	6.30	6.07
Promotional opportunity	3.37	3.91	2.65	3.04
Fringe benefits	2.50	2.51	2.21	2.51

*Significant at the .05 level or better.
The possible range for mean scores is between 1 and 10; the higher the score, the greater the
importance.

time in the organization. This argument is based on the notion that, in general, high-tenure workers hold better jobs than low-tenure workers. The longer people work in an organization, the more likely they are to receive more challenging job assignments, greater autonomy, and high-level extrinsic rewards. Definitive research on tenure's effect on work attitudes and perceptions calls for a longitudinal study. Nevertheless, a tentative assessment is possible using the data at hand. Data supporting this argument are presented in Table 18.5.

Work satisfaction among nurses tends to increase significantly with length of time on the job. The data further indicate that this increase is due to work rewards, as work values do not change substantially with job tenure. Moreover, the payoff is primarily in terms of intrinsic rewards. The findings reveal that task significance, task involvement, and task autonomy increase with increasing length of time on the job. Extrinsic rewards, on the other hand, do not appear to increase significantly with job tenure. While all nurses assign great importance to intrinsic rewards, these rewards are most readily available to the high-tenure nurses.

DISCUSSION

The foregoing analysis indicates that nurses express a moderate level of work satisfaction. At the same time, nurses have a significantly lower level of satisfaction than do other professional occupational groups. The

TABLE 18.3 Continued

	Occupation			
Police Officer (N = 440)	Clerical Worker (N = 102)	Factory Foreman (N = 68)	Factory Worker (N = 249)	F
7.35	6.72	6.56	5.89	16.03*
6.73	6.36	6.03	5.49	18.62*
5.91	5.66	6.29	5.30	15.22*
4.90	6.37	5.54	5.93	9.42*
5.90	5.12	5.07	5.55	4.09*
4.72	4.53	4.56	5.31	5.58*
7.07	7.38	7.62	8.07	12.50*
4.39	3.84	3.97	5.02	15.03*
2.37	2.83	2.48	2.36	9.99*

relatively low level of work satisfaction among nurses correlates with low levels of task autonomy, supervisory assistance, salary, and some lack of task involvement. Additionally, the data suggest that both work satisfaction and intrinsic rewards increase significantly with length of time in the organization. These findings seem helpful to hospital administrators and nursing educators.

Nurses enter the job with a specific set of work values. These values are influenced primarily by educational experiences, particularly nurse training. Recent studies suggest that the more-educated workers assign significantly greater importance to intrinsic rewards but less to extrinsic rewards than their less-educated counterparts (Wright and Hamilton 1979; Mottaz 1984). This effect of nursing education is clear from the data in Table 18.4. Nurses are trained to care for the health needs of patients; using these skills and abilities to make responsible decisions is extremely important to them. Thus, the importance of task autonomy is not surprising.

Today, the nurse works almost exclusively in the hospital. The internal structure of the hospital, like that of other large-scale organizations, is based on bureaucratic principals—a division of labor based on functional specialization, a hierarchy of authority, and a system of rules, regulations, and procedures governing task activities. As a result, the

TABLE 18.4

Mean and Analysis of Variance Results for Perceptions of Work Rewards by Occupation

Work Value	Occupation			
	University Faculty (N = 169)	Administrative Personnel (N = 167)	Elementary Teacher (N = 108)	Registered Nurse (N = 312)
Task autonomy	3.32	3.09	2.92	2.72
Task significance	3.23	3.08	3.25	3.12
Task involvement	3.24	2.87	3.21	2.98
Supervisory assistance	2.97	2.76	2.82	2.68
Co-worker assistance	3.14	3.01	3.30	3.05
Working conditions	2.49	2.53	2.44	2.48
Salary	2.00	2.32	1.97	1.97
Promotional opportunity	2.39	2.20	2.48	2.30
Fringe benefits	2.50	2.51	2.21	2.51

*Significant at the .05 level of better.

The possible range for mean scores is between 1 and 4; the higher the score, the greater the reward.

opportunity for nurse self-direction is very limited. Generally, nurses feel that their input regarding health care is not highly valued by either physicians or administrators. A survey of approximately 17,000 nurses found that 66 percent of the nurses sampled felt the administration unresponsive to their suggestions and 70 percent felt completely eliminated from the decision-making process (Godfrey 1978). This lack of autonomy reduces work satisfaction.

Another outcome of limited autonomy is that nurses are very dependent on supervisors in the performance of daily nursing tasks. Consequently, competent, friendly, and supportive supervision plays a major role in work satisfaction. However, a number of recent studies indicate that nurses are very dissatisfied with the quality of supervision they receive (Johnston 1976; Everly and Falcione 1976; Cronin-Stubbs 1977; Wolf 1981). Godfrey (1978) found that the major complaints regarding supervision include a lack of management and leadership skills, lack of support, lack of availability, failure to follow through on complaints, and abuse of authority. Several researchers attribute the problem of poor supervision to the failure of most educational programs and hospitals to provide nurses with the necessary management training (Godfrey 1978; Cronin-Stubbs 1977).

An additional problem concerns the task itself. Several studies indicate that a good deal of the nurse's time is spent on non-nursing activities (Godfrey 1978; Johnston 1976; Wolf 1981) like paperwork and housekeeping. Nurses feel this affects the quality of health care patients

TABLE 18.4 Continued

Occupation				
Police Officer (N = 440)	Clerical Worker (N = 102)	Factory Foreman (N = 68)	Factory Worker (N = 249)	F
2.75	2.87	2.97	2.14	141.16*
2.87	3.08	2.96	2.82	22.38*
2.76	2.81	2.57	2.17	78.05
2.58	3.02	2.72	2.93	16.81*
2.95	3.14	2.95	2.90	12.72*
2.34	2.64	2.52	2.61	5.22*
2.02	2.12	2.01	1.92	8.07*
1.97	2.30	2.42	2.15	15.07*
2.37	2.83	2.48	2.36	9.99*

TABLE 18.5

Means and Analysis of Variance Results for Work Satisfaction,
Work Rewards, and Work Values by Years of Job Tenure

Job Tenure (years)	0–1	2–4	5–7	8⁺	F	P
Work satisfaction	2.81	2.88	3.076	3.22	4.53	.005
Rewards						
Task autonomy	2.53	2.73	2.79	2.86	3.41	.020
Task significance	2.89	3.10	3.19	3.40	6.94	.000
Task involvement	2.78	2.99	3.02	3.17	2.93	.047
Supervisory assistance	2.80	2.83	3.06	2.83	1.79	.153
Co-worker assistance	2.97	3.03	3.12	3.10	.56	.641
Working conditions	2.25	2.26	2.39	2.50	1.25	.295
Salary	2.07	1.96	1.92	1.93	.49	.686
Promotional opportunity	2.26	2.29	2.30	2.38	.28	.839
Fringe benefits	2.50	2.58	2.43	2.50	.23	.876

receive. Johnston (1976) reports that nurses spend only a third of their time on health care responsibilities. Excessive time spent on non-nursing duties reduces task involvement in turn affecting work satisfaction. For the most part, people are happiest doing what they have been trained to do.

Salary also appears to be an important problem for nurses. Despite findings in earlier studies, recent research suggests that salary is a growing concern among nurses. In fact, a few of these studies find salary to be the major determinant of work dissatisfaction (Thompson 1981; Wandelt et al. 1981). When nurses compare their salary to that of other professionals in the hospital, namely physicians and administrators, they feel grossly underpaid and hence dissatisfied with work.

To increase work satisfaction and to reduce employee turnover, several working conditions require improvement. First and foremost, analysis suggests that it is necessary to focus on the task itself to enhance intrinsic rewards. This indicates some type of job redesign program aimed at developing more autonomous, meaningful, and interesting jobs.

In this regard, efforts should be made to increase task autonomy by providing nurses with greater opportunities to participate in the decision-making process, particularly in matters directly affecting them. The decentralization of nursing units would increase autonomy by allowing nurses to manage their own staffing, scheduling, and educational opportunities. Moreover, committees using input from nurses as well as other personnel could deal with larger organizational problems such as recruitment, retention, and salary procedures. More important, a similar strategy could apply to patient care. Wolf (1981) reports that some hospitals have experimented with a joint practice approach, whereby a doctor and a nurse together design a plan for the care of patients. Other hospitals have established joint practice committees for this purpose. Participation and involvement in the decision-making process conveys to nurses the notion that they are important contributors in the health care enterprise, rather than passive subordinates of administrators and physicians.

Another strategy for increasing intrinsic rewards is eliminating or greatly reducing non-nursing responsibilities so that nurses can spend more time on health care responsibilities. This approach would require employing additional domestic and clerical staff or using volunteers.

Despite the probable benefits of job redesign programs, this strategy has not been used as a panacea for low work satisfaction among nurses. For one thing, these programs tend to be extremely costly in terms of reorganization, retraining, additional staff, etc. Additionally, some aspects of any occupation are dull and repetitive in nature and hence difficult, if not impossible, to redesign. In this regard, realistic training programs are vitally important. All the duties, responsibilities, and authority associated with the job should be thoroughly discussed and understood in order to avoid unrealistic job expectations.

The evidence presented here further suggests that improvement in the quality of immediate supervision would help increase the level of work satisfaction among nurses. Strong supervisory assistance is necessary to provide a basis of support and confidence in task performance. Apparently, few hospitals train nurses for management roles. Instead, promotion to supervisory positions is based on nursing experience and skills. While these factors are important, leadership skills are as important in quality supervision. Thus, hospital or nursing administrators should probably provide management training for nurses promoted to supervisory positions. In the long run, these training programs are much less expensive than turnover costs.

Finally, a nurse's salary must adequately reflect level of training and importance in the health care system. Pay is a complex aspect of work, serving not only to justify the work activity itself, but also to convey personal worth and competence. Thus, it is not too surprising that perceptions of pay inequity result in lower levels of work satisfaction. At the same time, salary is not the most important source of satisfaction. Increases in pay without increases in intrinsic rewards and quality supervision may have little effect on work satisfaction.

In conclusion, the findings of this study must be viewed cautiously.

Further research on nurses in other metropolitan areas is necessary. Nevertheless, this research has hopefully provided insight into the nature of work satisfaction among nurses.

APPENDIX

MEASUREMENT

The factors in this study include overall work satisfaction, work values, and work rewards. Regarding the latter, nine work rewards frequently reported to have strong effects on work satisfaction were selected from the literature. The work of Katz and Van Maanen (1977) shows these rewards to represent three distinct areas of work: intrinsic task rewards, extrinsic social rewards, and extrinsic organizational rewards.

WORK SATISFACTION

Overall work satisfaction is defined as the worker's affective response to the total work situation. This scale was constructed in a four-point Likert format from three commonly used global items, slightly revised for the present study. the items are as follows:

1. Generally speaking, I am satisfied with this job.
2. If I had the opportunity to start over again, I would choose the same type of work I presently do.
3. Taking into consideration all things about my job, I am very satisfied.

The reliability of this scale was assessed by Cronbach's alpha which yielded a reliability coefficient of .772. With regard to validity, a factor analysis of the items, along with those of several other work dimensions, revealed that the items formed a clearly distinct factor.

Intrinsic Task Rewards

Three intrinsic rewards associated with the task were selected for the analysis. They are task autonomy, task significance, and task involvement. Task autonomy refers to the degree of self-direction in task performance. Task significance refers to the degree to which the task is perceived as a significant contribution to the work process. Task involvement refers to the degree to which the task is considered interesting and rewarding in itself. The scales used to measure these three factors were constructed by the author and reported in a previous article (Mottaz 1981). Each scale consists of seven four-point Likert-type items. Cronbach's alpha produced a reliability coefficient of .917 for the autonomy scale, .790 for the task significance scale, and .875 for the task involvement scale. Validity was evaluated through factor analysis yielding distinct factors.

Extrinsic Social and Organizational Rewards

Six extrinsic rewards associated with the work context were included in the analysis. The items used to measure these factors were drawn from several widely used scales reported in Robinson et al. (1969) and slightly modified for present purposes. Each scale consists of four to six four-point Likert-type items. Social rewards include two factors: (1) supervisory assistance—the degree to which supervisors are perceived as supportive and helpful in job matters, and (2) colleague assistance—the degree to which colleagues are perceived as supportive and helpful. Cronbach's alpha yielded reliability coefficients of .822 and .821 for the two scales, respectively. Organizational rewards include four factors: (1) adequate working conditions—the extent to which there are adequate resources, supplies, equipment, and time, (2) pay equity—the extent to which workers feel their salary is comparable to that of others performing the same or similar jobs, (3) promotional opportunity—the extent to which the job provides opportunity for advancement, and (4) adequate fringe benefits—the degree to which the worker feels the pension plan, medical coverage, and time off are sufficient. The reliability coefficients reported for the four scales are .712, .832, .815, and .732, respectively. Validity was assessed through factor analysis again yielding distinct factors.

Work Values

Respondents were asked to rate each of the nine work rewards discussed above in terms of importance. Responses ranged from 1 to 10. The higher the score, the greater the importance.

Demographic Characteristics

Several demographic factors possibly related to work satisfaction were included in the research. These factors are gender, age, educational level, total income, marital status, work shift, and length of time on the job.

NOTE

1. The measurement procedures for research variables appear in the Appendix.

REFERENCES

Brief, Arthur P. "Turnover among Hospital Nurses: A Suggested Model." *Journal of Nursing Administration* 6 (1976): 55–58.

Campbell, A., P.E. Converse, and W.L. Rogers. *The Quality of American Life: Perceptions, Evaluations, and Satisfactions.* New York: Russell Sage, 1976.

Cronin-Stubbs, Diane. "Job Satisfaction and Dissatisfaction among New Graduate Staff." *Journal of Nursing Administration* 7 (1977): 44–49.

Diamond, L.K., and D.J. Fox. "Turnover among Hospital Staff Nurses." *Nursing Outlook* 6 (1958): 388–91.

Donovan, Lynn. "The Shortage: Good Jobs Are Going Begging These Days, So Why Not Be Choosey?" *RN* 43 (1980): 20–27.

Everly, G.S., and R.L. Falcione. "Perceived Dimensions of Job Satisfaction for Staff Nurse." *Nursing Research* 25 (1976): 346–48.

Godfrey, M. "Job Satisfaction or Should That Be Dissatisfaction?" *Nursing* 8 (1978): 89–102.

Gruneberg, Michael. *Understanding Job Satisfaction.* New York: John Wiley & Sons, 1979.

Herzberg, F. *Work and the Nature of Man.* Cleveland: World Publishing Co., 1966.

Johnston, R. "Nurses and Job Satisfaction: A Review of Some Research Findings." *Australian Nurses Journal* 5 (1976): 23–27.

Kalleberg, Arne L. "Work Values and Job Rewards: A Theory of Job Satisfaction." *American Sociological Review* 42 (1977): 124–43.

Katz, R., and J. Van Maanen. "The Loci of Work Satisfaction: Job Interaction and Policy." *Human Relations* 30 (1977): 469–86.

Katzell, R.A. In *Man in a World of Work*, edited by H. Borow. Boston: Houghton-Mifflin, 1964.

Locke, Edwin A. "What Is Job Satisfaction?" *Organizational Behavior and Human Performance* 4 (1969): 309–36.

——. In *Handbook of Industrial and Organizational Psychology*, edited by M.D. Dunnette. Chicago: Rand McNally, 1976.

McCloskey, Joanne. "Influence of Rewards and Incentives on Staff Nurse Turnover Rate." *Nursing Research* 23 (1974): 239–47.

Mottaz, Clifford J. "Some Determinants of Work Alienation." *The Sociological Quarterly* 22 (1981): 515–29.

——. "Education and Work Satisfaction." *Human Relations* 37 (1984): 985–1004.

——. "The Relative Importance of Intrinsic and Extrinsic Rewards as Determinants of Work Satisfaction." *The Sociological Quarterly* 26 (1985): 365–85.

Mowday, R.T., L.W. Porter, and Richard Steers. *Employee-Organization Linkages. The Psychology of Commitment, Absenteeism, and Turnover.* New York: Academic Press, 1982.

Munro, B.H. "Job Satisfaction among Recent Graduates of Schools of Nursing." *Nursing Research* 36 (1983): 350–55.

Neumann, Edna. "Job Satisfaction among Nursing Service Personnel." *Communicating Nursing Research* 6 (1973): 165–76.

Perry, Henry B. "The Job Satisfaction of Physician Assistants: A Causal Analysis." *Social Science and Medicine* 12 (1978): 195–212.

Price, James L., and Charles W. Mueller. *Professional Turnover: The Case of Nurses.* New York: S.P. Medical and Scientific Books, 1981a.

———. "A Causal Model of Turnover for Nurses." *Academy of Management Journal* 24 (1981b): 543–65.

Robinson, J.P., R. Athanasion, and K. Head. *Measures of Occupational Attitudes and Occupational Characteristics.* Ann Arbor: University of Michigan, 1969.

Saleh, S., et al. "Why Nurses Leave Their Jobs—An Analysis of Female Turnover." *Personnel Administration* 27 (1965): 25–28.

Seybolt, J.W., C. Pavett, and D.D. Walker. "Turnover among Nurses: It Can Be Managed." *Journal of Nursing Administration* 8 (1978): 4–9.

Seybolt, J.W., and D.D. Walker. "Attitude Survey Proves to Be a Powerful Tool for Reversing Turnover." *Hospitals* 54 (1980): 77–80.

Slavitt, Dinah B., Paula L. Stamps, Eugene B. Piedmont, and Ann Marie B. Haase. "Nurses' Satisfaction with Their Work Situation." *Nursing Research* 17 (1978): 114–20.

Thompson, Linda. "Job Satisfaction of Nurse Anesthetists." *American Association of Nurse Anesthetists Journal* 49 (1981): 43–51.

Vroom, V. *Work and Motivation.* New York: Wiley, 1964.

Wandelt, M.A., R.M. Pierce, and R.R. Widdowson. "Why Nurses Leave Nursing and What Can Be Done about It." *American Journal of Nursing* 81 (1981): 72–77.

Weisman, C.S., C.S. Alexander, and G.A. Chase. "Evaluating Reasons for Nursing Turnover." *Evaluation and the Health Professions* 4 (1981): 107–27a.

Wolf, G.A. "Nursing Turnover: Some Causes and Solutions." *Nursing Outlook* 29 (1981): 233–36.

Wright, J., and R. Hamilton. "Education and Job Attitudes among Blue-Collar Workers." *Sociology of Work and Occupations* 6 (1979): 59–83.

19 The Medical Staff of the Future

Stephen M. Shortell

To develop effective hospital-physician relationships in these troubled times requires the ingenuity of a rose gardener working in a very poor climate. The old methods of providing care and attention no longer work. Under pressures of cost containment, increased competition, continued changes in technology, and social and public expectations, physicians have become increasingly concerned about their roles as professionals, as artisans of their craft, as entrepreneurs, and even as bureaucrats. Hospitals are feeling the same pressures even more acutely. The result is a climate ripe for mistrust, conflict, negativism, and entropy. But it is also ripe for establishing a new kind of "garden," one that provides a fertile basis for developing long-term productive relationships. The key lies in the willingness and ability of hospitals and physicians to give up old ways of thinking and behaving and to build a new kind of social contract—a social contract based on paradox, ambiguity and change, risk, and the pursuit of "responsible excellence." The ability of hospitals and physicians to develop such a contract is a key factor that will shape the delivery of health services over the remainder of the century. . . .

Cost-containment pressures, increased competition, the "corporatization" of health care, and the growth of health care teams are at one and the same time pushing hospitals and physicians closer together and yet farther apart. These factors give rise to the . . . characteristics of paradox, ambiguity and change, risk, and responsible excellence. . . .

Excerpted from the article in *Frontiers of Health Services Management* 1 (February 1985): 3–48, with permission, Health Administration Press.

316

SHAPING THE FUTURE: CREATING GOOD NEWS

ASSUMPTIONS

The designs and guidelines to follow in shaping the future delivery of health care are based on six assumptions, shown in Figure 19.1. The first assumption is that prospective payment in some form will continue to exist and, in fact, will be expanded to cover nearly all payers of care for services provided on both an inpatient and an ambulatory care basis. Such payment systems may or may not be based on the current DRG approach and will certainly *not* be based on the current DRG classification system. DRGs will undergo continual refinement, particularly through the incorporation of clinical staging criteria[1] and improvements in disease severity assessment.[2] However, the underlying concept of prospective payment will remain and will create continuing incentives for hospitals and physicians to provide more cost-effective care.

The second assumption is that the corporatization of American health care will continue to grow. This growth will take place both horizontally and vertically. Freestanding hospitals will join multiunit hospital systems, and multiunit systems will continue to aggregate into megasystems

FIGURE 19.1

Assumptions Shaping the Future Delivery of Health Care

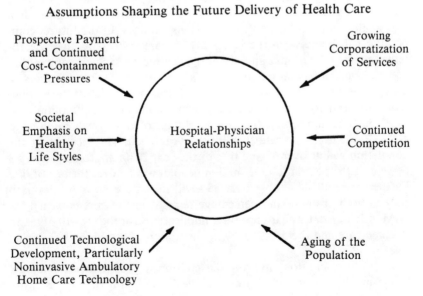

such as those currently represented by American Healthcare System (AHS) and Voluntary Hospitals of America (VHA). There will be fewer systems (or at least slower growth in the number of systems), but the systems will be larger. Further, the hospital systems will integrate forward into ambulatory primary care, home care, ambulatory surgery, hospice care, chemical dependency units, renal dialysis, long-term care, and related initiatives. Backward integration into supplier services will also occur through joint ventures with pharmaceutical and hospital supply firms—in addition to the currently prevalent group purchasing arrangements. A significant portion of this corporate growth will be of a for-profit nature, initiated by *both* investor-owned and voluntary systems. Joint ventures between investor-owned companies and voluntary not-for-profit hospitals will become commonplace.

This growing corporatization raises a number of medical staff issues, including relationships to the corporate office, involvement in decision making, degree of autonomy at the local level, delineation of privileges, and related issues. Current data indicate that only 15 percent of multiunit systems have a single medical staff organization, almost all of these being geographically concentrated systems.[3] Data also indicate that more centralized systems in which individual local hospital boards have little autonomy are less likely to have physician involvement in the local board.

A third assumption is that competition will continue and, if anything, intensify. Up to now, competition has been primarily between individual and small groups of hospitals for inpatient services. In the future, competition will be between the larger health care systems as they vie for larger shares of national and not just local markets. Such competition will focus much less on inpatient care and more on new product/service lines, including a variety of initiatives related to ambulatory care, long-term care, and home health care, as well as nonrelated health initiatives.

A fourth assumption is that the percentage of elderly will continue to grow. Predictions indicate that by the year 2000, 12.2 percent of the population will be over 65 and that by the year 2030, approximately 18.3 percent of the population (55 million people) will be over the age of 65.[4] Further, the old old—those over 85—will increase even more dramatically in both absolute and percentage terms over the next 60 years. As previously noted, this has important implications for the growth of team-oriented care and the accompanying disruption of established physician roles.

A fifth assumption involves the continued growth of technology. While much of this will continue to be in the form of high-intensity lifesaving technology (for example, the artificial heart), the most important developments may lie in the growth of noninvasive, smaller-scale technologies that can be used in ambulatory care settings and patients' homes. The changing locus of technology will force changes in the relative dependencies of hospitals, physicians, other health professionals, and patients on each other.

The final assumption is that the growing interest in healthier life-styles will continue. In varying degrees, hospitals, physicians, and other health professionals will be involved in this continuing trend. At the same time, much of it will take place outside the formal health care system. This development will change the way in which consumers view their health and, in turn, their views of hospitals, physicians, and other care givers. Providers will be asked to assist more in actively promoting health rather than treating disease or curing illness. The locus of decision making will be centered more on the consumer and less on the hospital or physician. . . .

ALTERNATIVE HOSPITAL–MEDICAL STAFF ORGANIZATIONAL DESIGNS

There are six principles underlying the creation of effective medical staff organizational designs. These are: (1) the need to recognize differences in professional socialization and training, (2) the need to maximize effective problem identification, (3) the need to maximize effective communication, (4) the need to maximize the generation of useful alternatives, (5) the need to maximize effective implementation, and (6) the need to maximize professional and organizational learning. These principles become the criteria against which to evaluate the ability of alternative designs to embrace or incorporate the characteristics of paradox, ambiguity and change, risk, and comparative advantage.

Three important differences in socialization and training between physicians and administrators need to be recognized: (1) the differences between the micro perspective of the physician and the macro perspective of the administrator;[5] (2) differences in the "rules of evidence" used for evaluating decisions; and (3) differences in time orientation. Physicians are trained to provide the best possible care to *individual* patients—the micro focus. A high degree of *autonomy* is required in order to effectively discharge one's clinical responsibilities to individual patients. Administrators are trained to think in terms of organization-wide issues and the larger political economy within which health care is delivered— the macro perspective. Dealing with these issues requires more collaborative, or less "autonomous," decision making. Both groups need to have a greater understanding of the strengths and limitations of each other's perspective and requirements.

While medicine as practiced remains largely an art, a major portion of medical education continues to emphasize the scientific component. As such, physicians look for "hard data" and indicators of cause-and-effect relationships in evaluating clinical alternatives. Since they also tend to carry this orientation over to other aspects of their lives, they frequently become perplexed and frustrated in dealing with administrators who, by necessity and by the nature of administrative reality, are forced to base decisions often on "softer" qualitative information — often without knowing in advance what the cause-and-effect relationships are and sometimes even without having full agreement on the desired outcomes.

This problem is compounded by the difference in time orientation. Physicians generally operate on a short-run time perspective based on patient-treatment contingencies, while administrators typically operate on a longer-run time perspective based on three-year and five-year strategic plans and one-year operational plans. Thus, physicians become impatient with what seems to be unresponsiveness to their requests. Effective designs will be those that help each group see and understand the different mind-sets operating in regard to "rules of evidence" and "time frames" for decision making. Identifying the relevant problems is particularly important because often physician-administrator conflict arises from a premature rush for solutions. The controversy and conflict this generates could be minimized by taking more time in mutually identifying relevant problems. Effective designs will be those that will assist administrators and physicians in identifying the most important problems and arriving at a fuller understanding of these problems.

Communication is at the center of all relationships. Administrators and physicians need to improve their individual interpersonal skills, but in addition, organizational designs that facilitate communication can be put in place. In similar fashion, designs exist that tend to promote creativity in developing alternative solutions. Another common problem aggravating physician-administrator relationships lies in implementing what has been agreed to. Each party needs to understand the incentives, both financial and nonfinancial, facing the other party. Again, an effective design will be one that facilitates implementation.

A final issue concerns the professional and organizational learning that lies behind all of the above principles. Administrators and physicians need to develop a commitment to mutual learning. Physicians need to keep up with the latest advances in knowledge and refine their skills. Administrators require the same for themselves and their organizations. The real problem in undertaking new initiatives is not the possibility of failure, but rather the failure to learn from the experience. These principles — recognizing differences in socialization and training, maximizing problem identification, improving communication, developing creative alternatives, and facilitating implementation — all result in a greater probability that learning will occur. It is the learning that results from *both* success and failure that makes possible corrective actions and future improvements. It is also essential to developing mutual trust and respect.

ALTERNATIVE DESIGNS

The present environment calls for:

- More physician involvement in hospital-wide decision making, particularly involving those physicians with positive attitudes toward the hospital and who are willing to take action.[6]
- Longer appointments for chiefs of staff, including, for example, two years as president-elect, two years as president, and two years as past president, in order to assure greater continuity of leadership and involvement in decision making.
- Full-time or part-time paid medical directors.
- More stringent review of privileges, involving assessment of cost-effectiveness and longer probationary periods before awarding full privileges.
- By-laws that better reflect community needs; that is, by-laws that attempt to match the composition and practices of the staff to the defined needs of the community.

These actions are necessary, but they are insufficient: they are primarily Band-aids. They represent mere trimming of the garden, while what is needed is more radical pruning or replanting. To be sure, such pruning will involve more bloodletting for both physicians and administrators entangled on the thorns of past behavior. But what is needed is fundamental change in the design of the relationship itself.

Organizational design may be defined as the grouping of activities to achieve the organization's goals and objectives. It explicitly includes the allocation of authority, responsibility, accountability, roles, power, decision making, information flow, and rewards. It is a dynamic process involving the recognition that inherent in any design is a set of solutions and a set of problems.[7]

Hospitals are *incompletely designed organizations*. The nonphysician part of the hospital is typically organized along *functional* lines; that is, nursing, finance, personnel, materials management, dietary, housekeeping, and so on. However, it is an incomplete functional organization in that it does not contain within itself the curing component — namely, the medical staff. The physician portion — the traditional medical staff organization — is typically organized along *divisional* lines; that is, the division of medicine, surgery, obstetrics, pediatrics, and so on, with various subspecialists concentrated within each division. However, the typical medical staff is an incomplete divisional design in that, while it contains relevant clinical specialists, it does not contain the relevant clinical and administrative support services — nursing, personnel, finance, medical records, and so on. This, of course, has resulted in the classic dual hierarchy of authority originally noted by Smith[8] and explored more recently by others.[9] While these differences have long been noted and the reasons for them (social, political, historical, and economic) well understood, proposals for reconciling them have been flawed by an inadequate understanding of the twofold "incompleteness" noted above. The usual recommendations are to develop more integrating committees and task forces, to involve more physicians in hospital management and governance, and, in turn, to involve more hospital managers, nurses, and other health professionals in medical staff activities. (Indeed, recent studies suggest a marked increase in these activities.) For example, the average number of medical staff committees has grown from 8 in 1973 to 14 in 1982; the percentage of hospitals with physicians as voting members of the board has increased from 67 percent in 1973 to 98 percent in 1982; and the percentage of physicians on the executive committee of hospital boards has increased from 26 percent in 1973 to 44 percent in 1982.[10] However, these mechanisms, as noted above, are insufficient to meet the current challenges.

Aside from the current traditional staff structure, there are three primary alternative models to consider. The first is to make the hospital a totally functional organization which deals at arm's length with the totally independent medical staff organization or corporation. We call this the *independent-corporate* model. The second is to make the hospital a "completed" divisional organization by integrating the major functional areas within medical divisions. We call this the *divisional* model. The third is to leave present structure (hospital and physician components) as it exists, but create a parallel medical staff organization structure whose function is to provide the integration and long-run strategic planning required by both components. We call this the *parallel* model. The following sections develop these models in some depth, taking into account the degree to which they might meet the earlier defined criteria for developing more effective relationships between physicians and administrators.

THE INDEPENDENT-CORPORATE MODEL

The independent-corporate model is shown in Figure 19.2. As indicated, the medical staff becomes a separate legal entity which negotiates with the hospital for its services in return for receiving the hospital's functional patient care and administrative support services. There are no *hospital-generated* medical staff by-laws, credentialing, quality assurance, or related mechanisms as such. These responsibilities are taken over exclusively by the group of independent physicians that enters into a contract with the hospital. Depending on their relative bargaining power,[11] hospitals may, of course, require that such physician groups have in place certain commonly accepted standards and review criteria. Licensure laws and regulations may also impose such requirements. But the difference from current practice is that this would be solely the responsibility of the independent group of physicians. Obviously, in a competitive market it would be to the physician group's advantage to develop quality assurance systems that could be used as a selling point to develop contracts with the more desirable hospitals in the community. In fact, again depending on the degree of competitiveness in local markets, there would exist incentives for physician groups to develop certain quality and cost standards that go beyond those set by the Joint Commission on Accreditation of Hospitals and other licensing and regulatory bodies.

The independent-corporate model may seem farfetched. However, some hospitals and their medical staffs are giving it serious consideration. Further, it is a model which has had a rather long history in the delivery of prepaid health care, where it is recognized as the *group model* HMO. The classic and longest-standing example is the Kaiser Health Plan, which contracts with the Kaiser-Permanente Medical Group. To an increasing extent, many hospitals are moving towards this kind of relationship with their medical staffs in terms of preferred provider organization arrangements. However, these arrangements are usually added to or overlaid on the traditional medical staff organization structure. The independent-corporate model involves complete legal separation of hospital and physician.

It is important to consider the possible advantages and disadvantages of this model from the viewpoint of both physicians and hospitals. From the physicians' perspective, there are significant advantages in autonomy. Legal decisions (*Darling* v. *Charleston Community Memorial Hospital*) and new JCAH accreditation requirements[12] according hospital governing boards and administrations more responsibility for the quality of care have curtailed the ability of the medical staff to independently develop, implement, and monitor standards of medical practice. Estab-

FIGURE 19.2

The Independent-Corporate Model

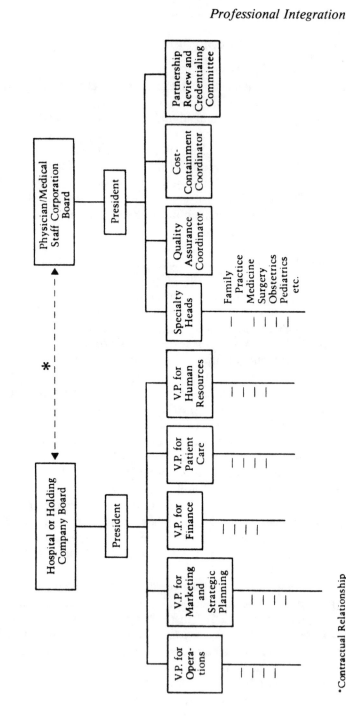

*Contractual Relationship

lishing an independent legal entity would once again give physicians sole responsibility for developing their own governing by-laws, quality assurance, and credentialing mechanisms. Hospitals and accreditation/ licensing groups could still influence these developments and, perhaps, impose even stricter criteria for entering into a contractual relationship; but the influence would be less direct than what currently exists. This would be particularly true in multihospital communities, where physician groups could attempt to play off one hospital against another.

Another potential advantage to physicians from the independent model is that it would eliminate the tying of privileges to volume of use or the cost-effectiveness of the individual physician's practice. In fact, under this model, there would be no "privileges" as such. Rather, the hospital would enter into a contractual relationship with the physician group or establish exclusive contracts with several groups based on identifiable product or service lines. All eligible, qualified members of the group would have "usage" rights to the hospital, and it would be up to the physician group to police its members regarding use, cost, and quality of care. Of course, hospitals would reserve the right to review these data as well (although it might be in a more aggregate form and not on a physician-by-physician basis) and to terminate or renegotiate the contract within a mutually agreed-upon time frame.

A third advantage to physicians from the independent model is that they would be exempt from the accreditation, licensing, and regulatory apparatus directed at hospitals. Nothing, of course, could prevent these same bodies from turning their attention to the independent medical staff corporations or groups, but in the short run some autonomy would be bought. Further, many physicians would feel somewhat more comfortable dealing with these "third parties" directly through their own group leadership than being "represented" by the hospital.

The main disadvantages to physicians involve legal and organizational change issues. Incorporating as a separate legal entity may mean that hospital-based physicians could not purchase malpractice insurance at the same rates that they receive through the hospital. This is a major concern because the number and size of claims and the amounts of premiums are again increasing.[13] The organizational change issue involves possible resistance on the part of many physicians to dissolving their hospital ties. This is particularly true of older members of the staff and others who may have established considerable loyalty to the hospital. It may also be true of those physicians (approximately 25 percent) who are currently compensated by the hospital. While many physicians may be frustrated with current relationships and see some clear-cut advantages to separate status, it may be difficult for the medical staff as an *entire group* to decide to pursue independent status. As previously noted, physicians differ greatly by specialty, age, and philosophy of practice, and these differences may impede achieving the degree of consensus needed for establishing an independent body. For example, under the independent model there might be fewer checks and balances on physician behavior, with power unduly concentrated in the clinical chiefs of the corporation. This could result in problems for younger physicians, women physicians, physicians of minority ethnic backgrounds, and foreign-trained physicians.

From the hospital's perspective, the disadvantages of the independent model would appear to outweigh the advantages. In brief, the hospital loses control over the medical staff. The hospital may also find it more difficult to coordinate the caring and curing functions. In independent arm's-length transactions, the primary means of integration is the financial arrangement and other conditions built into the terms of the contract. These require time and effort to police. In contrast, when a group is part of the organization, one can more easily use leadership skills, communication, information, decision-making structures, culture, rewards, and people as integrating mechanisms.

A possible advantage is that the hospital becomes a "cleaner," functionally oriented organization. Without the voluntary medical staff, the caring and administrative support functions of the hospital may be more efficiently and effectively organized. In particular, the power, authority, influence, and perhaps effectiveness of the nursing staff may increase.

It is also useful to consider the independent-corporate model in terms of the six underlying principles developed earlier and the characteristics of paradox, ambiguity and change, risk, and comparative advantage. First, the independent-corporate model explicitly recognizes differences between physicians and administrators through the creation of the separate groups. But the creation of these two separate groups does little in terms of embracing the paradox and ambiguity of such relationships. It is a design that attempts to simplify the world, but in so doing places tremendous demands on both groups for developing effective interorganizational relationships. In fact, the design does little to address the remaining underlying principles involving the ability to identify problems, facilitate communication, generate alternatives, promote implementation, and maximize learning. Achievement of these objectives would depend greatly on the interest and skills of the leaders involved in implementing the terms and conditions specified in the contractual relationship. This might be particularly problematic for the physician group because of the difficulty involved in having one physician trying to represent many different specialty viewpoints.

On the other hand, the independent-corporate model could facilitate risk taking and the promotion of comparative advantage. Each group acting alone and in its own perceived best interest might be more willing and better able to try new and innovative approaches to developing more cost-effective care. Thus, hospitals might more readily develop urgi-centers, ambulatory surgery centers, home health agencies, and related ventures without being encumbered by the elaborate committee structure of the traditional medical staff organization. In similar fashion, physicians might develop new initiatives without having to touch base with hospital officials regarding whether or not physician plans fit in with the hospital's overall plans or its capital or operating budgets.

In regard to comparative advantage, the independent-corporate model might allow each side to more clearly understand its comparative advantage — specifically, the community-wide caring and administrative support function of the hospital and the individual-patient-centered curing function of the physicians. By maintaining an arm's-length relationship, each group might be better able to develop relationships that build on each other's strengths while enjoying greater freedom to initiate new ideas. The disadvantage may be in the inability to *jointly* respond quickly to changes in the environment and new market opportunities. The independent-corporate model maximizes each group's ability to respond more quickly to individual opportunities but not to those requiring collaboration.

Table 19.1 presents a comparison of the potential advantages and disadvantages of alternative medical staff organizational designs. The second column summarizes the possible pros and cons of the independent-corporate design. For the most part, it would appear that the disadvantages outweigh the advantages. Given the degree of change from present practice which this design represents, it is unlikely to be adopted by many hospitals or physicians, although it may be a viable model for a few hospitals and their medical staffs in selected multihospital communities. It also serves as an example of what hospital-physician relationships might look like in the future if viable alternative models are not developed.

THE DIVISIONAL MODEL

Figure 19.3 shows the divisional model of medical staff organization. This model is characterized by the placement of such functional areas as finance, nursing, personnel, and marketing within each division, organized around groups of several specialties as shown in Figure 19.4 or broken down more finely among product or service line groupings as

TABLE 19.1

Potential Advantages and Disadvantages
of Medical Staff Organization Designs

	Design			
Criterion	*Traditional**	*Independent-Corporate*	*Divisional*	*Parallel*
Recognizes and deals with professional differences	–	+	+	+
Facilitates identification of problems	–	–	+†	+‡
Facilitates communication	–	–	+†	+‡
Facilitates generation of alternatives	–	–	+†	+‡
Facilitates implementation	–	–	+†	+‡
Promotes learning	–	–	+	+
Incorporates paradox	–	–	+	+
Incorporates ambiguity and change	–	–	+	+
Incorporates risk	–	+	+	+
Promotes comparative advantage ("responsible excellence")		+	+	+

*The minuses *are not* meant to suggest that the traditional medical staff organization structure *cannot* meet these criteria; rather, they are meant to suggest that, relative to other models, it is more difficult for the traditional model to meet them.

†The divisional design may lose some of these advantages when dealing with organization-wide issues.

‡Meeting these criteria depends on the maintenance of consistent and ongoing communication with the formal operating organization.

shown in Figure 19.5. All three could also be combined with the product/ service lines feeding into the traditional specialty division groupings, which in turn could be combined into the larger divisional groupings shown in Figure 19.4. Divisions could be further organized on a geographical basis as in the case of multiunit hospital systems. The important feature of the divisional design is that each division has the necessary functional support services to do its tasks and is responsible for the management of those functions. The hospital may continue to have vice-presidents for finance, planning, and human resources, but these individuals would act more in a staff capacity to coordinate and support individual finance, planning, and human resource managers within each division. These divisional managers would report directly to the chiefs of

FIGURE 19.3

The Divisional Model — Traditional Specialties

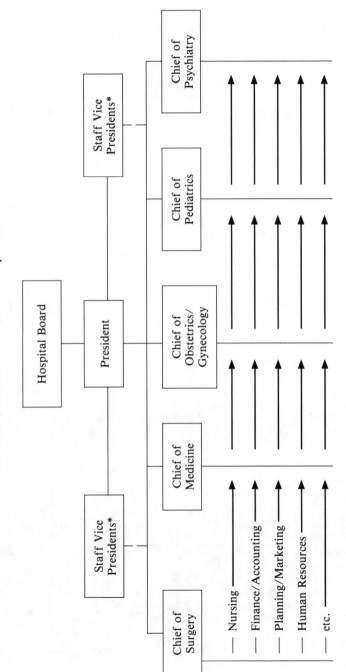

*Hospital or corporate-wide vice presidents for nursing, finance, planning and marketing, human resources, etc. They are staff positions reporting directly to the president. They serve in a consultative or advisory position to the division chiefs, as indicated by the dotted line.

FIGURE 19.4

The Divisional Model – New Groupings

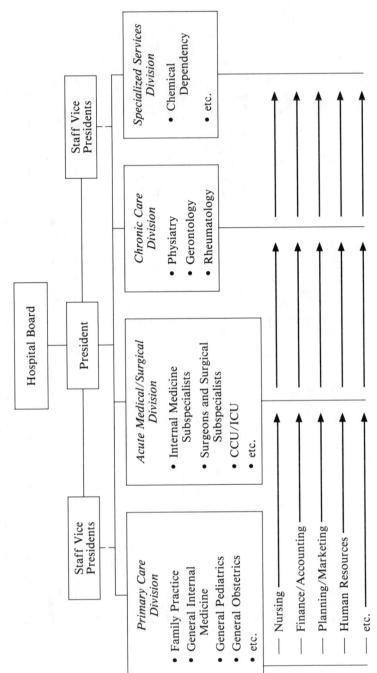

FIGURE 19.5

The Divisional Model — Traditional Specialties

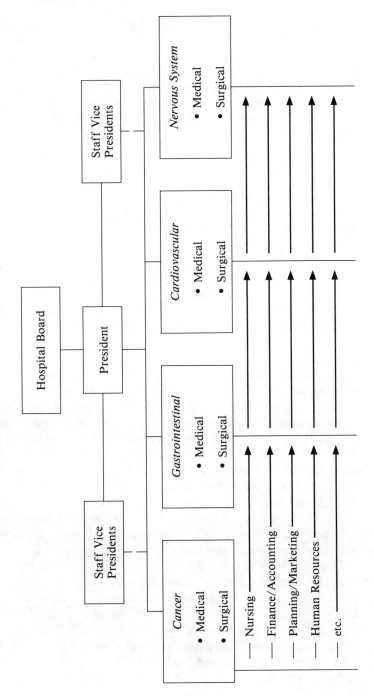

each clinical division and not to the respective vice presidents. However, in a matrix design, lateral reporting relationships could also be established. Divisional designs are currently found among some large teaching hospitals such as Johns Hopkins Medical Center in Baltimore[14] [see Chapter 14] and Rush-Presbyterian-St. Luke's in Chicago.[15]

The divisional model represents the opposite end of the continuum from the independent-corporate model. While the independent-corporate model deals with the issue of incompleteness by separating the two groups (so that each becomes "whole" unto itself), the divisional model deals with the issue by completely integrating or incorporating the functional aspects with divisional management. It represents a specific form of Scott's conjoint model for coordinating professional work.[16] The hospital becomes on paper a totally integrated curing/caring organization. There is no longer any need for the traditional voluntary medical staff organization structure because the functions typically provided by that structure (review of privileges, credentialing, quality assurance, staff services, and so on) are now performed by the clinical divisions themselves and incorporated directly into the line reporting relationships of the hospital. There may be cross-divisional task forces or coordinating committees to handle some organization-wide quality assurance functions or to meet accreditation requirements, but the basic unit of the organization is the division.

The major advantage of the divisional model for physicians is increased authority and control. Each division is headed by a physician-clinical specialist from that division. This individual controls all the resources needed to provide cost-effective care within the division. There is no need for negotiating with the hospital functional areas. The division chief, in turn, reports directly to the president of the hospital, who may often be, but need not be, a physician. Thus, there is strong physician influence and direction throughout the organization. From the physicians' viewpoint, a major disadvantage is the new set of management skills, attitudes, and time required to make a divisional organization effective. Not all physicians want to invest the time and energy required and not all are able to adapt to a divisional form.

From the hospital's perspective, a major advantage of the divisional model is the potential to better integrate the clinical and support services of the organization. This is particularly advantageous in connection with DRG-based prospective pricing, where divisions could be organized around product/service lines or clusters of given DRGs. Organization by division also enables the hospital to respond quickly to rapidly changing market forces. By grouping resources within specialized divisions it becomes possible for each group to react more quickly to alter its own service line. It also makes each group directly accountable for managing its resources and for bottom-line financial performance. The Hopkins experience suggests that the divisional model can result in better control over resources, improved efficiency, and more flexibility in adapting to new payment systems.[17] Such a design may also greatly facilitate the merging and use of clinical and administrative data required by the new payment systems.

The major disadvantage from the hospital's perspective is the loss of control by hospital administration and, in particular, by the nursing staff. The divisional design decentralizes power and authority, as well as dissemination of information to the operating clinical divisions and, in the process, transfers more influence to physicians and their support staffs charged with operating those divisions. This issue may be especially critical where the problems faced by the hospital are of an interdivisional nature requiring coordination and cooperation across divisions. For example, some surgeons and radiologists may have more in common with each other than with their divisions. The greater the number of divisions the greater the likely magnitude of the problem. The nursing staff, understandably, may be expected to be upset with the divisional design because of having to report through a physician clinical chief in each division rather than through their own administrative hierarchy composed of the vice president or director of nursing. This issue was of considerable concern in the Hopkins design, but the long-run experience suggests that nurses are satisfied with the new design and that they have increased influence and responsibility in patient care decisions and other areas of concern. In particular, they believe that the quality of communication has improved.[18]

The divisional design has a number of advantages relevant to the earlier-noted criteria. It explicitly recognizes differences between physicians and managers; but, unlike the independent model, it attempts to deal with these differences through education, training, and socialization experiences within the division itself. The objective is to arrive at a complementary blend of skills based on clinical and management teams that work within each division. Such teams can also enhance the identification of problems within the division. However, this may be at the expense of identifying organization-wide problems—issues that cut across divisions. This is a potential problem within divisional designs generally and pertains to issues of communication, the generation of alternatives, and implementation as well. However, divisional designs facilitate these processes when the issues involved are pertinent to specific divisions. Where interdependence exists, the organization requires strong top management which can see the larger picture and can appropriately coordinate and integrate as necessary divisional plans and objectives.

Of particular note is the capacity of the divisional design to facilitate learning, in that all of the relevant specialties (both clinical and administrative) are concentrated in a given unit. This not only facilitates clinical continuing education programs but also enhances *market responsiveness*—an increasingly important consideration for hospitals and their medical staffs.

Divisional designs would also appear to provide useful forums for considering issues of paradox, ambiguity and change, risk, and the promotion of comparative advantage. What might seem paradoxical for the hospital as a whole may not seem so when considered on a division-by-division basis. For example, the primary care division may use a visit-based productivity incentive scheme to recruit more physicians and increase market share, while a specialty division may develop an incentive scheme emphasizing cost containment and maximization of net revenues. Thus, the hospital may be simultaneously pursuing two strategies which appear to be contradictory but which make sense given each division's goals and objectives within the hospital's strategic plan.

Divisions are also able to deal with ambiguity and change by virtue of having housed within them the relevant expertise to deal with the situation. Relative to an independent-corporate design, it is easier for groups of individuals within specific divisions to develop alternative assumptions[19] about important but ambiguous events—for example, the future impact of DRGs combined with the physician surplus. Explicit consideration of such assumptions can generate more creative alternatives for dealing with such events.

The decentralization of information, communication, and expertise inherent in divisional designs can also promote more prudent risk taking. Each division knows more about its product/service line, its environment, its strengths and weaknesses, and its competition than the organization as a whole. This level of decentralization and concentration of expertise also permits a quicker assessment of risk and consequent decisions regarding "go or no go."

Finally, the divisional design can promote comparative advantage through the concentration of appropriate expertise and experience. It provides clinicians with the administrative support needed for providing patient care while providing administration with more direct clinical input into the hospital's service line and overall strategic planning. These possible advantages are summarized in the third column of Table 19.1.

THE PARALLEL MODEL

The parallel model may hold the most promise for many hospitals. As defined in the organizational literature, the parallel model involves the creation of a separate organization for purposes of conducting certain activities which are not handled well by the formal organization.[20] Individuals who are appropriate in terms of skills, experience, and interests are selected from the formal organization to participate in the parallel organization. The parallel organization differs from an ad hoc task force or committee in that it is intended to be relatively permanent. It differs from a formal matrix design (where a single person reports to two superiors) in that is has no dual authority reporting channels. The individuals making up the parallel organization still maintain their operating responsibilities in the formal organization, but some part of their time (for example, 25 to 50 percent) is freed up to work in the parallel organization. Often, a steering committee is formed to make sure that the ideas of the parallel organization are integrated into the operating organization.[21]

In the context of hospital medical staffs, the suggestion is that an organization be developed that runs "parallel" to the current traditional medical staff organization structure as shown in Figure 19.6. The purpose of the parallel organization would be to deal with major strategic issues facing both the hospital and its medical staff. Examples include development of new product/service lines, initiation of joint ventures, examination of the hospital's teaching responsibilities, and efforts to improve organization-wide productivity and quality. Representatives from the medical staff, nursing staff, other health professionals, and administration would be selected to serve in the parallel organization. Expertise, interest, credibility with peers, and interpersonal skills would be among the primary criteria for selection. Members would be given time off from their daily operating responsibilities and provided with additional compensation in order to serve in the parallel organization.

The advantage of such an arrangement is that it is able to deal with complex, ambiguous, and poorly structured problems that cannot be handled by the current medical staff structure with its numerous committees, turnover in leadership, and generally "bottom-up" approach. Examples of parallel organizations include IPAs, PPOs, HMOs, and related joint ventures. Ellwood's MeSH plans, involving the development of a separate association with fifty-fifty participation of hospitals and physicians, represent another example.[22] St. John's Hospital in Santa Monica, California, has established a separate "Associated Physicians" organization to deal with alternative delivery systems and related issues

FIGURE 19.6

The Parallel Model

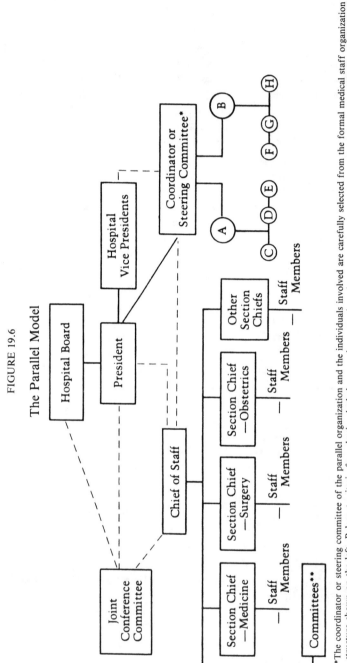

*The coordinator or steering committee of the parallel organization and the individuals involved are carefully selected from the formal medical staff organization structure shown on the left. Relevant criteria for selection include: maturity, expertise relevant to the mission of the parallel organization, credibility to both administration and medical staff, communication, listening skills, and creative abilities, and representation from different specialties, committees, and age groups. In the example shown, individuals A and B serve as co-coordinators for two subgroups made up of individuals C, D, and E and F, G, and H. It should be noted that members from nursing, other health professions, and administration may also be members of the parallel organization. The parallel organization may have as its major charge the development of a strategic plan for providing more cost-effective health care to current and future markets in ways that are consistent with the hospital's mission and medical staff interests.

**Executive Committee, Credentialing Committee, Quality Assurance Committee (Utilization Review, Medical Audit, Tissue), Medical Records, Pharmacy and Therapeutics Committee, Infections Committee, etc.

facing the staff.[23] Fairfax Hospital in Virginia has developed a similar structure,[24] and other hospitals are following suit. However, the parallel organization model discussed here goes beyond these examples to include incorporation of more significant medical input into the overall strategic planning and management process of the hospital. MeSH plans and physician associations represent stepping-stones to a more fully developed parallel model.

From the physicians' perspective, a major advantage of the parallel model is the opportunity for more significant input into those issues that affect their long-run future. The traditional medical staff organization is structured to deal with short-run daily issues of quality assurance, utilization review, credentialing, review of privileges, and related matters. It represents the "operating" organization of the medical staff. The parallel structure would address issues relevant to the hospital's long-range plans involving environmental assessment, competitive analysis, assessment of organizational strengths and weaknesses, and the development of new service lines based on such analysis. Physicians with appropriate skills, interests, and expertise would be drawn from throughout the staff to participate in this process. They may or may not be formally elected leaders of the operating organization, although it is essential that continued communication take place between the two groups. In particular, the parallel organization would have the major advantage of involving younger members of the staff years before they would usually have the opportunity to play such leadership roles in the traditional operating medical staff organization structure. The parallel organization thus serves as a potentially excellent vehicle for developing future medical staff leadership.

From the physicians' perspective there are three potential disadvantages. One is the amount of time involved. The second is the danger that physicians serving in the parallel organization would lose credibility with their peers and thus become ineffective. The third is that the parallel organization might begin to usurp some of the daily operating responsibilities of the traditional medical staff structure. The time issue can be addressed by appropriate compensation and meaningful involvement; that is, evidence that the ideas developed by the parallel organization are taken seriously. The credibility and usurpation issues can be addressed by appropriate leadership from the steering committee and the leadership of the hospital and medical staff.

The primary advantage of the parallel model for the hospital is that it provides a more effective way of involving physicians in the overall management process of the organization than is possible with the traditional structure. The hospital may also have somewhat more control over the process in encouraging selected physicians to become involved in the parallel organization—although clearly this would need to occur with close consultation and involvement of the medical staff. A major advantage of the parallel model over the divisional model is that it enables the hospital and its medical staff to deal with organization-wide issues that cut across divisions, thus avoiding potential "balkanization." It also involves a less pervasive change than that which occurs in totally reorganizing the hospital along divisional lines. At the same time, the parallel model maintains the present traditional medical staff organization structure and permits it to do what it does best with respect to overseeing daily clinical activities. The parallel model has advantages over the independent-corporate model in that it avoids the disassociation of the medical staff from the hospital and the potential disadvantages associated with that model noted earlier.

Potential disadvantages include the start-up time involved, the amount of training and support required, and the danger that the parallel organization might be perceived as a threat by other organizational members. Again, these issues can be effectively addressed by committed hospital and medical staff leadership, assuming that such leadership exists or can be cultivated. Without it, the parallel model is doomed to failure.

The parallel model also seems to hold considerable potential advantages with respect to the ten criteria defined earlier. It explicitly recognizes differences between physicians and administrators by establishing a separate mechanism in which physicians, unfettered by the traditional medical staff organization, can work with selected representatives from administration and nursing, as well as other health professionals, on longer-run issues of importance. It provides a forum in which the various parties can take time to get to know one another and develop trust and understanding of one another's viewpoints.

Problems and issues can be better defined and elaborated, particularly in response to long-run concerns, because the composition of the organization is based on relevant interests and expertise of key individuals from both the medical staff and the hospital. The time and flexibility provided by the structure also promote problem identification and clarification. Frequently, this is not possible with the traditional medical staff and hospital organization because of the barriers created by different divisions and committees and the pressing demands of daily responsibilities.

The parallel model has particular advantages in enhancing communication, generating alternatives, and facilitating implementation of new programs *across* organizational boundaries *provided* that consistent, ongoing communication is maintained with the operating organization, that is, the formal medical staff organization and the hospital's functional organizational structure. Without such consistent, ongoing communication the parallel organization faces the hazard of becoming an "elitist" group which can only impose its views on the operating organization, or a "splinter" group having little credibility or influence with the operating organization. Ongoing support from the hospital board, top levels of hospital administration, and medical staff leadership, along with consistent and continuous communication between the operating organization and the parallel organization, is essential to its success. A steering committee of appropriate selected individuals can be helpful. This process is also facilitated by remembering that the members of the parallel organization continue to hold responsibilities in the operating organization — whether as members of the formal medical staff organization or as members of the hospital functional organization hierarchy. This dual responsibility not only enhances communication and credibility but also provides for the early testing of new ideas generated by the parallel organization. Members can sense what might work and what might not work and can begin to take early steps, with respect to education and information, to facilitate those ideas which hold promise. In particular, the parallel model is well suited to the generation of alternatives based on examination of alternative assumptions.[25] In the example shown in Figure 19.6, the two subgroups could be charged with developing alternatives based on two different sets of assumptions regarding assessment of one's competition, different demand forecasts, changes in the regulatory environment, and likely new technological developments.

For many of the reasons noted above, the parallel model also facilitates professional and organizational learning. This is primarily due to the cross-disciplinary nature of the organization, the somewhat longer time frame involved, and the opportunity to test ideas in the operating organization as they develop.

In what ways does the parallel organization increase the ability to deal with paradox, ambiguity and change, risk, and the promotion of comparative advantage? First, it is important to recognize that the parallel model is itself somewhat paradoxical. Members are a part of the formal organization and yet are also part of another organization. They retain responsibility for many of their daily activities and yet are charged with developing new ideas and programs that may disrupt those very responsibilities. This is precisely the kind of forum in which paradox can be recognized, examined, and embraced as appropriate. By having the time to work together the various parties can see in advance where their interests may be compatible and where they may be incompatible; where collaboration makes sense and, equally important, where competition is the preferred vehicle.

In order to deal with ambiguous situations, one needs a longer-run strategic orientation to change.[26] Ambiguous situations have three characteristics: (1) the future is unpredictable, (2) the organization's choice of desirable outcomes is unknown, contradictory, or confusing, and (3) there is little understanding of what ought to be done to make the future more predictable (that is, the cause-and-effect relationships), how to arrive at greater consensus regarding desired outcomes, or how to bring those outcomes about in the event that some consensus can be reached. It is precisely the kind of situation that requires deliberative discussion over a period of time by a cross-section of relevant organization members. Thus, a particular strength of the parallel model is its ability to deal with ambiguous change situations which cut across organizational boundaries. These situations cannot even be considered in the independent-corporate model, and are extremely difficult to address with the divisional model or the traditional medical staff organizational model.

The parallel model enables one to approach ambiguous change situations through what Hitt calls the "staging" of issues.[27] Such staging involves three components: (1) anticipating issues so that they are discussed before the need to resolve them becomes urgent, (2) facing controversial issues far enough in advance of implementation that the problems will seem remote and less threatening, and (3) providing appropriate structures for making decisions. The parallel model provides a forum for meeting each of these criteria. In addition, it provides a mechanism for clustering issues in such a way that interdependencies are recognized and underlying assumptions and principles explored. As Hitt notes, ". . . a variety (of issues) builds constituency support for the overall plan."[28]

The parallel model enhances the willingness and ability of the organization to take risks in three ways. First, it provides more informed judgment on the nature of the risk because of the input of relevant expertise from different levels and groups of both the medical staff and the hospital. Second, the longer time orientation permits parallel organization members to think about new possibilities, to obtain new kinds of external information, and to consider new ways of doing things unencumbered by the constraints of daily operating responsibilities and current practice. Third, it provides for early implementation assessment of "risky ventures" through the ongoing discussion and exchange with members of the operating organization.

Finally, the parallel model is conducive to the promotion of comparative advantage. While the independent-corporate model accomplishes this by a clear separation of interests and the divisional model by close but perhaps overly narrow integration of interests, the parallel model retains some features of both. Like the independent-corporate model, the parallel model involves a separation of interests, but here the separation is between short-run operational concerns and longer-run strategic concerns and not between the hospital and the medical staff. Like the divisional model, the parallel model involves integration, but here it is based on relevant subgroups of both the medical staff and hospital, unconstrained by divisional issues. Thus, the assessment of comparative advantage can take place on a wider scale and within the context of long-run and not just short-run concerns. The potential advantages of the parallel model are summarized in the fourth column of Table 19.1.

It is clear from an examination of Table 19.1 that the divisional and parallel models of medical staff organization have potential advantages over the traditional and independent-corporate models. The essential requirements for implementing the divisional model include strong physician-managers (it is conceivable but politically unlikely that the division chiefs could be nonphysicians), strong administrative and ancillary support staffs within each division, and mechanisms for facilitating interdivisional communication and cooperation. There is some indication that the divisional model may be favored by university-based teaching hospitals where the teaching and patient care functions can be integrated within each division and where a significant percentage of the staff is full-time. However, it may also have advantages for other teaching hospitals and for hospitals that see merit in organizing more of their services as clusters of diagnostic categories, such as those represented in product line or service line management.

Essential requirements for implementing the parallel model include a willingness to release selected medical staff members and hospital staff from some portion of their operating responsibilities to spend time in the parallel organization; appropriate financial incentives; strong and ongoing support from top levels of the board, administration, and medical staff leadership; a commitment to the long run; and the need for continuous and ongoing communication with the operating organization. This model may have particular advantages for medium-sized hospitals (250 to 500 beds) and those belonging to multiunit systems. With respect to the latter, the parallel organization provides a forum for the hospital to handle its own future in relation to corporate-system–wide policies and a forum to provide input into those policies. Specifically, it may provide a link between strategic and operational decision making, a major need for most multiunit systems.

Some hospitals may find advantages in mixing the models. For example, the hospital may organize the medical staff largely along divisional lines but establish a parallel organization composed of representatives from each division to work with hospital administration on organization-wide issues. It is also important to recognize that the parallel organization itself is a mixed model in that it retains the traditional medical staff organization structure for handling daily hospital staff activities but adds a parallel component to deal with longer-run strategic issues. Still another variation would combine elements of the independent-corporate model and the parallel model. In this case, the independent physician corporation and the hospital would separately designate representatives to form a "bipartisan" parallel model for purposes of managing ongoing relationships and addressing strategic issues. This hybrid form might be termed the *integrated-corporate* model to distinguish it from the totally independent-corporate model.

It is also important to reiterate that the advantages and disadvantages discussed above are largely *potential* and not realized. Realizing these advantages depends not only on the specific implementation issues discussed above but also on the willingness of physicians and administrators to follow certain guidelines that will enhance the effectiveness of any of the models selected. . . .

CONCLUSION

We are often told that problems represent opportunities in disguise. The current environment of cost containment, regulation, competition, changing public expectations, and the growing for-profit role in health care should not be seen as eroding the professional values of medicine. Rather, these forces are directly challenging them. Whether the ultimate outcome is growth or erosion depends on the response.

These same forces are also challenging the values of hospital and health care administrators. What really are the values of physicians and administrators? Can new values be embraced? Should they be? Can administrators, physicians, and other health professionals play a leadership role as guardians of quality of care to the public and in helping to raise the moral consciousness of everyone confronted by the ethical issues posed by the new medical marketplace?

This article highlights the major forces influencing the future relationships between administrators and physicians and suggests a number of criteria by which future relationships can be assessed. Several new models for structuring hospital–medical staff relationships are developed and assessed in terms of the suggested criteria. . . . It is hoped that they will stimulate discussion, experimentation, and evaluation. They are not likely to provide neat solutions — for the problems posed to the hospital industry today are not amenable to "neat" solutions.

ACKNOWLEDGMENTS

The author is grateful for the helpful suggestions of Dr. Susan Adelman, David Hitt, Anthony Kovner, Dr. John Mamana, Dr. Henry Simmons, and Dr. Cyril Wiggishoff, who reviewed an initial draft of this paper. Appreciation is also expressed to Nancy Rodkin for research assistance and Joann Kaiser for manuscript preparation.

NOTES

1.   Gonnella, J. S., and M. J. Goran. "Quality of Patient Care — A Measurement Change: The Staging Concept." *Medical Care* 13 (June 1975): 467–73.

2.   Horn, S. "Validity, Reliability and Implications of an Index of Inpatient Severity of Illness." *Medical Care* 14 (1981): 354; Jacobs, C. *PAT (Physician-Administrator-Trustee) Conference on Quality/Cost Control* (Chicago: Inter-Qual, 1983).

3.   Morlock, L. L.; J. Alexander; and H. Hunter. "Governing Board and CEO/Medical Staff Relationships as a Function of Hospital Participation and Multi-Institutional Arrangements." Working paper, Health Services Research and Development Center, Johns Hopkins University, 1984.

4.   Vladeck, B. C., and J. P. Firman. "The Aging of the Population and Health Services." *Annals of the American Academy of Political and Social Science* 468 (July 1983): 133.

5.   Blanton, W. B., Jr. "Understanding Differences Between Medical Staff and Administration." *Hospital Medical Staff* 10 (December 1981): 15–21.

6.   Moore, T. F., and E. A. Simendinger. "How to Involve (the Right) Physicians in the Leadership Process." *Hospital Forum*, May–June 1983, pp. 61–66; Cunningham, R. M. "Get All the Working Parts Together." *Hospitals*, November 16, 1980, pp. 70–74.

7.   Kimberly, J. R.; P. Leatt; and S. M. Shortell. "Organization Design." In *Health Care Management: A Text in Organization Theory and Behavior*, ed. S. M. Shortell and A. D. Kaluzny, pp. 291–332. New York: John Wiley and Sons, 1983.

8.   Smith, H. L. "Two Lines of Authority Are One Too Many." *Modern Hospital* 84 (March 1955): 59–64.

9.   Harris, J. E. "The Internal Organization of Hospitals: Some Economic Implications." *Bell Journal of Economics* 8 (1978): 467–82; Pauly, M. V., and M. Redisch. "The Not-for-Profit Hospital as Physicians' Cooperative." *American Economic Review* 63 (March 1973): 87–100; Shortell, S. M., "Physician Involvement in Hospital Decision-Making." In *The New Health Care For-Profit: Doctors and Hospitals in a Competitive Environment*, ed. Bradford H. Gray. Washington, D.C.: Institute of Medicine, National Academy of Sciences, 1983, pp. 73–101.

10.   Noie, N. E.; S. M. Shortell; and M. Morrisey. "A Survey of Hospital Medical Staff — Part One." *Hospitals*, December 1, 1983, pp. 80–84.

11.   The model is most applicable to multihospital communities, where both physicians and hospital have some degree of choice.

12.   Joint Commission on Accreditation of Hospitals. *JCAH Accreditation Manual*. Chicago: JCAH, 1985.

13.   Richman, D. A. "On the Present State of Medical Malpractice." *Hospital Medical Staff*, January 1984, pp. 13–20.

14.   Heyssel, R. M. "The Faculty Role in the Competitive Academic Health Center." Paper delivered at the Annual Meeting of the Association of Academic Health Centers, Palm Springs, Calif., 1981.

15.   Sinoris, M. E.; T. H. Esmond; R. Newman; et al. "The Program Matrix: New Approach to Hospital Planning and Decision-Making." Unpublished monograph. Chicago: Rush-Presbyterian-St. Luke's Medical Center, 1980.

16.   Scott, W. R. "Managing Professional Work: Three Models of Control for Health Organizations." *Health Services Research* 17 (Fall 1982): 212–40.

17.   Heyssel, "Faculty Role."

18.   Ibid.

19.   Mitroff, I. I. *Stakeholders of the Organizational Mind: Toward a New View of Organizational Policy Making*. San Francisco: Jossey-Bass, 1983.

20.   Stein, B. A., and R. M. Kanter. "Building the Parallel Organization: Creating Mechanisms for Permanent Quality of Work Life." *Journal of Applied Behavioral Science* 16 (1980): 371–86.

21.   Kanter, R. M. "Managing Transitions in Organizational Culture: The Case of Participative Management at Honeywell." In *Managing Organizational Transitions*, ed. J. R. Kimberly and R. E. Quinn. (Homewood, IL: Richard D. Irwin, 1984), pp. 195–217.

22.   Yanish, D. "Hospitals Work with M.D.'s to Smooth MeSH Partnerships' Rough Edges." *Modern Healthcare* 14 (February 15, 1984): 58–62.

23.   Corlin, R. F. "Health Care in a Brave New World." In *Executive Briefing for Hospital Medical Staff Leadership: Creating New Incentives for Physician-Hospital Cooperation*. San Diego, Calif.: American Hospital Association, Division of Medical Staff Affairs, February 23, 1984.

24.   J. Mamana, personal communication, June 1984.

25.   Mitroff, *Stakeholders*.

26.   Quinn, J. B. "Managing Strategic Change." *Sloan Management Review*, Summer 1980, pp. 3–19.

27.   Hitt, D. H. "Grounding the High Intensity in Physician-Hospital Relationships." *Hospitals*, April 16, 1984, pp. 91–95.

28.   Ibid., p. 92.

V

Adaptation

A hospital is a living organism, made up of many different parts having different functions, but all these must be in due proportion and relation to each other, and to the environment, to produce the desired general results. The stream of life which runs through it is incessantly changing; patients and nurses and doctors come and go, today it has to do with the results of an epidemic, tomorrow with those of an explosion or a fire, the reputation of its physicians or surgeons attracts those suffering from a particular form of disease, and as one changes so do the others. Its work is never done; its equipment is never complete; it is always in need of new means of diagnosis; of new instruments and medicine; it is to try all things and hold fast to that which is good.

—John Shaw Billings
Address on the opening of the
Johns Hopkins Hospital,
May 7, 1889

ILLUSTRATION V

Organization Transformation Process

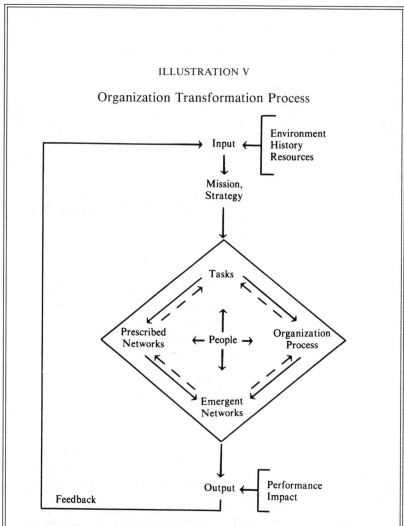

Mission, Strategy: Includes the organization's purpose, its basic approach to achieving its objectives.
Tasks: The functions by which the organization's work is accomplished.
Prescribed networks: The explicit organizational social structure, including subunits, authority networks, and structural mechanisms.
Organization processes: Mechanisms (communication, decision making, conflict management) that enable the prescribed networks to function.
Emergent networks: Structures and processes that emerge in the organization, although they are not formally prescribed.
People: Includes characteristics of organization members, including background, managerial style, motivational patterns.

Adapted from John R. Kimberly and Robert H. Miles, *The Organizational Life Cycle,* 1980, p. 173, with permission, Jossey-Bass, Inc., Publishers.

Commentary

Anthony R. Kovner
Duncan Neuhauser
with Connie Evashwick

Adapting the organization to external and internal stimuli may be the most difficult of the challenges facing the contemporary health services manager. This is true today more than ever before, particularly given the rapid rate of change in the health care environment. Section V addresses the relationship between organization and environment, in which adaptation is the key issue.

The word "adaptation" suggests a theoretical view of organizational survival as dependent on a specific direction of change, that is, change in directions that provide a closer fit between organization and environment. This close fit allows the organization to extract resources from society in exchange for a socially valued organizational product.[1]

The key paradigm here derives from marketing. With the exception of the drug industry, marketing is a new concept in the health field. It is sometimes said that modern marketing methods started a century ago with Lydia Pinkham's patent medicine company. (Lydia Pinkham was the first American woman to become a millionaire on her own.) Marketing has one central and powerful insight: it is easier to find out what people want and design the product or service to meet those desires than it is to create a product and convince people they want it. Medical care has overwhelmingly followed the latter rather than the former principle. That medical care provider-experts know what unknowledgeable patients need reflects a non- or antimarketing perspective. Finding out what patients or prospective patients want and organizing in response to those desires is the marketing perspective.

Organizations vary in their sensitivity to environmental conditions and in the extent to which the environment impinges upon internal operations. Health services organizations exist in particularly complex environments, and failure to be responsive to a variety of conditions threatens their viability. Four aspects of health care microcosm are especially important: scientific technology, community service, funding, and personnel.

Scientific technology is one of the important elements in the environment of most organizations. Technology affects the goals and values of an organization and, to a large degree, determines its internal structure. An auto body shop that repairs clients' damaged cars is set up quite differently from a plant that produces hundreds of new automobiles daily. Similarly, a medical clinic that diagnoses and treats individual patients exhibits different space and staffing patterns than does a screening unit that takes a standard chest x-ray of dozens of persons a day.

Health services organizations differ from many other contemporary industries in that the technology—medical, biological, chemical, and sociological—is changing continuously and rapidly. Kidney dialysis, which was once an experiment, becomes a major program offered by a hospital in its role as a regional referral center. Institutionalization of the mentally disturbed and one-to-one patient-physician therapy are replaced by a community drop-in center and group therapy, leaving a 1,000-bed hospital empty. Lithotriptors are today's hot new technology.

The health services manager needs to be aware of the latest changes in health care technology. New developments tend to be lauded as contributions, whether direct or indirect, to high-quality patient care—a goal that all health services organizations espouse. Yet evidence on the value of the innovation may be sparse. Furthermore, advances are occurring so rapidly and in so many areas that there is inevitably competition among programs or professionals within health services organizations. The health services manager must select and incorporate developments that contribute to the goals of the particular organizations while resisting immediate and unquestioned acceptance of all technological changes.

A second factor that makes health services organizations highly sensitive to their environments is their "community service" character.[2] Community service is a combination of three elements, all or only one of which may apply. First, either directly or indirectly, these organizations provide a service. Second, the service has nearly universal applicability and value. At one time or another, most people need and seek some type of health care. Third, in contrast to many organizations that sell products, the medical ethic holds that clients in need of emergency service, at least, will not be turned away.

Health services organizations are often identified with particular communities, either an entire town, a distinct neighborhood, or a suburb. As an institution serving a particular population, the organization is inevitably affected by the tenor of the community, and the community typically takes pride in its medical care organizations.

Many health services organizations are public institutions, ranging from hospitals run by municipal governments, to health planning agencies initiated by the state, to neighborhood health centers operated by citizen groups. The goals of such organizations may include, through law or through charter, meeting the health care needs of all the individuals of a community service area.

The power that community groups may have over health services organizations was demonstrated in the 1960s. The social movement of the decade reinforced the general belief that health care was a basic human right. Consumer participation in management decisions and organizational operations came into vogue. Employment of local resources was widely advocated and actively promoted by the federal government. The late 1970s saw rapidly growing interest in health services marketing. Another important change has been the growth in competition among health services providers and the belief by some that this is the way to allocate services efficiently. The "competition versus regulation" debate indicates two alternative ways to structure the "health services industry."

Even with this debate, health services organizations continue their close relationship with all levels of government. Many health services organizations are funded by government: approximately one-third of all hospitals are run by municipal, county, state, or federal governments. Vaccination programs, screening drives, community health centers, and drug and alcohol treatment centers are only a few of the programs that are paid for partly or totally with government monies. Thus organizations are subject to the whims of legislators, the economic realities of government budgets, and, at times, even the day-to-day functions of government bureaucracy. A city hospital, for example, may be required to have each purchase order for equipment approved by the city's comptroller, as if the hospital were an integral department of the city government.

Funding for such organizations may be uncertain from year to year, since the availability of money may depend upon the annual budget preparation and appropriations. A new program may depend upon a public referendum approving new taxes. Federal grants and appropriations also may have a direct effect on the organization. Cutbacks or changes in funds for medical research and education, for example, have caused many medical schools and teaching hospitals to revise their training programs. Since the advent of Medicare and Medicaid, the federal government has paid an increasing proportion of the bills for health care.

Organizations depending upon such funds rely upon federal and state agencies to process claims promptly and accurately. Changes in payment policies may seriously alter the financial status of an organization, often reducing cash flow.

As part of this dependence on government funds, health services organizations are subject to a plethora of government regulations. Standards for building construction, hiring and firing of employees, staffing patterns, purchase contracts, quality of care, membership on governing boards, and fixing of reimbursement rates are among the myriad factors over which federal, state, county, and municipal governments have regulatory authority. The effect of malpractice litigation is also massive. A manager must be keenly aware of the requirements pertaining to the organization and of changes in relevant regulations. Forward-thinking managers will keep up with trends in government regulations and, in a long-range planning process, will attempt to anticipate future government changes.

Another factor that makes health services organizations subject to external pressures is the number and range of persons working in the health field. A large organization, such as a specialty referral center, will have both a large number of employees and a seemingly inexhaustible variety of professional, allied, skilled, and unskilled personnel. The problems a manager encounters in dealing with physicians and physician organizations were discussed in Section IV. In addition, managers must usually relate to several unions and handle demands from nonunion groups of skilled and unskilled employees.

Until 1975, the National Labor Relations Act did not apply to employees of nonprofit organizations such as hospitals. With the growth of the health services industry and the concurrent change in the law, labor leaders are intensifying efforts and the concurrent change in the law, labor leaders are intensifying efforts to unionize health workers. In response, professional organizations are taking a more active role as bargaining authorities. The manager needs to be increasingly aware of the demands of labor and professional organizations in order to maintain control of internal structure and policies.

Health services organizations exist in a highly complex, volatile environment. Rapidly changing scientific technology, increased community expectations of service, increased competition, intense purchaser pressure from government and agents of large employers, and increasing pressures from organized professional and labor groups necessitate environmental awareness and effective responsiveness on the part of the organization. Managers may have little control over conditions external to their organizations. However, they must mold their organizations' internal operations and goals to be compatible with these forces. From the beginning, the context must be an integral part of considerations in developing the organization. Once established, the organization must constantly revise and review its estimate of the elements of the environment to ensure that the organization remains in touch with current developments and anticipates future trends.

The theory and literature on adaptation in medical care have only begun to be developed during the past two decades. This development will be discussed in the context of the four facets of organizations explored in this section. Two aspects of adaptation should be kept in mind; initial, or static, adaption of the organization to its environment; and continuous internal change by the organization to adjust to environmental changes.

Performance Requirements

The four performance requirements are discussed below in relation to adaptation. Table V.1 shows how each of the authors of the readings in this section approaches these requirements.

TABLE V.1

Perspectives on Performance Requirements and Adaptation

Readings	Goal Attainment	System Maintenance	Adaptive Capability	Values Integration
Sheps	Multiple goals		Seems lacking in academic medical center	Need for differentiation
Shortell, Morrison, and Robbins	Strategy serving mission		Importance of research	Balance health as economic & social good
Robinette	Meeting customer-client desires	Competitive environment	From charitable to competitive	Changing the paradigm
Size	Cooperative mission	Shared services	Rural hospital cooperative	Consistent with local values

GOAL ATTAINMENT

By definition, an organization is begun with the purpose of fulfilling one or more specified goals. Conditions in the environment may cause major modification of these goals, either from the outset or at some point in the organization's life cycle. The Infantile Paralysis Society is a classic example of an organization that underwent an abrupt change in its formal goals because of an occurrence that was essential to the organization's purpose yet beyond the organization's control.

The Infantile Paralysis Society was founded in the late 1940s as a fundraising institution designed to contribute to research on and treatment of this disease. At the time, polio was a severe epidemic; consequently, the society quickly spread across the nation and developed strong grass roots support. With the introduction of the Salk vaccine, the incidence of polio diminished rapidly. Within a few years, infantile paralysis went from a life-threatening disease that could infect the childhood population throughout the United States to an easily prevented disease. Mass immunization programs ensured that most children received the vaccine.

The leaders of the Infantile Paralysis Society were shrewd and adept enough to recognize that their large, well-developed organizations could be reoriented rather than disbanded. The goals were publicly changed from the prevention and treatment of polio to the prevention and treatment of all paralytic diseases of childhood. The organization continues today as the March of Dimes.

An organization may modify its goals in response to subtle, but powerful change in the political or social environment. Recently, federal funds for basic research have been curtailed. Funds for family practice and community medicine, on the other hand, have increased. As a result, medical schools and teaching hospitals found it expedient to alter the emphasis of their training programs from subspecialty research-oriented medicine to family-practice general medicine.

The literature on organizational goals is fairly extensive. However, relatively little analysis has been done on systematically identifying factors in the environment that affect the setting of goals.

SYSTEM MAINTENANCE

Although system maintenance is the steady state and adaptation is change, the dividing line between the two is not always clear. Considerable adaptive capability may be required to keep an organization going, and the organization's ability to adapt is in need of continuing maintenance.

Robert Guest recounts a case in organizational self-renewal in which an inefficient, low-morale industrial plant became, within a fairly short period, an efficient, high-morale corporate training ground. He emphasizes the effect of a new manager on the personnel and structure of the organization.[3] A new manager alone would not have solved the company's problems, and the formal structure was in fact not altered at all. The changes occurred because of the cooperative attitude that the new manager promoted. He used the plant's poor reputation as a tool to spark a new attitude of determination and enthusiasm among the workers. Guest emphasizes the social and behavioral aspects of a change that occurs within an organization in response to environmental pressures (in this case, top management). Guest's account is a good example of the accomplishments of a manager working under serious environmental constraints. Unable to influence the environment, the manager used his authority to alter the internal organization to accommodate external demands.

To a greater or lesser degree, all change is disruptive to an organization. The manager's role is to facilitate change in a way that minimizes distress to employees and disruption of productivity. This is particularly important in a health services organization, where a slip in performance for any reason can threaten a patient's life.

A manager may have minimal control over factors in the organization's environment, but he or she does control how the organization's internal operations (structure and personnel) respond to environmental pressures. Environmental conditions may affect all or part of an organization: the structure, the personnel, the work flow. Furthermore, numerous external events may occur simultaneously, affecting the organization in a different way. The manager must evaluate the single and combined effects of the changes in the environment to determine priorities among necessary internal changes and to implement multiple changes in a skillful and timely manner, while at the same time keeping the organization functioning smoothly.

ADAPTIVE CAPABILITY

Adaptive capability is inherent to organizations. Organizations may be defined as firms working together to achieve specific societal goals. As the needs of society change, the purpose of the organization changes, and the organization must adapt internally to meet its new role. The differences between earliest organizations and contemporary organizations are the complexity of the external environment, the growth of internal technology, and the rate of change. Technology of all types is developing rapidly and will continue to do so. Organizations and entire countries are increasingly interdependent in their relationships. Unity-of-command bureaucracy, once a standard pattern for organizational structure and control, is being replaced by patterns such as the matrix organization. Some believe that the growth of professionalism heralds the death of bureaucracy and that soon few organizations will exhibit the traditional pyramidal structure.

Change in the health services field has never been more rapid. Observers cite three reasons for this: (1) the increase in the number of physicians, (2) the growth of large multi-institution systems, and (3) the growth of competition based on both price and quality.

The increase in physicians means that new physicians will have a harder time starting a solo private practice and will be more willing to work in different settings, such as HMOs and emergicenters. Hospitals and other health organizations are grouping together in part to increase their access to lower-cost capital for renewal and expansion. The choice of health plans for employees and their dependents has made both price and quality important. Increasingly, people are choosing systems of care rather than individual physicians.

Merely understanding all of these changes is a challenge for health services managers. The individual manager may not be able to have much effect on these external changes. Instead, the manager's job may be to keep the organization stable, working to attain its stated goals while at the same time making internal changes to keep the organization in tune with external conditions.

The managerial task of adapting an organization is difficult enough in a relatively stable environment and with relatively well-defined roles for employees. In the health services field, with rapid changes in personnel and roles, implementing internal change will require extensive education and value reorientation among a wide range of employees. Examples of these changing roles include the nonclinician manager of clinical services and the increased interest of physicians in management careers.

More than ever before, managers must be effective in fostering change. One can expect to see, in the years ahead, a rapid increase in the number of health services organizations that will fail to survive without refocusing their goals. Effective measures of organizational performance are usually lacking because they do not evaluate the organization's ability to recognize and react to the need for change. In the future, the manager's skill in responding to changes in environmental pressures may be one of the major measures of successful organizational performance.

VALUES INTEGRATION

Change almost inevitably involves values.[4] A change in goals may result from, or cause, a change in beliefs about the organization's purpose. A change in output or performance measures may require concomitant change in workers' beliefs about what merits reward. A change in daily operations and structure may force acceptance of a change in worker attitudes and habits. Change may be forced upon an organization because of a shift in society's beliefs. Managers must understand the social values that pertain to their organizations and must be responsive to shifts in these values. Similarly, a manager's efforts to implement change in the internal organization may necessitate changing the values of the organization's employees and constituents.

A social and political system that values creativity, initiative, and freedom of the individual may be most conducive to organizational change. In America, change has been valued for itself. (Consequently, change often is not critically evaluated to determine whether it is indeed an improvement over existing conditions.) Society's values, then, temper the forces in the environment, the organizational goals, and an organization's policy toward change.

On an individual level, the values of an organization's members determine to a great degree how the organization can most readily accomplish change. Most theorists of change acknowledge and address the attitudes of the workers as the key to successful change. Organizational development has become a standard way of achieving change. This technique is based on involving and changing the attitudes of the workers first, then changing the organizational structure and work flow. The values and goals of the individual may conflict with the values and goals of others in the organization. This conflict may have to be resolved for all to be satisfied in goal attainment. For some, one of the main purposes of change is to resolve individual and group conflict.

As mentioned above, the community, the government, and the labor force are critical components of the environment of a health services organization. During the 1970s, the general public paid considerable attention to health care. The elderly, the poor, and members of labor unions were especially active in promoting financial and service programs to facilitate the availability and accessibility of health care. The passage of Medicare and Medicaid in 1965 marked the beginning or formal acceptance of health care as a right of the individual and a responsibility of society. In the 1980s, however, managers found new expectations and demands placed upon their organizations as a result of the election of new officials who wished to limit the role of government.

Within the organization, health services managers face constant change, due especially to rapidly changing technology. The manager must know and be able to reorient the attitudes and values of the employees to incorporate change smoothly. This is particularly difficult in organizations with old and established traditions and employees. For example, where physician assistants are introduced, tasks and roles must be carefully defined, and the attitudes of the health care team members and patients must be geared toward acceptance, cooperation, and enthusiasm. If physician assistants are not viewed as persons who will contribute to and enhance others' performance, they will not be fully used, no matter how well their role is specified in a job description. The nonclinical manager may often be charged with not understanding the values of clinical professionals. Overcoming such charges may require great tact. Skillful and well-trained managers who understand the process of change may be able to handle the problems of clinical practice better than health professionals who lack such understanding.

THE READINGS

Sheps speaks to the problems of managing academic medical centers and the need to develop more unity in institutional decision making, particularly regarding specific purposes and priorities, the content of activities, and the size, effectiveness, and fiscal implications of its programs. This calls for restructuring governance so that the hospital and the medical school are governed by two separate interacting organizations of equal strength. Of course, it is easier to recommend such changes than to make them happen, but the reader should wonder why Sheps's clear, sensible, and urgent recommendations have not been implemented more widely.

Shortell, Morrison, and Robbins discuss strategy formulation content and implementation, focusing upon research questions and sample hypotheses. For example, they hypothesize that "the greater the degree of competition, the greater the use of new market and new product service strategies." Their work is a good example of the usefulness of theory to practitioners, as many of the authors' hypotheses give the manager a wide array of approaches to try and guidance for using them in different situations. Thus the manager can draw on the theoretical underpinnings for the strategy, in addition to his or her skills and experience.

Robinette proposes that the new competitive environment for health care necessitates a fundamental rethinking of organizational values. He argues that patients should be viewed as customer-clients, and his management thinking goes along with that view.

Size gives one example of how some rural, nonprofit hospitals in Wisconsin are grouping together to provide shared services and to achieve economies of scale based on continuing traditional values.

ADDITIONAL TOPICS OF INTEREST

There is a large body of literature on the use of small-group processes for promoting change. Another rapidly growing area of interest is the study of technology assessment: the introduction and evaluation of new and sometimes costly medical technologies. Authors are now writing conceptual and theoretical summaries of important areas such as multi-institutional systems, governance, and organizational life cycles. There is also literature available on individuals and organizations that are the most likely to adopt new activities, as well as the organizational impact of changes in architecture, new types of professional personnel, and automated problem-oriented medical records. Professional associations, including the American Hospital Association and the American Medical Association, play a major role in mediating between provider organizations and professionals, and government. The selected bibliography below offers suggestions for further reading on topics related to adaptation. Readers should also refer to the annotated bibliography at the end of the book.

NOTES

1. The title of this section might make it appear that we are combining organizational level and performance requirement because "adaptation" is so similar to "adaptive capability." However, adaptation refers to the structural interface between organization and environment, and adaptive capability refers to the functional linkage between goal attainment and system maintenance.

2. This is somewhat analogous to the economic concept of "social good," which is defined as a product that yields advantages to society in general as well as to the individual who purchases it, but whose side advantages are not evident in marketplace prices.

3. Robert Guest, *Organizational Change* (Homewood, IL: Irwin, Dorsey Press, 1962).

4. Though attitudes, beliefs, and habits are distinct from each other, they will be subsumed here under the general concept of values, which we are treating as the characteristics of an organization held uniquely by individuals composing the organization.

SELECTED BIBLIOGRAPHY

Coddington, Dean C., and Keith D. Moore. *Market-Driven Strategies in Health Care*. San Francisco: Jossey-Bass, 1987.

Goodman, Louis J., and Larry J. Freshnock. "Why Medical Groups Fail." *Medical Group Management* 25 (November-December 1978): 10–14.

Grieco, Anthony J. "Home Care/Hospital Care/Cooperative Care, Options for the Practice of Medicine." *Bulletin of the New York Academy of Medicine* 64 (May 1988): 318–26.

Kotler, Philip, and Roberta N. Clarke. *Marketing for Health Care Organizations*. Englewood Cliffs, NJ: Prentice-Hall, 1987.

Kropf, Roger, and James A. Greenberg. *Strategic Analysis for Hospital Management*. Rockville, MD: Aspen, 1984.

Longest, Beaufort B., Jr. "An External Dependence Perspective of Organizational Strategy and Structure: The Community Hospital Case." *Hospital & Health Services Administration* 26 (Spring 1981): 50–69.

Longo, Daniel R., and Gary A. Chase. "Structural Determinants of Hospital Closure." *Medical Care* 22 (May 1984): 388–402.

Luke, Roice D., and James W. Begun. *The Management of Strategy in Health Care Management*. 2d ed. New York: Wiley, 1988.

McMillan, Norman H. *Marketing Your Hospital*. Chicago: American Hospital Association, 1981.

____. *Planning for Survival*. Chicago: American Hospital Association, 1978.

Milio, Nancy. "Health Care Organizations and Innovation." *Journal of Health and Social Behavior* 12 (June 1971): 163–73.

Peters, Joseph P., and Simone Tseng. *Managing Strategic Change in Hospitals*. Chicago: American Hospital Publishing, 1983.

Pfeffer, Jeffrey. "Size, Composition and Function of Hospital Boards of Directors: A Study of Organizational-Environment Linkages." *Administrative Science Quarterly* 18 (September 1973): 349–64.

Starkweather, David B. *Hospital Mergers in the Making*. Ann Arbor, MI: Health Administration Press, 1981.

Weiner, Joshua M., ed. *Swing Beds: Assessing Flexible Health Care in Rural Communities*. Washington, DC: Brookings Institution, 1987.

20 | Implementing Change within the Academic Medical Center

Cecil G. Sheps

The basic problems of developing an appropriate and effective program of patient education can be put in the general context of the underlying, fundamental challenge of developing appropriate and effective recognition, in practice, that patients bring more than their organs to the medical care system. They bring their psyches, their somas, their whole life envelopes, so to speak. Understanding the patient so that one can understand his illness, developing the patient's understanding so that the patient can become an ally, not to mention his own protagonist, is really not a new idea. It is almost 50 years since the medical literature began to demonstrate that this is indeed a vital concept. The remarkable thing about this is that, in terms of effective application, so little has really happened since then. There has been some progress, but patient education, like all of social medicine, remains at the periphery. It is at the periphery because a massive space-filling lesion has developed, one which is made up of the advances in human biology and its consequent technology. This reminds me of the doctor in Moliere's "The Imaginary Patient" who, when informed that he had confused the locations of the

Reprinted from *Bulletin of the New York Academy of Medicine* 61 (March 1985): 175–83, with permission, New York Academy of Medicine.

Presented as part of the *Conference on The Role of Academic Medicine in Patient Education* held by the Committee on Medicine in Society in cooperation with the Committee on Medical Education of the New York Academy of Medicine at the Tarrytown Conference Center, Tarrytown, N.Y., June 6 and 7, 1983. This conference was supported by a grant from Pfizer Pharmaceuticals.

liver and the heart, blithely replied: "Yes. It used to be so, but we have changed all that."

If we are going to put into place a comprehensive and optimally effective patient education program, it must be planned, managed, coordinated, and evaluated. This means that it should be an *institutional* program. It is not the kind of thing that one can assign to a little unit somewhere in the basement of the hospital because it must permeate and emerge from virtually every element of activity of the medical center. That this has been rarely done explains the frequent references at this conference that we do not have enough models in our academic medical centers to stimulate widespread program development. A pertinent observation was made succinctly and poignantly by a medical student in one of the discussion groups who said, "Medical students come to medical school identifying with the patient and they leave the medical school identifying with the doctors."

The basic issue here is one of the balance of goals and objectives in our academic medical centers coupled with the fact that, though physicians do not have to provide all of patient education, without their interest, leadership, authorization, and validation, it will not get very far. This means that we must look to academic medical centers for the future full development and achievement of the objectives of patient education. If we really want this to take hold and to develop well, we must recognize that it is in academic medical centers that the greatest responsibility lies. If these centers do not lead the way, progress, if any, will be slow and halting.

My views and statements about our academic medical centers are based on my experiences in them. They also stem from a national study which I directed, reported on in 1965 — a study of the relationships between hospitals and medical schools.[1] The capstone of my experience, observations, and analysis of these centers was the work that I did with another member of the New York Academy of Medicine, Irving J. Lewis, which culminated in a book published in 1983 entitled *The Sick Citadel*.[2]

The academic medical center has great power. Its power, its strength, its responsibilities, and its problems are, in our view, inadequately understood by the leading figures of the centers themselves, not to mention the government and the public. The most important thing about this is to understand the interdependence of the public and academic medical centers because, without each other, our whole health system breaks down. Academic medical centers are at the core of the nation's health care system; they feed it, fuel it, and they overtly run a substantial part of it. They increasingly control tertiary care and at the same time are the doctor to much of urban America—rich and poor alike. They produce physicians for the future and profoundly influence the shape, content, and emphasis of current and future medical practice.

The salient fact is that academic medical centers consist of some 126 medical schools affiliated with approximately 1,000 hospitals, which together constitute 40% of the general hospital beds of the nation. In these centers, 60,000 postgraduate residents are in training who give a significant amount of care to the nation's ill. In short, their broad range of functions in research, education, patient care, and community service, and their prestige empowers them to determine the scope and emphasis of our health services. Functioning in both academic and nonacademic environments, heavily dependent on tax funds, they must live in these two worlds. They carry out certain unique responsibilities and tasks that universities and their faculties do not readily welcome, not to mention cherish. The central health policy issue affecting these centers is their capacity and willingness to respond to considerations of the public interest as health priorities and public needs change over time. Of course, the special concern, and appropriately so, in the centers is to preserve their academic strength, as they see it in their own terms. The public interest, however, while accepting this, extends into the nonacademic world of society's health needs and the justification for support of these centers. They are, indeed, a vital national resource. This very fact warrants consistent thorough-going public scrutiny of the centers. As Victor Fuchs said to the Association of American Medical Colleges in 1979, "Even a sympathetic friendly observer . . . cannot help but get the impression that academic medicine's interest in health policy begins and ends with two commandments: First, give us money, and second, leave us alone."[3]

Collectively and individually, these centers are big business. Many have annual budgets of more than $200 million dollars. In most cases the present public posture of an academic medical center is that it is aggrieved, threatened, misunderstood, subjected to new demands without adequate resources to meet them, and, in some instances, to unreasonable demands for controls. At the same time, government approaches the centers, not as unified institutions which badly need improved governance, management, and public accountability, but as separate groups of hospitals, schools, and other facilities.

Patient education, like primary care, geriatrics, chronic care, and disease prevention are substantially neglected in today's academic medical centers, where the overriding emphasis is on acute specialty care and biomedical research. Medicine carries much mystery for the general public. It is time that the veil be lifted from academic medical centers so that their activities can be altered to reflect more adequately the public interest called for by the public funding upon which the centers depend for survival. Specific major changes in these centers are needed. The misfit between social demand and institutional response will be eliminated only after long periods of adjustment in academic medical centers in education, research, and patient care, and our nation's political behavior vis-à-vis these institutions. Above all, the public must understand the center's role and its responsibility to function effectively in its community and region as well as in the university at the same time that it enlarges and strengthens its expectations of them. And I suggest that our interest in patient education is a very good test of this.

The medical faculty is not a coherent body. Plato has said that what is honored in a country is what is cultivated there. The faculty is composed of a large number of groups and individuals with distinct and specialized interests and commitments. The strength and power of each is a function of his relative prestige and the amount of money available to them. This money comes from many different sources, much of it directly from outside agencies with special interests rather than through an institutional budget with allocations determined by the university or the medical school. The prestige of the faculty and the school largely depends upon the judgment of its peers outside the institution, that is, researchers and clinical leaders of similar institutions who exercise their judgment on the quality of research and specialty training grant applications. These peer judgments largely determine academic prestige. A medical faculty that does comparatively well by these judgments is assumed to be doing equally well in its medical education program. I believe, however, that this does not necessarily follow. The assumption has been that what the faculty does in research and specialty care will, in sum, naturally provide medical students with a full range of exposure, involvement, and teaching appropriate for their fundamental preparation for practice in the community. I submit that we have very little scientific evidence to establish the basis for this assumption which has now become dogma. I am happy to note that a few prestigious leaders in medical education with better qualifications than mine in academic clinical medicine have, in recent years, expressed the same view. I need only to refer you to Eichna's 1980 paper[4] and to a statement of a professor in a clinical field at Harvard at graduation ceremonies in 1980, that the one essential that those graduates would not be prepared for was how to be a doctor.[5]

How does this come to be since everybody involved really means well and works hard? I suggest to you that the underlying pathology is described best by the French term, *déformation professionelle*, the deformity that comes from the fact that the predominant emphasis in our medical faculties is upon being highly specialized, deeply technical, and therefore narrow—for which no corrective, balancing institutional context is provided.

The faculty tends to feel that such criticisms ignore the depth and high quality of their performance in research, patient care and, hence, teaching. They point out that their students and residents emerge with much greater knowledge of disease and skill in diagnosis and treatment than did those of earlier generations. This I understand, accept, and appreciate. It is, however, beside the point addressed in these criticisms, namely, that their educational program for the M.D. degree is not as well suited as it should be to meet the health needs of the public and the tasks of the physician in practice.

What is taught is what is best known and of greatest interest to the faculty, not necessarily what is needed as basic preparation for practice. I do not argue that the type of training now offered in teaching hospitals is irrelevant, but rather that students also need certain other important elements that now get little or no attention. It is not that the faculty does not care about their patients, but that they tend to care for them in a narrow and limited way. It makes no sense to separate human health and disease from the human being and the environment in which people live. The scientific approach requires the evaluation of *all* the facts that operate in a system addressed by a specific inquiry. To collect and evaluate a large series of physiochemical facts about a person and not to match them with relevant social, psychological, and economic facts is grossly incomplete, not to mention unscientific. Let us not forget the pertinent analogy in King Lear. Regan had the eyes of Gloucester, King Lear's faithful follower, plucked out, then ordered him from the castle with these words, "Let him smell his way to Dover." Unless our academic medical centers broaden the base of their commitments and activities to give psychosocial elements as much continuing attention as is now given to biological aspects, medicine's crisis and the public's disappointment and chagrin will continue to deepen.

How does this come about? Who is in charge? Who is responsible from the administrative point of view? I suggest that the present governance and organization of a typical academic medical center is not properly adapted to solving the issues that face it at all levels. From the president of the university to the medical school dean and department chairmen, no one seems satisfied that the most appropriate and effective organizational framework has been found. The uneasiness and frustration now growing in these centers results, in significant measure, from their inability to approach, analyze, and evaluate fundamental issues and to develop solutions in an expeditious, open-minded, and unified manner. Their current structure and process of decision-making protects the independence of the component principalities of the faculty. They fortify the status quo, rendering searching assessment and reassessment most unwelcome and extremely difficult to achieve. And there is much more involved in this than the fiscal stewardship of large sums of money or the acquisition of more.

Current governance fosters short-term solutions instead of the long-term comprehensive planning that is needed. Highly skilled professionals accustomed to autonomy and independence do not take well to administrators, even when they are deans, though they share a common background in terms of basic scientific training. The medical faculty, firmly rooted in the accepted and apparently successful traditions of the recent past, prefers to concentrate on *their* immediate special needs, as *they* see them. The administrators, on the other hand, more aware of societal pressures, cannot set aside long-term goals and the total institutional view, and tend to see more clearly the need to ensure that the academic medical center as an *institution*, will, in the long run, carry out its social contract as effectively as possible.

What is sorely lacking is a greater certainty about who is in charge. Greater unity is needed in institutional decision-making regarding specific purposes and priorities, the content of activities and the size, effectiveness, and fiscal implications of its programs. If an academic medical center is to carry out its social obligations effectively, it must cease to be a loose federation of independent duchies and principalities. These independent units of substantial size and power each representing different, often competing, objectives with more than one source of financing and control *are* the problem. The manner of financing and governance which has developed in this country, and the fact that they currently function in centrifugal fashion, frustrates efforts to centralize policy decision-making in the centers where it is needed—at the top level—in terms of their purposes, financing, and control. We must build a stronger institutional structure for policy development, operational support, and fiscal control. What is needed is flexibility, unity, and greater strength in decision-making at top managerial levels. Then the centers will be able to blend academic functions and social purposes into an overall coherent and effective program.

The issue of developing a more appropriate balance of objectives is crucial if academic medical centers are to attain a secure financial base as they direct their efforts more clearly to the health needs of the population. The basic questions are: Who are we, what is our purpose, and where are we going? Answering these vital and discomfiting questions necessitates open-minded, concentrated attention in the centers to decide which are the unique tasks which they must perform fully to carry out their responsibilities to the public. The response needs to be defined in the context of the essential role these centers need to undertake in education, research, patient care, and community service. The latter is not synonymous with care provided by them to the patients who are able to present themselves. This would lead to a clear statement of the optimum role of their facilities and services in functional integration with other facilities and services so as to satisfy the health needs of the region in which the centers are located. From this context a host of issues emerge which the governance of the center must address.

As the administrative head of the medical school, the dean presides over the full range of activities of the school. This often includes some 20 academic departments with significant subsections, which often total 40 or more, all of them requiring funds, space, and supporting services. The dean is involved in an enormous range of policy, procedural, and operational issues. A large portion of expenditures of the departments, not uncommonly more than half, sometimes more than two thirds, are made out of funds from external sources which they obtain. Hence the departments and sections view these funds, which they have generated, as belonging solely to them and not available, in any significant fashion, to support other school activities. The activities supported by external funds need space and supporting services, thus requiring institutional concurrence and support from the medical school and often the hospital. For these reasons, the faculty believes they must dominate policy-making and management. The formal relationship between faculty and administration of the school is expressed through both permanent and ad hoc arrangements. There is usually a school executive committee, called by various names, of at least 15 to 20 people, most of whom, if not all, are departmental chairmen. They bring a set of formal constituencies to the executive committee by representing the departments they lead. One can hardly expect such a group to relate itself readily to overall institutional needs. Instead, and understandably, they are concerned with protecting and strengthening the activities for which they are responsible.

To borrow John Gardner's phrase, "I'm not sure whether I am a critical lover or a loving critic," but let me now address the question, "What can be done about it?" I suggest three major considerations in implementing needed changes in our academic medical centers. The first is that the governance of the academic medical center needs to strengthen its executive power and capacity. Greater responsibility needs to be placed in the Board of Trustees for public accountability, which, in turn, should place it, with full accountability, in the hands of the top administrative officers.

Second, the academic medical center must develop planning and budgeting systems adequate to strengthen institutional decision-making and priority-setting, increase flexibility to utilize and shift resources to meet institutional priorities, and relate short-term gains to long-term obligations.

And third, the academic medical center is uniquely situated in the health care system to take the lead by undertaking a broad community service mission which it can fulfill simultaneously with its major additional obligations in research and teaching. It has the prestige, the technical capacity, and much of the needed resources. The problems of ill health and an uncoordinated system are all about them. If the centers would lead, the consequences would be substantial. First, the university patient care complex would be brought more clearly into the community care system, where it belongs. Second, research and education would be closely related, but not limited, to the needs of the community at hand. Third, the three familiar goals of research, education, and patient care would now be supplemented by a clearly defined fourth goal, that of community service. This means that the center would give high priority in its teaching, research, and patient care programs to the major health problems of the population of its area and to practice in the community. It would evaluate the relative importance of different health problems by their prevalence, the amount of disability and premature death they produce, and the age at which they take their toll. It would then take the lead in developing service programs by applying the latest knowledge and most relevant skills to these challenges. Acceptance of this goal of community service, as distinct from treating individual patient episodes, would then clearly highlight the need for proper attention and prominence to such challenges as primary care, geriatrics, chronic care, and patient education.

How can the effective implementation of this new mission and a new model be promoted? First, we must recognize the basic differences between the management and financing tasks of the teaching hospital and other patient care community programs, on the one hand, and those of research and education on the other. This calls for the restructuring of the basic governance framework of the academic medical centers so that the large range of "joint products" for which they are responsible are appropriately selected and adequately developed, nurtured, and controlled by two separate, interacting, organizations of equal strength. The organization of the academic medical center should consist of two clearly designated administrative management structures of equal strength and authority which act jointly, where necessary, under a unified overall university administration — one for patient care, the other for the academic activities of research and teaching. It is like a marriage where two people have decided that they need each other and that it is worth their while to share and live together, who find that their needs and interests are not the same at every moment. If they are both strong, they can accommodate to each other on a daily basis and maintain the effectiveness of their partnership. If one, however, is always dominant, then the best potential of that partnership does not develop and mature.

Second, if the medical school is to be an effective partner in achieving the four goals of the center and participate responsibly, then the position of its dean as an executive needs clarification and substantial reinforcement.

Third, we must be really serious about the appointment and promotion of an adequate number of faculty members whose skills and interests are in teaching and patient care, and stop the pretense that every faculty member is a triple threat person, equally interested and competent in research, teaching, and patient care. And I suggest that there *are* ways to measure quality of performance in patient care and in teaching.

I believe that such changes would provide adequate strength and insight to achieve the goals of the academic medical center. These goals are interdependent but distinct and cannot be substituted one for the other. There need to be strong protagonists and a surrogate for each of these goals that can speak for them and work out the necessary accommodations among them in an institutional context which fosters open discussion in which an appropriate balance of institutional programs and responsibilities can be developed and maintained.

This will not be achieved from the inside alone. It needs the understanding and the attention of the university through its trustees. It also needs the understanding of government and the public, whom government represents. It needs public expectation, public demand, and consistent financially adequate public support. The public interest, at the same time, must be informed and insistent.

I suggest to you that a new world in health services is waiting to be born. This is a difficult process, but if we want it to come about we must understand the underlying processes involved. As G.K. Chesterton said, in talking about Christianity, "It's not that it's been tried and found wanting. It's been tried and found difficult, and therefore abandoned."

REFERENCES

1. Sheps, C.G., Clark, D.A., Gerdes, J.W., et al.: *Medical Schools and Hospitals: Interdependence for Education and Service* Evanston, Ill., Assoc. Med. Colleges, 1965, *J. Med. Educ.* 40: September 1965.

2. Lewis, I.J. and Sheps, C.G.: *The Sick Citadel: The American Academic Medical Center and the Public Interest.* Cambridge, Oelgeschlager, Gunn, and Hain, 1983.

3. Fuchs, V.R.: Public policy and the medical establishment: Who's on first? *J. Med. Educ* 50: 5, 1979.

4. Eichna, L.W.: Medical education, 1975–79. *N. Engl. J. Med.* 303: 227–234, 1980.

5. Falkman, J.: Is there a doctor in the house? *Harvard Med. Alumni Bull.* 54: 37–40, 1980.

21

Strategy Making in Health Care Organizations: A Framework and Agenda for Research

Stephen M. Shortell
Ellen M. Morrison
Shelley Robbins

The American health care system is in transition. The transition is captured in both language and symbols. Observers speak of an "industry" rather than a "system" and there has been movement from a "cottage industry" to corporate consolidation, from health care as a social good to health care as an economic good, from a production orientation to a marketing orientation, from advertising as anathema to billboards dotting highways emphasizing the advantages of one provider over another. To this one might add a fundamental managerial transition from an emphasis on operational management to an emphasis on strategic management, or, if you will, from the image of the administrator as a "caretaker" to the image of the administrator as a "risk-taker".

The reasons for the transition are well known — prospective payment, competition, technological developments, and new consumer expectations. These factors have created a more hostile environment for health care organizations. Similar dynamics have occurred in the banking, trucking, airlines, and communications industries. The difference

Excerpted from the article in *Medical Care Review* 42 (Fall 1985): 219-27, 231-41, and 253-58, with permission, Health Administration Press.

between the winners and losers is likely to be their ability to *strategize*, that is, to develop and implement plans to position themselves so as to take advantage of the rapidly changing market, product, technological, and social environments relative to their competitors. As Greer, Greer, and Meyer (1983, p. 74) have noted in regard to medical technology, "organizational strategies are likely to emerge increasingly as explicit benchmarks for medical equipment decisions. These strategies cannot be directly extrapolated from either the march of science or financial exigencies. They merit the explicit attention of researchers and policymakers."

The purpose of this article is twofold. First, to call the attention of health services researchers to the importance of this emerging area of inquiry. Second, to provide an overview of several approaches to the issues including discussion of developing theories, key concepts, researchable questions, sample hypotheses, and suggested measures. We begin by providing a conceptual overview of the topic followed by discussion of strategy formulation, strategic content and strategy implementation. Within each of these sections, important research questions, concepts, measures, and approaches are suggested.

AN OVERVIEW

There are as many ways of studying strategy as there are definitions. We define strategy as:

> the plans and activities developed by an organization in pursuit of its goals and objectives, particularly in regard to positioning itself to meet external environmental demands relative to its competition.

This definition is generally consistent with that of Chandler (1962). It is a somewhat blander treatment than suggested by the original Greek derivation of the term "stratego" meaning literally "to plan the destruction of one's enemy with maximum force".

Neither definition, however, captures the dynamic nature of strategy as suggested by Mintzberg (1978) and Miles and Snow (1978). They view strategy as a *pattern* in a "stream" of important decisions made over time. Further, *strategic* decisions are those concerned with defining the long-term relationship between the organization and its environment (Salter and Weinhold 1979).

As defined above, the main dimensions of strategy as shown in Table 21.1 can be considered in terms of: (1) levels, (2) outcomes, (3) time frame, and (4) basic approaches. Corporate-level strategies address the

TABLE 21.1

Strategy Dimensions

Levels	Outcomes	Time Frame	Basic Approaches
Corporate	Intended	Past	Strategy Formulation
Business	Realized	Present	Strategic Content
Functional	Unrealized	Future	Strategy Implementation
	Emergent		

issue of what businesses the organization should pursue. Should a given hospital become involved in long-term care, ambulatory surgery, outpatient renal dialysis, or outpatient diagnostic imaging? Business-level strategies focus on how the organization should compete in the businesses they have selected (Hambrick 1980). For example, should the hospital penetrate existing markets, develop new markets, refine existing product-services, develop new product-services, grow from within, or grow through acquisition and joint ventures with others? Functional-level strategies determine the bases upon which the organization will support the corporate and business-level strategies (Wheelwright 1984). For example, what kinds of pricing policies, market research strategies, capital formation plans, and human resource strategies will be needed by a hospital or multiunit hospital system which decides to provide long-term care services?

While important research questions can be addressed at all three levels (corporate, business, and functional) the biggest payoff for health care organizations lies in exploring the relationships among the three levels (Schendel and Hofer 1979). This is because health care organizations are undergoing pervasive changes in all three areas simultaneously.

In addition to levels, strategies can be conceptualized in terms of outcomes. Mintzberg (1978), for example, suggests that strategies be considered as intended, realized, unrealized, and emergent. *Intended* strategies are those that a given organization says it intends to pursue. This may be reflected in annual reports and related documents, and what is communicated in interviews with organizational leaders. However, intended strategies may be realized or unrealized. this distinction is critical to understanding the relationship between strategy and performance. For example, a hospital's strategy to expand its out-of-hospital services through a program of vertical diversification may be unrealized because of its inability to work out cooperative arrangements with key physicians. Realized strategies may be expected to have a positive effect on performance, *assuming* that the "correct" strategies were selected relative to the nature of the problem addressed. Intended strategies that are realized are called *deliberate* strategies by Mintzberg (1978).

Emergent strategies, in contrast, are realized strategies that were never intended by the organization. They represent spontaneous adaptive and largely unconscious strategies that may have arisen as a function of rapidly changing external forces. For example, a medical school may be presented with an opportunity to develop a partnership with an investor-owned hospital company which can provide capital to meet the medical school's teaching and research missions.

Time frame is the third significant dimension of strategy. It is important to know whether strategies currently pursued are similar to past strategies and the degree to which they are likely to prevail in the future. Without such information, it is possible to mistakenly attribute a particular performance outcome to a current, as opposed to past, strategy because there is usually a lag between the adoption and implementation of a strategy and its impact on performance indicators, such as profitability, market share, cost, access, and quality of care. One might also mistakenly assume that a health care organization's current strategy is what it intends to pursue in the future. Thus, it is important to assess the relative permanence of an organization's strategy, something which can be done through retrospective historical analysis (Mintzberg and Waters 1982) and longitudinal prospective studies (Shortell, Wickizer, and Wheeler 1984).

There are also three generic approaches to the study of strategy: (1) *the formulation of strategy,* (2) *the content of strategy, and* (3) *the implementation of strategy.* The central question of what strategies (that is, content) are more or less effective for health care organizations can be influenced in important ways by both how a strategy is formulated and how it is implemented. While different investigators have different interests and practical research design limitations often preclude studying all three approaches simultaneously, the ultimate goal should be to integrate knowledge of these three areas of health care strategy making.

STRATEGY FORMULATION

The need for health care organizations to adopt an overall strategic approach to management has only recently been recognized (Domanico 1981; Longest 1981; Flexner, Berkowitz, and Brown 1981; Fournet 1982; Files 1983; Luke and Kurowski 1983) and only a small percentage of health care organizations have actually adopted a strategic management approach (Kropf and Goldsmith 1983). We define strategy formulation as the *process* that is used to assess or reassess the organization's mission, philosophy and goals, and to develop plans to achieve the organization's goals and objectives consistent with its mission and philosophy. The emphasis is on the process by which strategic plans are developed. Relevant questions include: (1) How does the organization review its goals, mission and philosophy? (2) How does it conduct environmental assessment and competitive analysis? (3) How does it assess its internal strengths and weaknesses? (4) How does it assess its specific programs' strengths and weaknesses? (5) How does it recognize when existing strategies should be changed? (6) Who is primarily involved in the process? and (7) How centralized versus decentralized is the process?

Longest (1981) provides a useful framework for considering these kinds of questions. As shown in Figure 21.1, strategy formulation is viewed as a dynamic interactive process between the environment and the organization. The key players are the organization's strategists, those stakeholder leaders who perceive changes in the environment and set in motion a process for matching the organization's distinctive competence with the demands of the environment. While strategists or key stakeholders play a dominant role in the strategy formulation process, a complex combination of strategies, tasks, structure, technologies, and people affects the implementation of strategy. The focus in this section is on the formulation process; implementation issues are addressed in a subsequent section.

APPROACHES, CONCEPTS AND DEFINITIONS

Fredrickson (1984) identifies two basic conceptual approaches to strategy formulation, the *synoptic* and the *incremental*. The synoptic approach assumes that purpose and integration are critical to an organization's long-run success and, as such, great emphasis is given to preplanned, comprehensive, rational decision making (Ansoff 1965; Schendel and Hofer 1979; Lorange and Vancil 1976). Incremental models emphasize less comprehensive approaches, which tend to break down problems into subproblems and tend to be somewhat more opportunistic (Lindblom 1959; Mintzberg 1978; Quinn 1980). As others have noted (Nutt 1977; Mintzberg 1978), some organizations may use both approaches depending on such factors as the nature of the environmental demands faced and the stage of the decision-making process.

It is also important to consider why organizations initiate strategies in the first place and why they change strategies over time. We suggest four reasons for strategy creation and change: (1) the perception of perfor-

FIGURE 21.1

The Strategy Formulation Process

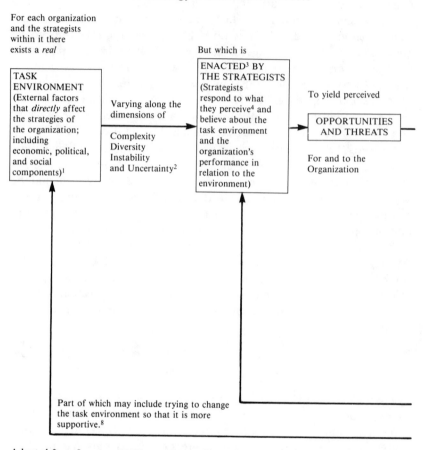

Adapted from Longest (1981), pp. 54–55, with permission, Health Administration Press.
    1. R. N. Osborn and J. G. Hunt, "Environment and Organizational Effectiveness," *Administrative Science Quarterly* 19 (June 1974): 231–46.
    2. S. M. Shortell, "The Role of Environment in a Configurational Theory of Organizations," *Human Relations* 30 (March 1977): 275–302.
    3. K. E. Weick, *The Social Psychology of Organizations*. Reading, MA: Addison-Wesley, 1969; and K. E. Weick, "Enactment Processes in Organizations." In *New Dimensions in Organizational Behavior*, eds. B. M. Staw and G. R. Salancik, 267–300. Chicago: St. Clair Press, 1977.
    4. R. B. Duncan, "Characteristics of Organizational Environments and Perceived Environmental Uncertainty," *Administrative Science Quarterly* 17 (September 1972): 313–27.
    5. B. B. Longest, Jr., "The Relationship Between the Environment Facing Community Hospitals and Their Strategy." Working Paper No. 17, Center for Health Services and Policy Research, Northwestern University, Spring 1978.

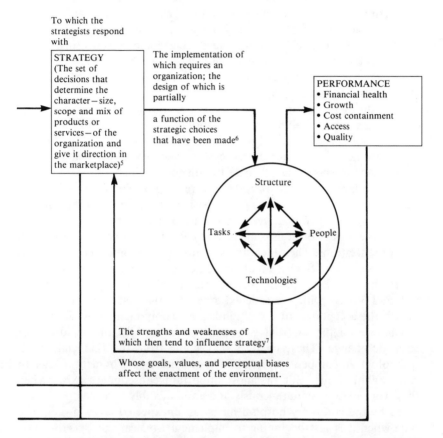

To which the strategists respond with

STRATEGY (The set of decisions that determine the character—size, scope and mix of products or services—of the organization and give it direction in the marketplace)[5]

The implementation of which requires an organization; the design of which is partially

a function of the strategic choices that have been made[6]

PERFORMANCE
• Financial health
• Growth
• Cost containment
• Access
• Quality

Structure

Tasks · · People

Technologies

The strengths and weaknesses of which then tend to influence strategy[7]

Whose goals, values, and perceptual biases affect the enactment of the environment.

6. A number of researchers have shown that the design of the organization is influenced by the choice of strategy. Some of these include: P. F. Drucker, *Management: Tasks, Responsibilities, Practices.* New York: Harper & Row, 1974; A. D. Chandler, Jr., *Strategy and Structure.* New York: Doubleday, 1962; J. Galbraith, *Designing Complex Organizations.* Reading, MA: Addison-Wesley, 1973.

7. Examples of research demonstrating this include: L. E. Fouraker and J. M. Stopford, "Organizational Structure and the Multinational Strategy," *Administrative Science Quarterly* 13 (June 1968): 47–64; J. G. March and H. Simon, *Organizations.* New York: John Wiley & Sons, 1958; R. Cyert and J. G. March, *A Behavioral Theory of the Firm.* Englewood Cliffs, N.J.: Prentice-Hall, 1963.

8. J. Pfeffer and G. R. Salancik, *The External Control of Organizations: A Resource Dependence Perspective.* New York: Harper & Row, 1978. Especially Chapter 7, "The Negotiated Environment," and Chapter 8, "The Created Environment."

mance gaps, (2) the perception of dissonance gaps, (3) changes in the external environment, and (4) changes in organizational leadership.

Organizations initiate or change their strategies when they perceive a difference in performance either between themselves and relevant competing-comparison organizations and/or between their current performance and their desired performance. These differences may involve market share for specific services, target occupancy rates, profitability, quality of care standards, or related indicators. Such discrepancies create incentives for initiating new strategies and/or refining current strategies (Dutton and Duncan 1985).

In addition to performance gaps, organizations also experience dissonance gaps (Shortell 1985). Organizational dissonance exists when the organization's view of itself is challenged or its identity is threatened. Such a state may be created by performance gaps (for example, the historically successful health care organization which suddenly experiences a failure) or by environmental threats (for example, an antitrust suit). However, such gaps may also exist because the organization suddenly finds itself doing very new and different things. Numerous examples exist as hospitals branch out to become more diversified health care organizations. Their identity as a "hospital" becomes threatened and dissonance sets in. Such a situation creates incentives to reduce the dissonance through development of strategies which either promote integration and linkage with a broadened organizational self-concept or which permit the acceptance of loosely linked subcomponents (Weick 1976).

Changes in the external environment are a third major source of strategic change. These changes may come from the financial, legal, technological, competitive, regulatory, and other environments of health care organizations. But the most important consequence exists when these forces occur simultaneously and unpredictably. An example is provided by the voluntary hospital hit by an unexpected large lawsuit at a time when it is just beginning to implement Medicare prospective payment requirements, is responding to contemplated state rate-review legislation, and has just seen its market share of inpatient admissions decline 10 percent due to the presence of a newly acquired investor-owned hospital. Such decisions may require changes in several of the organization's strategies, perhaps involving a major strategic reorientation.

Finally, strategies often change when leadership changes. New leaders frequently have different views of the organization, its strengths and weaknesses, its environment, and its competition. In fact, when the old leadership leaves involuntarily, it may be precisely because the old strategies weren't working or because there were no apparent coherent strategies guiding the organization's activities.

In considering the above issues, it is important to focus on the organization's leaders because it is their perception of performance gaps, dissonance gaps, external environmental threats, and the need for changes in leadership which drive the strategy-making process. Unlike most other industries, health care organizations and hospitals, in particular, have a divergent and loosely linked set of stakeholders composed primarily of the board of trustees, administration, the medical staff, other health professionals, employees, third-party payers, and patients. Particular challenges are posed by physicians who through their clinical decision making may generate upwards of 70 percent of the organization's activities and costs; yet most physicians are independent practitioners, not hospital employees. Further, hospitals are staffed by a great diversity of other health professionals with considerable interest in maintaining and expanding their professional autonomy and identity. No longer solely the "doctor's workshop", some have also suggested that hospitals have become community health service centers (Sigmond 1966) and "coalitions of professionals" (Shortell, Morrisey, and Conrad 1985). This represents a distinct challenge to the strategy-making process. How does one involve physicians in the strategy-making process? Who should be involved? In what ways should they be involved? What about the involvement of other health professionals? What should be the relative roles of the board of trustees, administration, medical staff, and other groups? Does the mix and type of involvement influence the content of strategies adopted or the degree to which they are implemented? In brief, which of the organization's stakeholders should become its strategists and in what ways? . . .

STRATEGIC CONTENT

APPROACHES, CONCEPTS AND DEFINITIONS

In deciding what lines of business to pursue, health care organizations can consider six basic kinds of strategies. These include market penetration, new market development, product-service refinement, new product-service development, growth from within, and growth from without. Combining new product-service development with new market development results in diversification. *Market penetration* involves attracting more patients from one's current market using one's current mix of services. For example, a hospital may attempt to increase its share of surgical patients by adding more surgeons to its staff. *New market development* involves actively developing new markets for one's current mix of services. For example, a health maintenance organization may try to reach new geographic areas by extending its current ambulatory services in the form of satellite clinics. *Product-service refinement* involves modifying or upgrading current product-services. For example, a nursing home may increase its physician coverage as a way of upgrading the quality of care it provides. *New product-service development* involves the creation of new products or services not previously provided by the health care organization. Examples might include the development of a home care program, hospice, ambulatory surgery center, or outpatient substance abuse treatment unit. *Growth from within* involves additions to one's own facilities or building new facilities. For example, a multiunit hospital system may decide to build a nationwide network of primary care centers. *Growth from without* involves the acquisition of other facilities and/or entering into joint ventures to purchase, lease, or manage other facilities. For example, an investor-owned hospital company might purchase a chain of nursing homes as a way of entering the long-term care field.

In addition to the strategies described above, there are a number of functional strategies which may be developed to support the basic corporate- and business-level strategies selected. These primarily involve marketing, finance, and human resources. Examples of marketing strategies include: (1) the relative degree of emphasis to be given to the quality, price, and convenience of given product-services; (2) the degree to which promotion should be directed at physicians, consumers, or employer groups; (3) the degree to which "loss leader" pricing strategies should be adopted for selected product-services; and (4) the degree to which two or more product-services should be marketed separately or together. In the financial area, strategic decisions may center around: (1) the third-party mix of patients to be served (Medicare, Medicaid, Blue Cross, commercial, etc.); (2) payment policies upon admission; (3) the decision to be a low-cost provider (Porter 1980): (4) the degree to which investment decisions should balance short-run and long-run objectives; and (5) the relative use of debt or equity in financing capital outlays. Some strategic decisions relevant to human resources include: (1) whether the current mix of professionals is adequate in experience and expertise to provide new market and new product-service development strategies; (2) whether it is necessary to substitute lower-paid for higher-paid professionals; (3) whether additional training is required to upgrade the interpersonal and managerial skills of middle managers; and (4) whether reward systems need to be modified to encourage risk taking and to acknowledge truly outstanding performance.

It is important to note that marketing, financial, and human resource functions and strategies are interdependent and, indeed, in higher-performing health care organizations, one would expect to find these functional strategies to be consistent with each other in support of a given corporate or business strategy. For example, a hospital starting a new ambulatory surgery center may find it necessary to market not only to physicians but also to consumers and employer groups, to adopt strict payment policies upon admission for those without adequate insurance coverage, and to offer productivity-based incentives to physicians utilizing the center. These strategies would appear to reinforce each other in pursuit of the goal of maximizing the utilization and profitability of the new center.

Several tools are available to assist health care organizations in choosing among different strategies. Generally, these involve examining important characteristics of different service or product lines relevant to one's competition. Two examples are the Boston Consulting Group Market Share-Market Growth Matrix (Henderson 1973) and the General Electric Multiple Factor Matrix (Abell and Hammond 1979) shown in Figures 21.2 and 21.3. The BCG Market Share-Market Growth Matrix suggests that, for each important service, health care organizations consider both the percentage of market share that the service currently enjoys relative to the competition and the degree to which the service is likely to grow in the future. Services high on both dimensions may be considered "Stars"; those with high market growth potential but low market share are called "Wildcats" or "Question Marks"; those with low

FIGURE 21.2

Boston Consulting Group's Portfolio Matrix

		MARKET SHARE	
		High	Low
MARKET GROWTH POTENTIAL	High	"STARS" e.g., DX + RX radiology, DX + RX lab	"WILDCATS" (or "Question Marks") e.g., Home care, hospice, substance abuse centers
	Low	"CASH COWS" e.g., General medical-surgical services	"DOGS" e.g., Maternity, pediatrics

FIGURE 21.3

General Electric Multiple Factor Matrix

MARKET ATTRACTIVENESS

		High	Medium	Low
COMPETITIVE POSITION	High	MAINTAIN OR EXPAND Psychiatric care	MAINTAIN ICU/CCU	DELETE IF OTHERS CAN PROVIDE Outpatient clinic for indigents
	Medium	EXPAND Ambulatory surgery	EXPAND Industrial medicine	DELETE IF OTHERS CAN PROVIDE Obstetrics
	Low	DELETE OR DEVELOP JOINTLY WITH OTHERS Home care	DELETE OR DEVELOP JOINTLY WITH OTHERS Outpatient alcoholism program	DELETE IF OTHERS CAN PROVIDE Pediatrics

market growth potential but high market share are "Cash Cows"; while those with low market growth potential and low market share are considered "Dogs". Some possible examples of each are shown in Figure 21.2. The organization needs to generate enough revenue from its "Star" and "Cash Cow" lines of services to subsidize the "Wildcat" ventures until such time that the functional marketing, finance, and human resource strategies result in greater market share and the "Wildcat" service becomes a "Star" or eventual "Cash Cow".

The "Dog" services are of particular interest. In most other industries, such services or product lines would be deleted. But because of the social and humanitarian goals of most health care organizations, the decision to delete such services takes on added meaning. The central question is: Under what circumstances are these services maintained or deleted? If other providers are available to provide the service, the decision may be less difficult. But if a given organization is the only provider, then issues of community need become paramount. It is precisely such trade-off decisions that more health care organizations are having to make. It also underscores the importance of the portfolio approach because an organization which has a good balance of "Star", "Cash Cow" and "Wildcat" services will be in a better position to support low market share, low growth but "needed" services (i.e., "Dogs") than the organization which does not have such a balanced portfolio.

It is also important for health care organizations to add a third dimension to the BCG matrix, namely, profitability. Unlike most other industries, many health care organizations provide product-service lines that are not profitable. Under prospective payment pressures and the growing trend toward capitation payment for all services, the profitability of given services will play a significant role. A health care organization is more likely to retain a low market share, low market growth potential service if it is profitable, than if it is not. Failing this, the service may continue to be offered through a joint venture with another organization, or to be subsidized by the "Star" and "Cash Cow" services. Alternatively, if there are other alternative providers, the service may be deleted.

The General Electric Multiple Factor Matrix, shown in Figure 21.3 with examples, makes the element of competition more explicit than does the BCG Matrix. The BCG Matrix is oriented toward a cash flow approach, while the General Electric Matrix emphasizes return on equity (ROE). As shown in Figure 21.3, each of an organization's product-service lines is assessed in terms of its competitive position based on such factors as current market share, technical quality, experience, human resources, and ability to market compared to the competition. Market or industry attractiveness is assessed using such criteria as (1) community need, (2) likely future market share, (3) ability to make use of one's particular expertise, experience, and resources, (4) extent to which the service relates to other product-service offerings, (5) extent to which it relates to the organization's mission and philosophy, and (6) extent to which it is likely to be reimbursed by third-party payment.

As shown, the most desirable services are those with higher market attractiveness and competitive position. These should be maintained and, where possible, expanded (the high and medium cells). The right-hand column of services where market attractiveness is low represents opportunities for deletion, particularly if others can provide the service. This becomes the strategy of choice even if one's competitive position is high since the service is essentially unattractive to the organization from a market perspective. However, a note of caution is in order as one might still provide the service as a preemptive or preventive strategy so as to deter a competitor from entering the market, particularly if the competitor could use the service to establish a toehold in a given market from which other more competitive services could be developed.

The two left cells in the lower row (low competitive position but with either high or medium market attractiveness) represent opportunities for joint collaboration with others in order to improve one's overall competitive position. Such collaboration may be based on securing complementary resources, expertise, experience, access to desired markets, capital financing, and so on. It is also important that such ventures be undertaken with other organizations which share similar philosophies and missions and, thus, essentially are compatible. Examples include hospitals in different market areas that have joined together to sponsor HMOs and PPOs. If cooperative ventures in these lower cells cannot be developed, then serious consideration should be given to deleting the service since the resources could be better devoted to maintaining or expanding those services in the high and/or medium cells that reflect competitive position and market attractiveness. Again, an exception exists where the product-service is maintained as a defensive strategy of preempting other new entrants into a desirable market, or where one wishes to maintain a "presence" against existing competition in order to retain leverage to assist in introducing new products or services in the future.

There is an important relationship between the kinds of strategic planning tools, discussed above, and the kind of competitive analysis which is done. Porter (1980) has outlined a general approach to competitive analysis which involves the examination of barriers to entry and exit, the substitution of product-services, the bargaining power of buyers and suppliers, and the degree of competition or rivalry among existing firms. For example, several of the new low-tech programs or services such as home care, hospice care, and ambulatory surgery centers, have relatively low barriers to entry (in terms of capital outlays and regulatory and/or licensing criteria) so that it is easy for competitors to duplicate the service quickly. An example of exit considerations is raised by the relative ease or difficulty with which an acute care hospital can convert unused beds to skilled nursing care beds. With regard to the market power of buyers and suppliers, the buying power of health care organizations, relative to their suppliers, would appear to have increased given cost-containment incentives for hospitals to negotiate price discounts. Hospitals that belong to large multiunit systems are in a particularly strong position in relation to suppliers. Given the surplus of physicians, the power of hospitals to bargain with their medical staff members has also increased. Entry and exit barriers and relative bargaining power will, of course, be affected by the intensity of competition in a given market area.

OTHER FACTORS

Strategies are not developed in a vacuum and, therefore, consideration must be given to factors other than those noted above. Among the most important of these are environmental factors such as the degree of regulatory activity, degree of competition, and community sociodemographic characteristics. Among organizational characteristics to consider are size, location, amount of resources, ownership, whether or not the hospital is a member of a multiunit system, hospital age or life cycle, goals, and the hospital's ability to perceive and assess the environment and to learn from its past mistakes. These factors influence the kinds of strategies adopted and, in turn, their effect on performance. The overall framework incorporating these dimensions is presented in Figure 21.4 and examples of strategic responses are shown in Table 21.2.

While questions and hypotheses involving relationships among these variables are considered in the following section, it is helpful to define those dimensions or aspects which are not self-evident. *Scope* of regulatory activity denotes the number of different types of organizations covered under the regulation (Chapko et al. 1984; Shortell, Morrisey and Conrad 1985). For example, do state capital expenditure review programs or rate-review programs cover only hospital inpatient services, or do they also cover out-of-hospital services including HMOs, ambulatory surgery, nursing homes, and so forth? *Stringency or restrictiveness* refers to whether the regulatory programs are voluntary or mandatory, along with the degree of detail or rigor involved in the program including penalties for noncompliance. *Uncertainty* means the number and degree of changes in the regulatory program over time, or a reversal of policy so that the decisions and activities of the regulatory agency become difficult for the health care organization to predict. *Duration* refers to the length of time the regulatory program has been in existence in terms of the overall regulatory life cycle. For example, hospitals that have recently come under rate-review regulation may learn from the experience of those that have already undergone such regulation.

In regard to competitive environments, it is important to highlight that such competition may be taking place between one hospital-physician partnership and another hospital-physician partnership in the community. This, in part, reflects the strategic responses of both hospitals and physicians. Therefore, a double-headed arrow between the competitive environment and the strategic response set is shown in Figure 21.4, indicating that strategic responses at time T can influence the nature of the competitive environment at time T + 1.

The organizational strategic response set shown indicates that the

FIGURE 21.4

A Framework for Studying Strategic Responses of
Health Care Organizations

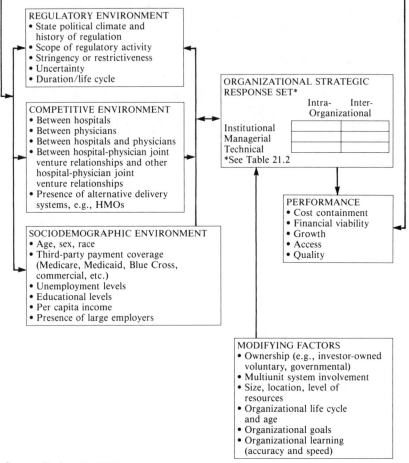

Source: Cook et al. (1983).

responses may take place at institutional, managerial, or technical levels
of the organization (Parsons 1956), both within the organization (intra)
as well as external to the organization (inter) (Cook et al. 1983).
Institutional-level responses refer to those that directly link the organization to its external environment. The managerial level allocates resources
in such a way as to link best the institutional and technical levels of the

TABLE 21.2

Strategic Response Set Examples (from Figure 21.4)

	Intraorganizational	*Interorganizational*
Institutional Level	Trustee education Lobbying	Acquisitions, mergers, consolidations, and divestitures
Managerial Level	Corporate reorganization Changes in levels of decision making— centralization vs. decentralization Addition of strategic planning and marketing functions Changes in medical staff organization	Shared managerial and administrative support services
Technical Level	Market penetration vs. new market development Product-service refinement vs. new product-service development Diversification (new product-service development *and* new market development)	Patient care joint ventures and shared arrangements with other organizations

organization, given the environmental demands placed upon it. The technical level focuses on the direct products or services delivered to clients.

Among the moderating factors, organizational life cycle requires explanation. It refers to the fact that new organizations may respond to external events differently than more highly developed or mature organizations (Greiner 1970; Kimberly and Miles 1980). It also refers to the fact that organizations may go through several cycles of birth, innovation, consolidation, maturity, retrenchment and rebirth, over time, as a function of their performance relative to their competition and environment and the ability to learn and grow.

The relationships outlined in Figure 21.4 also provide a framework for addressing some important issues in the organization theory literature at large. These involve primarily population ecology or natural selection models of organization versus contingency approaches. The population ecology or natural selection approach (Aldrich 1979; Hannan and Freeman 1977, 1984; Freeman, Carroll, and Hannan 1983; Delacroix and Carroll 1983) argues that environmental factors such as degree of market competition, hostility of the competition, and regulatory activity influence organizational success and viability. Strong organizations survive while weak organizations are "selected out" and fall by the wayside. In contrast, contingency theorists (cf., Thompson 1967; Lawrence and Lorsch 1969) emphasize the ability of organizations to adapt to their environments through appropriately linking or matching their structure and processes to the demands of the environment. Natural selection theorists agree that organizations can adapt but they believe that there are severe limits to adaptation in the form of inertial pressures (Hannan and Freeman 1984). They go on to suggest that such pressures may be influenced by whether the organization is essentially a generalist organization or a specialist organization (Aldrich 1979; Hannan and Freeman 1984). As previously noted, when the environment is relatively stable, the specialist organization will outperform the generalist because the specialist organization has focused and matched its resources to the particular market niche. But when the environment is turbulent and market niches are in flux, the generalist organization will do better than the specialist because the generalist has more diverse skills and resources to adapt to rapidly changing circumstances. The approach suggested in Figure 21.4 integrates population ecology-natural selection and contingency-adaptation perspectives by *highlighting the organization's strategies as the key linking concept.* The natural selection pressures are represented by the regulatory environment, competitive environment and sociodemographic variables. The organizational structure and/or process variables are represented by size, location, resource levels, system involvement, goals, and related variables. These, along with the nature of the selection pressures, are both seen as influencing the organization's strategic response set. The "correctness" of the strategies selected and the ability to implement them are viewed as an important determinant of organizational success and viability.

The above discussion is particularly relevant for those interested in studying health care organizations, because of the unprecedented degree of change in the composition of the industry within the past few years. Until recently, health care was unusual in comparison with other industries because of stability in the numbers and types of organizations comprising the industry—a fairly stable set of hospitals, physician offices, nursing homes, and long-established public health departments. But the past few years have seen a revolution in organizational forms. Not only are some hospitals failing (Mullner et al. 1982; Longo and Chase 1984), but many others have become members of multiunit systems (Ermann and Gabel 1984) or have restructured corporately (Goldsmith 1981). In turn, some systems have merged to become megasystems. Physicians continue to join large medical group practices or multispecialty clinics and to enter into joint arrangements with hospitals. Nursing homes increasingly have joined chains and some have joined multiunit investor-owned hospital companies. And a large variety of new organizations have sprung up on the scene including urgent care centers, ambulatory surgery centers, birthing centers, adult day health centers, hospices, health promotion centers, sports medicine clinics, and life retirement centers, to name some.

This flurry of organizational activity is a researcher's delight. In what specific ways are the natural selection pressures of prospective payment, competition, and changing consumer expectations affecting the viability of new forms of health care organizations? Why does it appear that some organizations are adapting better than others? Are generalist, diversified systems more likely to succeed than those that continue to specialize only in hospital care? Who are likely to be the long-run winners? And, most important, what does it all mean in terms of the provision of accessible cost-effective care to the community? . . .

STRATEGY IMPLEMENTATION

APPROACHES, CONCEPTS AND DEFINITIONS

The extent to which intended strategies are actually realized depends to a great extent on the degree to which they are successfully implemented (Barrett and Windham 1984). It is estimated that 90 percent of American companies fail to successfully implement their strategies (Keichel 1982). Successfully implemented strategies, in turn, are likely to have a positive effect on organizational performance. Implementation refers to the degree to which an activity is actually undertaken or the degree to which something is put into place.

Over the past 20 years, a vast literature on program implementation within the context of evaluation research has developed (Pressman and Wildavsky 1973; Williams and Elmore 1976; Scheirer 1981; Shortell 1984). This literature has emphasized the characteristics of the program being implemented, the characteristics of both the organization and people implementing the program including the type and amount of available resources, and the characteristics of the external environment that affect the ability of the organization to implement the program.

Much of this literature is relevant to the study of strategy implementation, as well.

In addition, there is a vast literature on the topic of organizational change and innovation (Zaltman, Duncan, and Holbek 1973; Daft 1978; Kanter 1982; Goodman and associates 1982; Kaluzny and Hernandez 1983) which is also pertinent to the study of strategy implementation. Similar to the program implementation literature, the change and innovation literature emphasizes the characteristics of the change or innovation itself, the characteristics of the organization and the people implementing the change or innovation (e.g., presence of an idea champion, existence of slack resources), the nature of the environment surrounding the change or innovation, and certain types of strategies for implementing change (e.g., education, persuasion, support, use of transition teams, etc.). Based on the program implementation and change innovation literature, we suggest three major blocks of variables which influence the strategy implementation process. These are characteristics of the strategies themselves, characteristics of the environment facing the organization, and internal organizational factors. These are shown in Figure 21.5.

The most important characteristics of strategy to consider for purposes of implementation are complexity, divisibility, reversibility, diversity or consistency, and degree of agreement. Complexity refers to both the number of different aspects of a strategy and the difficulty associated with them. For example, it is more complex for most health care organizations to undertake a strategy of diversification (involving both new market and new product-service development) than it is merely to continue penetrating current markets with current services. The more complex a given strategy or overall strategic portfolio, the greater the difficulty of implementation.

Divisibility denotes the degree to which a given strategy can be broken down into subcomponents and implemented on a piecemeal basis. For example, an overall acquisition strategy might be broken down into three subcomponents beginning with shared-service arrangements, leading to contract management and, finally, to acquisition. The greater the degree to which a given strategy or an overall strategic portfolio can be broken down into subcomponents, the less difficult it is to implement.

Reversibility means the degree to which a given strategy can be modified or dropped altogether if serious problems develop. For example, a strategy either of managing physician office practices or of becoming involved in the network of home health services may be relatively easy to reverse, since the capital costs and barriers to exit are relatively low. The greater the degree to which a given strategy or strategic portfolio is

FIGURE 21.5

Major Factors Influencing Strategy Implementation

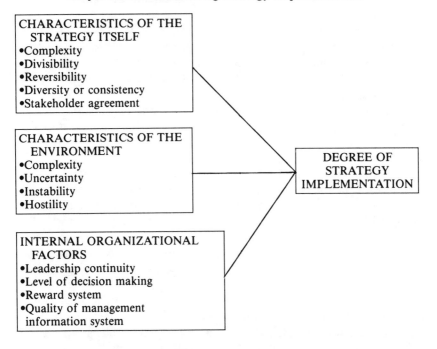

potentially reversible, the more likely it is to be accepted by those involved and, therefore, the lower the barriers to implementation.

Diversity or consistency refers to the degree to which a given strategy either represents a departure from the existing strategic orientation of the organization, or is consistent with the existing strategic orientation. A geographically concentrated, inpatient care oriented, multiunit hospital system, which decides to expand nationally into the long-term care field, would represent an example of a major departure from existing strategic orientation. The greater the degree to which a given strategy or strategic portfolio is characterized by diversity or departure from current strategic orientation, the greater the difficulty in implementation.

Another important characteristic of a given strategy is the degree of agreement among key organizational stakeholders regarding the strategy. (This could just as well be classified as an internal organizational characteristic, instead of a characteristic of a given strategy itself.) For example, a locally based health maintenance organization's decision to expand nationally is more likely to succeed if the key trustees and administrative and medical staff leaders are in agreement. And, in general, the greater the degree of agreement among key organizational stakeholders on a given strategy, the easier it is to implement.

Complexity, uncertainty, instability, and hostility are the four most important environmental dimensions likely to influence strategy implementation. The more complex the environment, the more difficult it is for the organization's stakeholders to discern the environment and its implications for the organization. For example, the current health care environment may be perceived by most health care organizations as complex, given the many changes which are occurring simultaneously in third-party reimbursement, competition, technology, aging of the population, and changing public expectations.

Uncertainty makes it more difficult for strategies to be implemented because of the inability to know what the future will bring. In such a situation, organizational members are less likely to implement a given strategy since they may think it will soon become irrelevant. For example, some physicians may be reluctant to implement hospital cost-containment strategies because they believe they are only short-run strategies that will have little relevance to future unknown regulatory initiatives.

Instability refers specifically to *rapidity* of change. In other words, future changes may be somewhat predictable (that is, certain) but occur so quickly that it becomes difficult for the organization to implement a given strategy. Hrebiniak and Joyce (1984) suggest that the short time horizons created by such rapid changes result in complex implementation, particularly when large strategic changes are required. For example, while many hospitals are currently pursuing ambulatory care and long-term care diversification strategies, extensions of prospective payment to physicians and out-of-hospital services may shortly make such strategies less effective than they would be otherwise.

Finally, hostility can have a negative effect on strategy implementation. It refers to the degree to which an external event or factor threatens the organization's well-being. Examples include medical staff opposition to hospital diversification plans, antitrust suits, unionization and strikes, and the degree of competition in local markets. For example, outright medical staff opposition to what may be perceived as the "corporate practice of medicine" made it much more difficult for many hospitals to implement a strategy of primary care services through the development of hospital-sponsored group practices (Shortell, Wickizer, and Wheeler 1984).

Internal organizational factors also influence strategy implementation. Among the most important are continuity of leadership, the level at which decisions are made, the degree to which rewards are attached to implementation, and the quality of the organization's management information system. While changes in organizational leadership may promote innovation and change, they tend to be generally disruptive when it comes to implementing current or recent strategies. Leaders who develop new strategic directions for the organization may encounter implementation problems because they lack knowledge of the organization.

The levels at which strategic decisions are made and the implementation details worked out can also influence the likelihood of successful implementation. Research from other industries suggests that, in a competitive environment, decentralization is positively associated with better economic performance (Negandhi and Reimann 1972; Khandwalla 1974; Galbraith and Nathanson 1978). Decentralization involves more people in the strategy-making process which is likely to facilitate quick implementation, and this may be particularly important in competitive environments. However, it is likely that the degree to which decentralization facilitates implementation depends on the type of decision involved. For example, capital acquisition decision strategies may be implemented better if they are decided centrally, while product and/or market strategies may be implemented better if made on a more decentralized basis involving people familiar with the local situation.

The degree to which rewards reinforce the adoption of specific strategies also influences implementation. Health professionals, in particular, need to see a link between implementation of a given strategy and their own professional aspirations and goals. For example, physicians are more likely to help implement hospital cost-containment strategies if they can see economic and professional benefits to themselves without a concurrent detrimental effect on the quality of care they provide. On another dimensions, rewards must also balance the short-run and long-run organizational objectives. For example, it would be inconsistent to reward financial managers in a health care organization on the basis of monthly accounts receivable performance, if both its long-term growth on investments and its diversification strategies are more relevant to the organization's success.

Finally, the quality of the health care organization's management information system is key factor associated with successful strategy implementation. In order to know how well a given strategy is working, feedback is required. Such feedback must get to the right people, in the right place, at the right time, and be understandable, accurate, and relevant to each person's major responsibilities. These are the criteria by which a management information system should be assessed. It is becoming more and more important for such a system to integrate both clinical and financial information and to be linked explicitly to the strategic planning process. A management information system provides the basis for taking corrective action and promotes overall organizational learning. Strategies implemented without an adequate tracking system often get scuttled along the way. . . .

SUMMARY AND CONCLUSION

This article has attempted to highlight the importance of strategy making as a subject for investigation by health services researchers and social scientists at large. Frameworks for studying strategy formulation, strategic content, and strategy implementation have been presented. . . . The new economically oriented environment of health care delivery is not likely to be transitory. It represents a permanent transition to an era in which managers, trustees, physicians, other health professionals, and the public at large need to balance the concepts of health care as an economic good and health care as a social good. The central construct around which this balancing will occur is strategy. This is true whether the issue be further changes in third-party payment and financing, the introduction of new technologies, or concerns about access and quality of care. Decisions involving these issues will be enhanced by more informed systematic research on strategy—its formulation, content, and outcomes.

ACKNOWLEDGMENTS

Supported in part by Grant No. HS-05159–01 from the National Center for Health Services Research, HHS, Grant No. 9181 from The Robert Wood Johnson Foundation, Princeton, N.J., and the A.C. Buehler Chair in Hospital and Health Services Management, J.L. Kellogg Graduate School of Management, Northwestern University. Appreciation is expressed to Joann Kaiser for manuscript preparation.

REFERENCES

Abell, D.F., and Hammond, J.S. (1979). "Market Attractiveness-Business Position Assessment." Chap. 5 in *Strategic Market Planning*, 211–27. Englewood Cliffs, New Jersey: Prentice-Hall.

Aldrich, H.E. (1979). *Organizations and Environments*. Englewood Cliffs, N.J.: Prentice-Hall.

Ansoff, H.I. (1965). *Corporate Strategy*. New York: McGraw-Hill.

Barrett, D., and Windham, S.R. (1984). "Hospital Boards and Adaptability to Competitive Environments," *Health Care Management Review* 9 (Fall): 11–20.

Chandler, A.D. (1962). *Strategy and Structure*. Cambridge: MIT Press.

Chapko, M.; Conrad, D.; Cook, K.; Shortell, S.M.; and Morrisey, M.A. (1984). "Development of a Multi-Dimensional Measure of Capital Expenditure and Rate Regulation for Hospitals." Working paper, Department of Health Services, University of Washington, June.

Cook, K.; Shortell, S.M.; Conrad, D.A.; and Morrisey M.A. (1983). "A Theory of Organizational Response to Regulation: The Case of Hospitals," *Academy of Management Review* 8 (April): 193–205.

Daft, R.L. (1978). "A Dual-Core Model of Organizational Innovation," *Academy of Management J.* 21 (June): 193–210.

Delacroix, J., and Carroll, G.R. (1983). "Organizational Foundings: An Ecological Study of the Newspaper Industries of Argentina and Ireland," *Administrative Science Quarterly* 28 (June): 274–91.

Domanico, L. (1981). "Strategic Planning: Vital for Hospital Long-Range Development," *Hospital & Health Services Administration* 26 (Summer): 25–50.

Dutton, J.E., and Duncan R.B. (1985). "The Creation of Momentum for Change through the Process of Strategic Issue Diagnosis." Working paper, Department of Organization Behavior, J.L. Kellogg Graduate School of Management, Northwestern University, January.

Ermann, D., and Gabel, J. (1984). "Multihospital Systems: Issues and Empirical Findings," *Health Affairs* 3 (spring): 50–64.

Files, L.A. (1983). "Strategy Formulation and Strategic Planning in Hospitals: Application of an Industrial Model," *Hospital & Health Services Administration* 28 (November-December): 9–20.

Flexner, W.A.; Berkowitz, E.; and Brown, M., eds. (1981). *Strategic Planning in Health Care Management*. Rockville, Md.: Aspen Systems Corp.

Fournet, B.A. (1982). *Strategic Business Planning in Health Services Management*. Rockville, Md.: Aspen Systems Corp.

Fredrickson, J.W. (1984). "The Comprehensiveness of Strategic Decision Processes: Extension Observations, Future Directions," *Academy of Management J.* 27 (September): 445–66.

Freeman, J.; Carroll, G.R.; and Hannan, M.T. (1983). "The Liability of Newness: Age-Dependence in Organizational Death Rates," *American Sociological Review* 48 (October): 692–710.

Galbraith, J.R., and Nathanson, D.A. (1978). *Strategy Implementation: The Role of Structure and Process*. St. Paul: West Publishing.

Goldsmith, J.C. (1981). *Can Hospitals Survive? The New Competitive Health Care Market*. Homewood, Ill.: Dow Jones-Irwin.

Goodman, P.S., and associates (1982). *Change in Organizations*. San Francisco: Jossey-Bass.

Greer, A.L.; Greer, S.; and Meyer, A.D. (1983). "The Diffusion of Medical Technology to Community Hospitals: An Institutional Analysis." Working paper, Urban Research Center, University of Wisconsin, Milwaukee, January.

Greiner, L.E. (1970). "Patterns of Organizational Change." In *Organizational Change and Development*, eds. G.W. Dalton, P.R. Lawrence, and L.E. Greiner, 213–29. Homewood, Ill.: Irwin.

Hambrick, D.C. (1980). "Operationalizing the Concept of Business-Level Strategy in Research," *Academy of Management Review* 5 (October): 567–75.

Hannan, M.T., and Freeman, J. (1977). "The Population Ecology of Organizations," *American J. of Sociology* 82 (March): 929–64.

_____. (1984). "Structural Inertia and Organizational Change," *American Sociological Review* 49 (April): 149–64.

Henderson, B.D. (1973). "The Experience Curve Reviewed. IV. The Growth Share Matrix of the Product Portfolio." Boston: The Boston Consulting Group.

Hrebiniak, L.G., and Joyce, W.F. (1984). *Implementing Strategy*. New York: Macmillan.

Kaluzny, A.D., and Hernandez, S.R. (1983). "Organizational Change and Innovation." In *Health Care Management: A Text in Organization Theory and Behavior*, eds. S.M. Shortell and A.D. Kaluzny, 378–417. New York: John Wiley & Sons.

Kanter, R.M. (1982). *The Changemasters: Innovations for Productivity in the American Corporation*. New York: Simon & Schuster.

Keichel, W., Ill. (1982). "Corporate Strategists Under Fire," *Fortune* 106 (December 27): 34–39.

Khandwalla, P.N. (1974). "Mass Output Orientation of Operations Technology and Organizational Structure," *Administrative Science Quarterly* 19 (March): 74–97.

Kimberly, J.R., and Miles, R.H. (1980). *The Organizational Life Cycle*. San Francisco: Jossey-Bass.

Kropf, R., and Goldsmith, S.B. (1983). "Innovation in Hospital Plans," *Health Care Management Review* 8 (Spring): 7–16.

Lawrence, P.R., and Lorsch, J.W. (1969). *Organization and Environment: Managing Differentiation and Integration*. Homewood, Ill.: Irwin.

Lindblom, C.E. (1959). "The Science of Muddling Through," *Public Administration Review* 19 (Spring): 79–88.

Longest, B.B. (1981). "An External Dependence Perspective of Organizational Strategy and Structure: The Community Hospital Case," *Hospital & Health Services Administration* 26 (Spring): 50–69.

Longo, D.R., and Chase, G.A. (1984). "Structural Determinants of Hospital Closure," *Medical Care* 22 (May): 388–402.

Lorange, P., and Vancil, R.F. (1976). "How to Design a Strategic Planning System," *Harvard Business Review* 54 (September-October): 75-81.

Luke, R.D., and Kurowski, B. (1983). "Strategic Management." In *Health Care Management: A Text in Organization Theory and Behavior*, eds. S.M. Shortell and A.D. Kaluzny, 461-84. New York: John Wiley & Sons.

Miles, R.E., and Snow, C.C. (1978). *Organizational Strategy, Structure, and Process*. New York: McGraw-Hill.

Mintzberg, H. (1978). "Patterns of Strategy Formation." *Management Science* 24 (May): 934-48.

Mintzberg, H., and Waters, J.A. (1982). "Tracking Strategy in an Entrepreneurial Firm," *Academy of Management J.* 25: 465-99.

Mullner, R.M.; Byre, C.S.; Levy, P.S.; and Kubal, J.D. (1982). "Closure among U.S. Community Hospitals, 1976-1980: A Description and a Predictive Model," *Medical Care* 20 (July): 699-709.

Negandhi, A.R., and Reimann, B.F. (1972). "A Contingency Theory of Organization Reexamined in the Context of a Developing Country," *Academy of Management J.* 15 (June): 137-46.

Nutt, P.C. (1977). "An Experimental Comparison of the Effectiveness of Three Planning Methods," *Management Science* 23 (January): 499-511.

Parsons, T. (1956). "Suggestions for a Sociological Approach to a Theory of Organizations—I," *Administrative Science Quarterly* 1 (June): 63-85.

Porter, M.E. (1980). *Competitive Strategy*. New York: The Free Press.

Pressman, J.L., and Wildavsky, A.B. (1973). *Implementation*. Berkeley: University of California Press.

Quinn, J.B. (1980). *Strategies for Change*. Homewood, Ill.: Irwin.

Salter, M.S., and Weinhold, W.A. (1979). *Diversification Through Acquisition*. New York: The Free Press.

Scheirer, M.A. (1981). *Program Implementation: The Organizational Context*. Beverly Hills, Calif.: Sage Publications.

Schendel, D.E., and Hofer, C.W., eds. (1979). *Strategic Management: A New View of Business Policy and Planning*. Boston: Little, Brown & Co.

Shortell, S.M. (1984). "Suggestions for Improving the Study of Health Program Implementation," *Health Services Research* 19 (April): 117-25.

———. (1985). "Successful Organizational Parenting: Testing Natural Selection and Adaptation Prespectives." Working paper, Program in Hospital and Health Services Management, and Department of Organization Behavior, J.L. Kellogg Graduate School of Management, Northwestern University.

Shortell, S.M.; Morrisey, M.A.; and Conrad, D.A. (1985). "Economic Regulation and Hospital Behavior: Effects on Medical Staff Organization and Hospital-Physician Relations," *Health Services Research*. In press.

Shortell, S.M.; Wickizer, T.M.; and Wheeler, J.R.C. (1984). *Hospital-Physician Joint Ventures: Results and Lessons from a National Demonstration in Primary Care*. Ann Arbor, Mich.: Health Administration Press.

Sigmond, R.M. (1966). "Professional Education for Tomorrow's Hospital Administrators—As Viewed by a Hospital Planner," *Hospital Administration* 11 (Summer): 23–39.

Thompson, J.D. (1967). *Organizations in Action.* New York: McGraw-Hill.

Weick, K. (1976). "Educational Organizations as Loosely Coupled Systems," *Administrative Science Quarterly* 21 (March): 1–19.

Wheelwright, S.C. (1984). "Strategy, Management, and Strategic Planning Approaches," *Interfaces* 14 (January-February): 19–33.

Williams, W., and Elmore, R.F. (1976). *Social Program Implementation.* New York: Academic Press.

Zaltman, G.; Duncan, R.; and Holbek, J. (1973). *Innovations and Organizations.* New York: John Wiley & Sons.

<table>
<tr><td>22</td><td>Adapting to
the Age of
Competition:
A Paradigm Shift
for Voluntary
Hospitals</td></tr>
</table>

22 | Adapting to the Age of Competition: A Paradigm Shift for Voluntary Hospitals

Tasker K. Robinette

You're not alone. Many administrators are having a hard time making the changes required to meet competition and new prospective pricing requirements. They know their institutions must learn to relate to physicians in new ways, diversify, add new programs, and eliminate old ones. They know they must attract new patients and cut costs without reducing quality. But they can't seem to successfully accomplish the changes necessary in their own institutions.

They find that the newer rational management techniques like strategic planning, marketing, productivity improvement, and incentives management don't work any better in their institutions now than management-by-objectives did two decades ago.

Why do some hospitals find it difficult to employ techniques so clearly demonstrated in business and in an increasing number of hospitals? Much of the answer lies in the way the board, administrator, medical staff, and middle management leaders in the typical voluntary, not-for-profit hospital see their institutions. It will take a paradigm shift to make these institutions adapt to the age of competition.[1]

A paradigm shift is a look at the familiar in an entirely different way.

Reprinted from *Hospital & Health Services Administration* 30 (May–June 1985): 8–19, with permission, Health Administration Press.

In *The Tao of Physics*, Fritjof Capra describes how a paradigm shift was required for the development of high energy physics.[2] In his later book, *The Turning Point*, he suggests the same paradigm shift for further progress in medicine, biology, psychology, economics, and environmental science.[3] The shift may be required to enable the typical voluntary hospital to adapt to the age of competition. Dr. Capra does not suggest that such a shift is easy. Albert Einstein, for example, developed the theory of relativity but never accepted the logical consequences of that most important theoretical construct; having been developed in a Newtonian age, the "model" in his brain was Cartesian rather than relativistic.[4]

I have a model in my brain developed over 35 years of experience with a typewriter. When I press a key, the same image always appears on the paper. I had to change that model to learn to use a computer. With the computer, what the keys do depends on the software I insert. A computer isn't a typewriter, even if it does have a similar keyboard. What it does depends on the program (paradigm) I use. I had to learn to see the keyboard in a new way.

Just as I made a paradigm shift to use a computer, other healthcare professionals must look at their hospitals in new ways if they are to adapt to the age of competition.

THE TRADITIONAL PARADIGM WON'T WORK

Most of us view the traditionally organized not-for-profit hospital as a charitable and humanistic institution established for patient care, community service, scientific research, and training and educational programs. We see it as an institution that does not seek money, except as required to support these purposes, and one that does not seek growth or political power for its own sake.

Most important, we view the hospital as a trust that must be managed on behalf of beneficiaries who are assumed not to be competent to participate in the management of the institution. Our job, we think, is to do for those beneficiaries what they would do for themselves if they knew what was in their best interest. Our job is not to offer them the health services they want. We assume that they would not exercise appropriate discretion if they had the right to choose because they do not have the required expertise. Therefore, we provide for them what we know they need.

Because we see the hospital this way, we organize and administer it as if it were a cross between a welfare and an educational institution. We utilize a modified Weberian form of bureaucratic organization at the top and a combination pyramidal and matrix organization for the body of the institution.[5] We view our employees (and they usually view themselves) as people motivated by the altruistic desire to help others and the intellectual desire to practice and advance their skill, technology, or profession. Our institutional purpose becomes the provision of financial and emotional support, space, equipment, and the supplies requested.

We expect administrators to coordinate the department heads, see that operating income meets operating expenses, and make sure the medical staff has everything it wants. The medical staff's purpose is to assure that doctors practice within established quality standards and individual physicians are not unduly interfered with. The board's purpose is to assure the hospital's continued existence, to encourage the medical staff to keep the hospital abreast of the latest medical technology, and to make sure the administrator does his job.

This view of the hospital as a care provider is the paradigm of the voluntary hospital of the past 30 years. It was a realistic view when

- capital funds came from grants, bequests, donations, and contributions;
- operating funds came from the reimbursement of costs;
- hospital employees were poorly paid and in short supply;
- there was a nurse and doctor shortage;
- HMOs were small and PPOs didn't exist;
- proprietary hospitals were mom-and-pop businesses owned by one or two doctors;
- the need for internal change was small and there were no major challenges from the external environment.

This was a useful paradigm as long as it fit the hospital's real-world circumstances. It is not, however, a paradigm that readily accommodates prospective pricing, overtures to attract new patients, or activities designed to permanently reduce costs. It is particularly unsuited to program and price competition.

How can a competitive strategic plan be constructed if the board is reluctant to compete, and the medical staff (which includes physicians who also hold privileges at competitor hospitals) will not maintain confidentiality?

Why diversify if we believe the people we serve don't need new kinds of services?

How can marketing provide any benefits if the leadership believes consumers are not competent to express preferences?

How can management-by-objectives be anything but a mystery if the hospital doesn't have clearly specified objectives?

What can we expect from productivity improvement if we believe that costs are already at their lowest possible levels?

How can incentive compensation fit in if we believe our employees are not motivated by money and are already doing their best?

Shifting the Paradigm

My answer to these questions is that we can't make these approaches work without shifting our paradigm. Hospitals must see themselves as customer satisfiers. Once we've made that shift, rational management techniques can work. At first glance, the difference between customer satisfier and care provider may seem insignificant, but it is a *fundamental* difference. When hospitals view themselves as customer satisfiers, rational management approaches suddenly make sense. Until they do, those approaches can look like witchcraft. That shift in the paradigm presents a whole new dimension of possibilities.

We are all familiar with the stories of hospitals on their last legs that were turned around in short periods of time after being sold to investor-owned corporations. No doubt there is some fiction and exaggeration in some of those stories, but there are also a great many verifiable cases in which hospitals have been turned from losers to big winners in short periods of time. In most of the cases I know, it wasn't cream skimming that did it. It was the fact that the new leaders viewed the hospital differently than did their predecessors.

The new leaders did see the hospital as a community trust. The change of ownership transformed an otherwise stagnant institution from a care-providing into a customer-satisfying organization. It became a business, and a whole new series of options opened. A similar shift of focus for a voluntary hospital that chooses to retain its existing form of ownership will be more difficult. Recent experience suggests that it may take from two to five years. But the necessary change in focus can be made, in parallel with the installation of rational management programs and with significant rewards.

The paradigm shift doesn't have to start at the top. The board and medical staff don't have to lead the change. The shift is possible even if the administrator plays a passive (but supportive) role. The necessary shift can begin at the assistant administrator or department head level.

The new paradigm doesn't have to replace the old. People can and do hold contradictory paradigms in their minds without apparent difficulty. This is the phenomenon noted by anthropologists in their observations of the conversion of primitive peoples to Christianity. Even though the natives became Christian, they usually continued to believe in and practice many rituals from their previous religion. New paradigms simply act as overlays on the old. The new perspective, if it has greater utility, gradually becomes dominant but never entirely replaces the old.

It would be convenient if we could persuade hospital leaders to look at their institutions in new ways simply by persuading them that a new paradigm is required. It would be nice if they would notice that the charitable components of nearly all voluntary hospitals have become vestigial, that almost no hospitals give free services if they can help it. But such paradigm changes don't happen that way. Most people resist a frontal attack on their world view. The best way to encourage change is to lead people into situations that make them challenge their own assumptions and discover new insights. This requires avoiding direct confrontation with the old paradigm and the use of negative words associated with hospital personnel (like business, selling, profit) and introducing the new perspective in an unobtrusive way.

Such change can be accomplished through strategic planning, productivity improvement, and marketing programs. It can be started by encouraging middle managers to analyze the strategy inherent in Medicare's prospective reimbursement program for hints of changes underway. In implementing the prospective reimbursement program, the government said, in effect, that it no longer considers hospitals to be charitable trusts whose costs it will underwrite in return for care provided to its beneficiaries. The government now views its role as a purchasing agent and the hospital's role as that of a seller of services. If a hospital wishes to sell services the government wants to buy and a price can be agreed upon, then a transaction occurs. The government has made it clear that this transaction will not be viewed as substantively different from other purchases it routinely makes. This customer-client concept is a *fundamental* paradigm shift.

A New View

Using this new perspective to take a look at some old relationships, we can see what difference the new paradigm can make. To present a clear example, I've eliminated the complications caused by outpatient and extended services, third-party, and regulatory organizations. I've also considered the case of a fictional, 100% inpatient voluntary hospital in which all patients are admitted by private physicians and all bills are paid by the patients. The steps involved in this example follow:

1. Let's first assume that a male adult who lives in our service area undergoes an incident of illness or injury and decides he needs

help to assure recovery. He is not without alternatives. He can go to a friend or relative, a pharmacist or nurse practitioner, a physician's assistant or chiropractor, a naturopathic, osteopathic, or allopathic physician, a group practice clinic, a family practice center, or an urgent-care center.

Let's say that he goes to a physician member of our medical staff. In doing so, the patient becomes the doctor's customer (or client). Like the patient, the doctor also has alternatives. He can treat the patient himself or seek the help of a specialist. He can treat the patient in his office or the patient's home. He can admit the patient to our hospital, another one nearby, or to a medical center in a distant city. Let's assume, however, that the doctor and his customer decide that admission to our hospital is their best alternative and the doctor proceeds to make the necessary arrangements.

2. On admission, the doctor in effect subcontracts to the hospital the provision of those services that he does not wish to perform himself. Thus, the doctor becomes the hospital's customer. Note that the patient is not (and never becomes) the hospital's customer. The hospital never works for the patient directly; it simply helps the doctor do what the doctors want done.

3. Now let's say the hospital assigns the management of the patient's care in the hospital to a person serving in the role of an account executive. It is this person's job to see that the hospital does for the doctor's customer everything the doctor wants done. In most hospitals, that account executive is a nurse and is usually the head nurse in charge of the nursing unit to which the patient is admitted.

4. Next, the doctor tells the account executive assigned to him what he wants done for his customer. He issues standing orders and specific orders for tests, diets, drugs, or therapeutic procedures. He issues verbal orders later confirmed in writing and approves activities by agreeing to departmental policies and procedures specified in the medical staff bylaws, rules, and regulations.

   Strictly speaking, what the doctor orders for his customer are the only things the hospital can do for *his* patient. The hospital cannot treat the patient as *its* customer and choose to provide services it deems necessary or that the patient requests. It can do *only* what the doctor orders or approves. In this example, the doctors are the hospital's only customers.

5. The nurse serving as account executive acts as the doctor's agent in the hospital. She fulfills this responsibility by doing some

things herself, by delegating others to nursing personnel, and by subcontracting with other hospital department heads for services that she and her nursing personnel cannot do themselves. The individual doctors who admit patients to a nursing unit are, therefore, the customers of the head nurses who (acting as doctors' agents) are the primary customers of the other department heads.

6. The heads of the ancillary departments do what the doctors want done, as interpreted by and under the supervision of head nurses. They can be viewed as responsible to the doctors for the technical quality of their work (the accuracy of tests and the intelligibility of reports, for example) and to the head nurses for the availability, timing, scheduling, responsiveness, and amenities of their services.

7. Now, the heads of the support departments serve the needs of the head nurses and the ancillary department heads who are their customers.

8. Finally, all other hospital employees provide services or products to the department heads and head nurses who are their customers.

For this example to be realistic, we would need to include third-party payors in our analysis and add outpatient and home-service clients to our customer list. Even then it would only be *one* way of looking at customer/client relationships within the organizational structure of the traditional voluntary hospital. But looking at the hospital this way reveals a number of realities and opportunities that otherwise might not be noticed.

A DIFFERENT PARADIGM MAKES A BIG DIFFERENCE

Because sick or injured persons do have options, doctors are not wholly free and must face competition. When we realize that doctors — not patients — are our customers and that doctors have options in the way they treat their customers, the need for improved relationships with doctors becomes evident. Because nurses are the key to our relationships with our customers, the head nurse position is seen in a new light, making us as careful of their attitudes and personalities as we have always been of their technical capabilities.

If head nurses are those whom we expect to accomplish what our customers want done, why should we not allow them more options? Why should they not be able to specify their requirements for ancillary services and take bids from suppliers outside the hospital as well as in? And if this is an option to be considered, why couldn't the same option be extended to them for the purchase of maintenance, laundry, dietary, and housekeeping services?

If head nurses had this authority, it would then become the challenge of the ancillary and support service department heads to assure the head nurses that no better or cheaper services were available to them from sources outside the hospital. It would then become the challenge of the employees within each department to continuously develop new and better ways to meet external competition. When we look at the hospital from this customer/client perspective, a whole new scheme of organization can be envisioned and, suddenly, rational management approaches begin to make sense.

STRATEGIC PLANNING MAKES SENSE

Strategic planning makes sense when a few can visualize a new direction and make confidential plans to attain it over a period of years. The medical staff, if it is recognized as a customer group, need not be involved at all for its interests to be protected. Businesses do not ask their customers what directions to choose, what products or services to make and sell. They observe their customers' choices and plan accordingly.

Once a strategic plan is in hand, management-by-objectives becomes not only easy but inevitable. When we recognize that we are offering services in a competitive market to customers who have many alternatives, it makes sense to find out what our customers want. If we are not offering the services our customers want, we must diversify. Finally, if our prices are higher than our competition, we must learn to cut our costs without damaging quality.

MARKETING *CAN* BE ATTRACTIVE

Marketing, which has for so long been a mystery to many voluntary hospitals, becomes crystal clear when we understand our true customer/client relationships. We must make doctors on our medical staff attractive to their prospective customers and make our hospital attractive to our doctors. It's not a matter of selling at all; it's learning to look at things through the eyes of our customers, then making adjustments in our own organization to increase our appeal.

Productivity improvement represents an obvious strategy for cutting the costs of the services we provide to our customers without reducing the quality of those services. It involves specifying our outputs, controlling the quality of those outputs, and then gradually reducing the inputs required to produce those outputs at the specified level of quality. This has seemed an impossible task when viewed from the perspective of the traditional paradigm. From the customer/client paradigm, the challenge doesn't seem nearly so insurmountable.

Outputs need not be the arcane mathematical constructs that have mystified us in the past. Viewed from the customer/client paradigm, they are what the customer thinks he is buying. The federal government gave us our first hint. It didn't want to buy patient days, visits, or relative value units. It wanted to buy 467 different all-inclusive packages of service. From the federal perspective, a hospital's output is now defined as everything done for a patient during his or her stay in the hospital. Within the hospital, outputs become what the doctors want to buy and what the head nurses, acting as their agents, order on the doctors' behalf.

QUALITY CONTROL IS SIMPLE

From the customer/client perspective, quality control is equally simple. Good enough means good enough in the judgment of the buyer, not the Joint Commission on Accreditation of Hospitals or one of the many technical or professional associations. This means setting quality standards for outcomes (outputs), not for processes and procedures, and in terms that would be readily understood and agreed to by those who make the decisions (the customers).

Once department heads and head nurses are confident that they know who their customers are, what they want to buy, and how they judge quality, the process of ranking enables the middle managers to reduce inputs to almost any level required to meet competition. They will make the necessary reductions when they have the authority and mandate and when they have the incentives that make it in their best interest to do so.

Finally, when we view employees as people who sell department heads units of output in return for money, status, and security, we can offer a higher price (incentive compensation) for more output or outputs of higher value.

All of this becomes possible, obvious, even easy, once the paradigm shift has been made. Without the paradigm shift, it is virtually impossible to make these rational management approaches work in the typical voluntary hospital.

SUMMARY

The typical American, voluntary, not-for-profit hospital was not designed to compete or withstand competition. Competition is foreign to its underlying concept, its reasons for being, its organizational structure, its values and traditions, and to the motivations that drive most of its leaders.

But you can't ignore competition when other hospitals begin to compete, when governments and third-party purchasers sponsor competition, and when alternative healthcare services proliferate. If you want your voluntary hospital to survive and to continue to progress, you have no alternative but to adapt it to the increasingly competitive environment. That takes thinking, planning, organizing, managing, and acting like a customer satisfier even as you retain the ownership structure and value orientation of a care provider.

If your hospital seems inordinately resistant to the kinds of changes you know are necessary, and you can't seem to make rational management approaches work for you, you may be defining your problem in reverse. Maybe you've been trying to adapt business techniques to an institution still seen by influentials as a private social welfare trust. Try shifting the paradigm. Help your influential leaders discover for themselves that the voluntary hospital must, for all practical purposes, operate like a business.

Don't confront them with the idea, or especially, that word! Introduce the new paradigm unobtrusively. Introduce it first into the mid-levels of the organization as part of the implementation of a strategic planning, marketing, or productivity-improvement program. From the mid-level, the concept can then filter upward and downward throughout the organization. At some time during the next two to five years you will probably find that it has become a dominant overlay on top of the traditional paradigm. You will know this has happened when your rational management programs really start to take hold. You'll be amazed at the difference it will make.

REFERENCES

1. *The Random House Dictionary* defines paradigm as "an example serving as a model." A paradigm shift, then, is a change in a cognitive map.

2. Fritjof Capra, *The Tao of Physics* (Boulder, CO: Shambhala Publications, Inc., 1976).

3. Fritjof Capra, *The Turning Point* (New York: Simon and Schuster, 1982).

4. *Ibid.*, paragraph 3, page 82.

5. Max Weber, *The Theory of Social and Economic Organization* (Glencoe, IL: The Free Press, 1947); "The Hospital as a Matrix Organization," *Hospital & Health Services Administration* 17 (Fall 1972): 8–25.

23 | The Rural Wisconsin Hospital Cooperative: An Evolving Systems Model Based on Traditional Community Values

Tim Size

Rural hospitals in Wisconsin are searching for an alternative to the two extremes of unsustainable traditional autonomy or "selling out" to other state or national corporations. As a result of that search, the Rural Wisconsin Hospital Cooperative has had substantial growth since it was begun in 1979 as a regional shared-service organization and advocate for rural interests.

In 1983, one of the nation's first rural-sponsored HMOs was licensed as a joint venture between local physicians and hospitals as the result of a Cooperative initiative.

The rural hospitals that are in the Cooperative have no illusion about the difficult years ahead. They realize that not all will continue as acute care hospitals and that most will be substantially changed. The Cooperative is seen as having the potential to be the vehicle to develop an alternative and perhaps better system built on values consistent with local primary care and community-controlled not-for-profit facilities. The future of these rural hospitals and communities lies in their own hands, not that of some distant forces.

WHY AND HOW WAS THE COOPERATIVE BEGUN?

The Rural Wisconsin Hospital Cooperative was incorporated in the summer of 1979 following informal discussions among several hospital administrators in southern Wisconsin. The purpose was to develop a corporation that could be a base and catalyst for the development of joint ventures and that was not controlled by any one hospital. The model of the dairy cooperative was chosen because it respected the autonomy of the sponsors and was a type of organization familiar to the community boards that would have to approve individual hospital participation.

After incorporation, a series of planning sessions was held to determine what cooperative activities were both of high interest and had a good chance of being implemented without major delays. A few early successes were seen as critical to establishing the credibility necessary to gain more substantive commitments from existing members as well as to attract additional members. During the fall of 1979, the decision was made that a paid staff person was necessary if the Cooperative was to develop as a serious enterprise. Consequently, each of the 10 members at that time pledged $5,000 for the first year. (To date, the annual assessment has continued to average less than $5,000.) An executive director was recruited and office space found in one of the hospitals.

At the same time, a second major function of the Cooperative was developed in response to a local health systems agency's committee report. Without input from the communities to be affected, a series of draft recommendations was released that suggested the consolidation or closure of most of the rural hospitals in southern Wisconsin. Public opposition was demonstrated by attendance in the hundreds at each of the hearings held around the region. The Cooperative led the charge (or was led by it) to successfully defeat an unfortunate example of top-down planning.

The Cooperative, at a very early point in its development, was given the opportunity to demonstrate the value of rural hospitals working together while simultaneously attracting substantial favorable public attention in many rural communities. The mission of the Cooperative being expanded beyond its initial one of shared services to include rural advocacy was made, not born.

STATEMENT OF MISSION AND GOALS

In early 1985, as part of the ongoing corporate planning process, the following was developed as an updated statement of Cooperative mission and goals. While it has the mandatory praise of motherhood, this statement clearly indicates a commitment to developing a more highly integrated system of rural health care.

> The Cooperative as hospitals acting together will promote the preservation and further development of a coordinated system of rural health care. Such a system will provide both quality and efficient care in settings that best meet the needs of rural residents in a manner consistent with their community values. Through its collective strength, the Cooperative is a catalyst to create necessary change in the delivery of rural health care. The Cooperative recognizes it has an important role in rural economic development. To meet this mission the following goals are established:
>
> > [The Environment] The Cooperative will utilize its collective strength to support rural health care and rural communities in both private and public sectors. It will represent the rural perspective on legislative and regulatory issues affecting rural health care and illness prevention with the political influence necessary to be an effective advocate. It will negotiate jointly, as appropriate, to maximize the effectiveness of its members in private sector affairs.
> > [The Corporation] The Cooperative will develop alternatives for rural hospitals and affiliated institutions to the increasing presence of competing health care corporations and systems.
> > [Products and Services] The Cooperative will develop and maintain efficiently operated services for its members. It will be a corporate vehicle to provide flexibility to individual institutions by incorporating a broader base of support for programs requiring substantial participation or risk sharing.

THE BASIC COOPERATIVE MODEL

Each Cooperative hospital has one representative (usually the administrator) and vote on the board of directors. The officers initially acted as a steering committee. A nonvoting affiliate membership was developed and offered to rural hospitals too distant to participate in most shared-service activities but interested in supporting the political function. Each hospital agreed to be assessed an equal sum for overhead and development expenses. Membership was restricted to rural hospitals, with an exception made for the University of Wisconsin Hospital and Clinics given its participation in the initial development.

Participation in particular shared services is voluntary and on a contracted fee-for-service basis. Public statements by the Cooperative are usually only made about areas of clear consensus among the rural members.

After several years, the steering committee became an executive committee and was expanded to include the immediate past president and a member-at-large. Recently, as the business of the Cooperative has become more time-consuming, the executive committee has become increasingly more involved in the overall direction of the Cooperative. However, all of the voting members acting as the board of directors continue to be the principal Cooperative authority.

The initial bylaws included two ideas that have not been implemented — to give additional votes to those members that bought more services and to create an executive board when the membership exceeded 16 members. The lack of interest in implementing these two provisions probably reflects a degree of comfort with a sense of common bond between the hospitals and concern for losing control through the development of an elite inner group.

REACTION WITHIN THE HOSPITAL COMMUNITY

The initial response to the development of the Cooperative appeared to be quite varied among the provider community in southern Wisconsin. Those rural hospitals participating felt a need for the organization and were cautiously optimistic about the Cooperative's long-range potential. Others were supportive but wanted to see how it did before joining or attempting to get their board's support for general assessment. Several rural hospitals indicated that they had no interest in being part of the Cooperative because they did not believe in the concept or did not believe they would receive sufficient benefit to justify the participation. While, to date, the Cooperative has grown substantially, rural hospital opinion about the Cooperative appears to continue to fit into one of these categories.

The Cooperative by nature is a relatively open enterprise and has continued to try to attract and welcome new members interested in working to develop a rural hospital system. To the credit of the hospitals that led the early development, new members are not asked to "buy in" and reimburse for past investments. The existing members realize that it is through strength in numbers that they can balance other major forces.

The Cooperative was first seen by some in the Madison press as an outreach tool for the university — a mechanism for the university to use "its" Cooperative to steer patients towards its specialty services. Since then the independence of the Cooperative from any particular dominance has been demonstrated. As major news outlets are usually located in cities and naturally describe many rural events from the home base perspective, the Cooperative has begrudgingly become accustomed to seeing regional initiatives portrayed as urban-inspired and led.

Among the other urban hospitals that noticed, the Cooperative was seen by some as a joke or at best as a nice but impractical idea. Over time, the practical implications of the Cooperative appear to have become clearer in terms of its roles as a potential competitor, ally and purchaser of service. The Cooperative's long-term prospects continue to be perceived as uncertain by some, particularly larger corporate interests that are the least comfortable with a model that is explicitly presented as an alternative to totally centralized control.

In general, if anyone in the medical community noticed, the Cooperative was considered an administrative activity unrelated to individual practices. Since its participation in the successful development of a health maintenance organization, HMO of Wisconsin, many rural physicians have expressed support for the Cooperative and appreciation for its early work. The HMO is notable for having brought physicians and hospitals to the same regional table to face their mutual threats and opportunities. Some urban physicians expressed discomfort with the Cooperative's role in assisting rural physicians to organize themselves independent from urban-based clinics and HMOs.

The initial reaction of the state hospital association was one of indifference given the original singular focus on shared services. Once the Cooperative became more visible politically and active as an advocate for rural interests, a natural concern and perhaps antagonism developed about the Cooperative. At worst, it was seen as having the potential to become an alternative trade association for rural hospitals or, at best, threatening the association's effectiveness as the role voice of hospitals with state government.

What has evolved is a reasonable working relationship between the Cooperative and the association similar to that which the association has had for years with a council of Milwaukee hospitals. None of the hospitals in the Cooperative has dropped its membership in the association, and on many issues, the Cooperative has given the association independent support. The Cooperative has provided a partial outlet for issues that are inherently divisive for rural and urban hospitals.

SHARED-SERVICE DEVELOPMENT

The difficulty of recruiting and retaining physical therapists was the specific problem that was the catalyst for the formation of the Cooperative. Appropriately, a physical therapy service was the first shared service implemented by the Cooperative, in the spring of 1980. A director was hired with the responsibility of recruiting and supervising other therapists while also individually providing direct service to reduce the overhead of developing the department. After five years of yeoman systems duty, the first director left, having succumbed to the allure of a single hospital in Alaska. To the degree possible, backup coverage has been provided during vacation and other absences by existing staff, as well as a number of hourly contracts with other therapists in the region.

While there is no easy answer in this area of relatively scarce personnel, a network approach has reduced duplicative efforts at recruitment and tended to reduce the isolation traditionally associated with rural placements. This model has been expanded to the areas of respiratory therapy, audiology, and speech-language pathology services.

During the first year, it became clear that a major issue with the Cooperative would be the "outmigration" of patients from rural counties to urban medical centers. Data presented by the local health systems agency indicated that a significant percentage of rural residents were not using their local providers for primary care. It was also clear that once they were in their cars, they overwhelmingly drove a little farther to urban providers for that primary care. The myth of blind community loyalty was seen as just that. It was understood that the threat for rural providers was not their neighbors but the aspirations for expansion by many regional medical centers.

Then it was called outmigration; now it is called the result of competition. It was agreed that if the Cooperative was to prove relevant to rural hospitals, it would need to address this issue head-on. It was agreed that a federally financed HMO feasibility study was an ideal mechanism to study the outmigration phenomenon.

With the assistance of a very capable health services administration graduate student, an application for an HMO feasibility study was quickly prepared. At that time, even the discussion of HMOs, particularly by nonphysicians, was politically sensitive. Thus, even the submission of an application to study HMO feasibility required authorization by the member hospital boards and medical staffs. While the Cooperative received authorization to submit the application and it was subsequently approved by Region V, President Reagan terminated funding for such studies.

Other sources of funding were pursued but with no immediate success. However, a general dialogue was begun with the W. K. Kellogg Foundation, which eventually led to a $150,000 grant being awarded in the fall of 1983. This money was used to fund the development of a cooperative infection control project that would determine the most efficacious and necessary approach to infection control in rural hospitals and nursing homes.

In 1980, a contract was made with a Madison-based legal firm to provide legal services to the Cooperative and interested Cooperative members. In addition to the financial benefits of contracting as a group for specialized health law and regulation expertise, there was the substantial advantage of having one firm in the state capital that would, over the next several years, gain an intimate understanding and focus on the reality of rural health care. This relationship has been, over time, one of the most valuable to the Cooperative.

In 1980, the Cooperative's executive director represented the member hospitals in a series of negotiations with several groups of pathologists that provided on-site consultation services and reference laboratory services. By a demonstrated willingness to work as a group, along with the Cooperative having advertised for staff pathologists, the hospitals were able to achieve more reasonable terms from their existing providers without changing individual sources of the service.

While the financial savings were substantial, a political cost was incurred, in that one major regional group of pathologists has continued to actively speak out against the Cooperative whenever the opportunity occurs. While this has clearly hurt the Cooperative on at least one occasion, it is a good example of a type of change that, without a Cooperative approach, rarely occurs in smaller hospitals.

Similar efforts have been more than slightly injurious to individual administrators who have tried to negotiate on their own more reasonable "hospital-based physician" contracts. Once it was clear that the administrator was trying to create change, the adversely affected parties would go on the offensive and could frequently create substantial political pressure on the false grounds of administrative intrusion into the practice of medicine. Discussion on the appropriateness of the particular contract or what it cost the rest of the medical staff in lost opportunities would then be successfully diverted and the status quo retained.

Since 1980, the Cooperative has continued to develop a number of shared services as need and opportunity allow; a current list includes:

Audiology Services
Biomedical Engineering Consultation
C. T. Scanning
Dietary Consultation
Health Maintenance Organization
Hospital Trustee Education
Insurance, Disability
Insurance, Health
Insurance, Life

Kellogg Infection Control Project
Legal Consultation
Middle Management Development
Mobile Nuclear Medicine
Patient Discharge Studies
Physical Therapy
Printing Services
Respiratory Therapy
Speech-Language Pathology Services

The development of insurance programs through the formation of a Multiple Employer Trust and the development of HMO of Wisconsin will be discussed later in this paper.

SUMMARY OF SHARED-SERVICE APPROACHES

It has become clear that there were several ways in which the Cooperative could function to create shared service opportunities for participating hospitals. The first and most obvious is the purchase and resale of a service such as the group purchase of legal services. (Given the availability in Wisconsin of strong group purchasing organizations for drugs and supplies, the Cooperative has not developed substantial activity in this traditional shared service area.)

A second method is the employment of staff by the Cooperative to provide specific clinical or administrative services, such as physical therapy or administration of the Trust or HMO. A third method is the use of Cooperative staff to act as an agent but noncontracting party for the hospitals, as in the case of the pathologist negotiations. A fourth method that will be noted later in this paper is the development of separate affiliated corporations, such as in the case of the HMO of Wisconsin. Obviously, several of these approaches may be applicable for any one project. Shared-service programs have grown because services were designed that met the needs of significant numbers of hospitals at a competitive price and due to the commitment of the hospitals to invest in the Cooperative by purchasing its services.

In 1983, the administration and development of shared services grew to the point where a director of shared services could be hired. As with all young corporations, the attraction of the right staff at the right time was critical. The Cooperative was again fortunate to attract such an individual. As all of us came from the traditional hospital sector, the development of a different corporate model has meant the learning of new administrative approaches. Individuals in a new business seem to thrive on ambiguity, long hours, and some benign neglect. They appear to be driven less by current rewards or praise and more by the excitement of a vision of what can be and the satisfaction of having the opportunity of being part of a significant creative process.

A real benefit of the Cooperative from the staff's perspective is that the primary market for shared services is also the corporate board. Every board meeting is, in part, a focus group of representatives of the Cooperative's principal customers. An openness by board and staff has kept new service failures to a minimum, and problem areas of existing services are usually identified at an early stage.

A problem that has been experienced with the board being made up of hospital administrators is that individual hospital responsibilities can conflict with Cooperative board responsibilities — what is in the interest of the group as a whole versus the perceived interest of an individual hospital. Perhaps it is more of a surprise that this has not been observed as a major problem.

A less well-defined problem is the cultural differences between the hospital administrators on the board and the Cooperative staff. Understanding continues to have to be built between individuals working within the corporate culture of established hospitals and Cooperative staff working within a new and rapidly growing corporation somewhat removed from local medical and community pressures.

Cooperative shared services are developed not to primarily create stockholder profits or as a loss leader for regional medical center outreach, but as a tangible means of supporting rural health care through a regional joint venture.

The idea was developed that rural hospitals were not less important versions of large hospitals but, in fact, had an equally important but unique role in the health care system. This was, and still is, an uncomfortable position for some rural hospitals because it is a position perceived as carrying with it the danger of being stigmatized as a lower class or lower quality hospital. The position of the Cooperative has always been that, while the rural hospital does not provide all services, what it does do, it can and must do well.

Rural hospitals have a natural advantage in the critical area of delivering accessible and personalized care compared to larger and necessarily more complex institutions. Personal and accessible care through rural hospitals is their competitive edge, a natural strength upon which specific shared services can be built.

ADVOCACY FOR THE RURAL REALITY

During its first year, in part due to the controversy about closing rural hospitals, the executive director was asked to become a member of the board of the Regional Health Systems Agency. Since then, the Cooperative has increasingly represented a rural community perspective to the Department of Health and Social Services (Health Planning, Medicaid), Office of the Commissioner of Insurance (HMO), Hospital Rate-Setting Commission (mandatory rate-setting), as well as to the legislature as a whole.

Again, these activities do not replace the state hospital association that frequently speaks on behalf of its rural constituency, but is, in effect, a supplement to that effort.

Advocacy within an industry as important as health care is not limited to formal governmental units. Primary linkages are also maintained by the Cooperative with the following groups:

- Wisconsin Association of HMOs
- Wisconsin Association of Manufacturers and Commerce
- Wisconsin Federation of Cooperatives
- Wisconsin Hospital Association
- Catholic Health Association of Wisconsin
- State Medical Society of Wisconsin
- Health Planning Council, Inc.
- Southern Wisconsin EMS Council
- Wisconsin Health Facilities Authority
- UW-Madison Med Flight Advisory Committee
- UW-Madison Health Services Administration Program
- Shared Magnetic Resonance Imaging Facility, Inc.
- Center for Public Representation
- Coalition of Wisconsin Aging Groups

What are the attributes of rural hospitals and communities that need to be considered when health care policy is being developed—both at the point of problem definition as well as proposed resolution? The following specific factors comparing most rural hospitals to many larger urban-based facilities have been noted over the last six years of Cooperative activity.

Organizational factors:

- fewer on-site administrative resources
- greater control by board
- higher visibility/accountability in community

- larger daily fluctuation in demand for services
- fewer cash reserves to absorb major changes
- lower Medicare reimbursement for same service
- greater Medicare domination of budget decisions
- greater Medicare cost-shift per private payer
- more difficulties in recruiting basic specialized skills
- greater dependency on individual physician activity
- closer hospital-physician relationships

Community factors:

- higher, if not double, unemployment rates
- lower (80 percent to 90 percent) family incomes
- fewer options for medical care within area
- not multiple hospital communities
- larger share of local employment opportunity
- greater importance as part of community pride
- greater importance as part of keeping or maintaining businesses
- less diversified and thus more vulnerable local economy

DEVELOPMENT OF A COOPERATIVE MULTIPLE EMPLOYER TRUST

In mid-1982, following the decision of the federal government not to fund the application to study the feasibility of a rural-based HMO, the Cooperative again addressed the issue of developing an alternative health care plan. The context was one of rapidly escalating employee health insurance premiums, a lack of carrier explanation of those increases and a continued desire to find a mechanism to deal with the patient outmigration problem.

A local consultant familiar with both the insurance industry and health care providers was engaged to facilitate the review of options. Bid specifications were drawn up and sent to major insurance agents and carriers active in Wisconsin. The response was not encouraging. Some companies doubted the Cooperative's ability to form a cohesive group for insurance purposes, others could not understand the need to develop a model that provided rural communities greater incentives to use local providers.

In the case of Wisconsin Blue Cross, it was clear that they had already developed a strategy based on a network of urban-based HMOs, now known as CompCare. To the degree Blue Cross had any interest in rural

Wisconsin, they were perceived as interested in it only as a secondary market for CompCare and its urban clinical and hospital partners.

In the end, it became clear that the development of a Multiple Employer Trust with its own self-insured health benefit plan was at that time the principal option. The Trust was developed, and coverage began in August of 1983 for approximately 3,500 employees and dependents of 11 Cooperative hospitals. Benefits were kept comparable for most of the hospitals. Premium collection, cash management, and coordination between the hospitals was the responsibility of the Cooperative; claims administration was subcontracted to a firm specializing in that service in Kansas City.

Approximately $350,000 in premium expenses was saved in the first year—a 16 percent reduction per hospital of what would have been paid to their existing carriers. These savings were in addition to the allocation of sufficient premium income in the first year to create the necessary reserves for claims that were incurred but not paid during that year. These reserves were distributed through a bid process to rural banks, thus contributing substantially to the investment capital available for other rural businesses.

DEVELOPMENT OF A RURAL-BASED HMO

While the Trust was being developed, it was understood that there was a high probability that eventually the Cooperative would have to come back to the need for a rural-based HMO. What was not anticipated was that in the spring of 1983, months before the Trust actually became operational, the HMO would be actively under development. While it was the environment, not the Trust, that led to the development of the HMO, the development experience gained by both the staff and the board was good training for the HMO development process.

In early 1983, it became clear that the governor and state legislature would be providing major incentives for HMO development in Wisconsin, primarily through modification in the manner it purchased health insurance coverage for state employees. It was anticipated that this would significantly accelerate the development of urban HMO plans around the state.

In fact, that occurred, and during 1983 the state capital (Madison) saw an increase in HMOs from two to five. Medical specialists in Dubuque (100 miles west of Madison) were forming an HMO with close ties to one of the major clinics in Madison—a dividing of the rural spoils was clearly in the wind. Similar efforts were underway in LaCrosse about 60 miles north of Dubuque. The three main urban areas impacting on southern and western Wisconsin were alive with action.

The Cooperative decided in May of 1983 that any possibility of an independent rural-based HMO had to be pursued at that point in time — that there was a window of opportunity that would quickly be lost once rural providers were divided up amongst the various urban-based plans. In June, a regional meeting of rural hospital medical staff and board representatives was hosted by the Cooperative with representatives of a Philadelphia consulting firm, American Health Management and Consulting Corporation. The firm was made available by St. Mary's Hospital in Madison in exchange for referral consideration by the HMO if it actually was able to be developed.

It became clear at that meeting that while no one was eager to take on the task of developing a rural HMO in such a brief time, it was necessary to do so. The decision was understood to be not whether HMOs were "good or bad," but whether individuals wanted to be a part of their own or eventually reduced to being merely an agent or employee of HMOs controlled by competing specialty clinics or insurance carriers.

The decision was made to proceed and to attempt to develop a rural-based HMO in time for the October HMO bidding "war" for state employees during their annual dual-choice selection of health insurance plans. It was understood that a minimum of eight hospitals and medical staffs would need to commit to incorporation by the end of the summer if the project was to be sufficiently feasible to proceed. Two task forces were created, the first to focus on HMO administration and the second on medical components.

The former evolved into HMO of Wisconsin, a licensed not-for-profit insurance company, and the latter into the Rural Physicians' Association, a for-profit corporation representing all physicians that provide services to the HMO. The Cooperative maintained its relationship to the HMO by contracting with it to provide all of its administrative services.

The HMO is governed by a board comprised equally of a physician and hospital administrator from each sponsoring hospital. The RPA is governed by representatives of physicians that admit at least half of their patients to rural hospitals. The actuarial risk associated with any insurance plan is shared by both the hospital and physicians.

By September 1, there were signed agreements from 11 hospitals with explicit support from their medical staffs to proceed. On the 1st, an application was submitted to the State Insurance Commissioner for a license, as well as a bid, to the State Group Insurance Board to be an eligible HMO for state employees during their October dual-choice period. The HMO was approved by October 1st by the Commissioner's office. By the end of October, the HMO had 2,600 members with which to initiate HMO operations on January 1st.

By the end of 1984, the HMO had attracted 8,500 members compared to the 3,500 budgeted. In mid-1985, the HMO had 15,000 members, close to 40 participating hospitals, and 1,500 physicians and was active in over 20 rural counties. Medical care not available in rural communities is purchased through contract with participating medical centers and specialists. It currently offers both a high- and low-option benefit package for groups of ten or more. Individual plans are available for dairy farmers—FARMCARE; a Medicare supplement package began to be offered early in 1985—65 PLUS. By the end of 1985, the HMO expects to have 24,000 members and to see continued geographic and product expansion.

CURRENT STATUS AND THE FUTURE

For the Cooperative, 1985 is a year of review and preparation for the future. In six years, the Cooperative has grown from scratch to become a significant economic and political force in rural Wisconsin. With 28 members in southern, central and western Wisconsin, it employs close to 50 people and with its associated corporations, has an annual budget of over $10 million and growing. It has become increasingly well known around the country as an alternative multihospital model for rural hospitals.

For the first time since its start, the Cooperative is fully staffed, and after two years of temporary quarters, all Cooperative office staff will be under one roof of 10,000 square feet of converted retail space.

In May [of 1985], the Cooperative was chosen as the "Innovative Rural Project of the Year" by the National Rural Health Care Association. Rural members of the Wisconsin legislature are supporting a special legislative citation for the Cooperative in recognition of its efforts on behalf of rural communities. While such public recognition is important to the credibility and support needed by the Cooperative, both the staff and the board have an acute appreciation of the difficult challenges ahead.

It is understood that the growth of the Cooperative and the development of the HMO and RPA are just the beginning of a process of debate and conflict. It is understood that these corporations are not end points but vehicles through which more significant cooperation can be developed.

It is hoped that rural providers can forge the necessary cohesion to survive and prosper during an era marked by increased urban competition and reduced government funding.

The spirit of rugged individualism continues fiercely in many rural communities and along with "high school sports rivalries" too frequently prevents neighboring communities from seeing the need to join forces for their mutual benefit. Many associated with the Cooperative believe that rural providers and communities can succeed if they decide to do so.

They must be willing to study their communities and determine what it is they want in their health care and then organize to provide it. The myth of undying loyalty by the local resident regardless of the service or cost must be put to its final resting place. Rural communities need to recognize those with whom they share common interests and values and then work together to build a better health care system consistent with those values.

VI

Accountability

Let's not be too hasty; speed is a dangerous thing.
Untimely measures bring repentance.
Certainly, and unhappily, many things are wrong
   in the Colony.
But is there anything human without some fault?
And after all, you see, we do move forward . . .
                        —Cavafy

ILLUSTRATION VI

Community Survey Form, Androscoggin Valley Hospital, Berlin, New Hampshire

AREA MEDICAL NEEDS SURVEY

Next fall the new hospital building will be ready for use. Our new quarters are larger so that we can provide more services and we're starting to plan what these new services should be, to best benefit the region we serve. You were selected at random to participate in a survey which will help us gather this information. Your answers and opinions will be used in our planning. A self-addressed envelope is enclosed for easy mailing.

THANK YOU!
Richard H. Greene
President

PART I—About our services . . . .

1. In the present hospital, we have the services listed below. Please check any which you or your family have used within the past three or four years.

_____ Children's unit	_____ x-ray
_____ Maternity	_____ Respiratory therapy
_____ Critical care unit	_____ Physical therapy
_____ Medical/surgical unit	_____ Social service
_____ Laboratory	_____ Full-time emergency department

2. In our new building, we will have room to add new services. As finances and other resources become available, we are considering one or more of the following. Please rank from 1 through 10 in order of importance as you see it. Give #1 to the most needed, #2 to the next, and so on.

_____ Alcoholism treatment center	_____ Senior citizens' health care needs
_____ Doctors' offices adjacent to hospital	
	_____ Community health education
_____ Cardiac rehabilitation for heart attack victims	_____ One-day treatment and outpatient clinics
_____ Psychiatric inpatient care	_____ Ambulance attendant training
_____ Registered nurses' training school in conjunction with the vocational technical institute	_____ Child health clinics
	_____ Others: _____

3. Education is an expanding role for most hospitals around the country. If you had a health problem, would you be interested in coming to the hospital for any of the following?

   (a) Nutrition and diet counseling   Yes_____ No_____

   (b) Diabetes instruction   Yes_____ No_____

   (c) Cardiac rehabilitation   Yes_____ No_____

   (d) Breathing rehabilitation   Yes_____ No_____

   (e) Others: _____ _____

Commentary

Anthony R. Kovner
Duncan Neuhauser

Organizations receive resources from society based on the acceptability of their products to users and purchasers. If health services are perceived as acceptable, then the organization will satisfy the concerns of groups such as purchasers, employers, or patients who are affected by organizational performance. Of course, people might not agree on what price and level of quality constitute satisfactory service. Satisfaction levels are obviously affected by the various services that are or might be available to persons who use or purchase them.

Accountability in health services organizations seems to be moving away from primary accountability to clinicians, who know best what services should be provided and in what ways, toward primary accountability to payers and to customers or potential customers. Health care is increasingly purchased wholesale rather than retail by purchasers or their agents, who will pay for specified benefits from certain providers at specified amounts. Agents for wholesale purchasers will exchange increases in patient volume for price discounts, assuming that retail customers are satisfied with quality and service.

The managers of health services organizations must be increasingly concerned with production costs on the one side and customer preferences on the other, the kind of circumstances that American business organizations have been facing for years. Two factors are vital in applying the concept of accountability: a specification of organizational performance that is mutually agreed upon in advance by the interested parties; and the capability of managers to control the resources and behavior necessary to achieve such specified performance.

Managers and evaluators can assess levels of organizational performance in a variety of ways. In order to improve service, managers can undertake marketing studies to find out what patients and prospective patients say they like and do not like about the organization's services. Managers can set up special organizational units to advocate for patients, such as patient relations coordinators, patient care committees, or advisory committees. They can reorganize work so that fewer people provide more services for each patient, as in primary nursing. They can reevaluate organizational routines periodically in terms of patient outcomes or convenience, as well as provider convenience. Special units or committees can be organized for assuring quality of care. The manager can tour the facility regularly, talk with staff and patients, and observe how services can be improved and made more convenient. The manager can make it easier for patients to complain by establishing a hotline to his or her office or to that of another manager. The manager can analyze patient complaints, their resolution, and follow-up and can talk to complainants personally after discharge. The manager can let patients know what they should expect when they come for services and what behavior is expected from them. Similar sets of activities can be conducted to improve employee perceptions and employer accountability to employees.

The manager can report regularly to purchaser and employee representatives on performance, plans, and problems. Members of such constituencies can be included on policymaking and advisory committees. Management information systems can be developed to gain access to data needed for planning and evaluating services; information should include population served, population using various services, quantities of service, cost of service, quality of service, and patient satisfaction. Summaries of reports of regulators and accreditors can be shared with constituent groups. Organizational goals and performance can be analyzed, as can information relating to such system maintenance concerns as trends in turnover, overtime, and absenteeism; fundraising; profit and loss; and new capital equipment. The process of decision making itself can be examined and improved, either as a process, given certain ends, or as a structure, by including constituent groups who are affected by or who can affect the organization policy decisions. By making itself accountable, the organization incurs substantial costs in terms of management time, monies spent on information systems, and conflict raised about present and future direction. But the organization may also reap substantial benefits: plans that are more acceptable to constituents and therefore more feasible to implement, the commitment of key providers of services, and a sharper focus on the organization's mission so that goal attainment is more easily obtained and justified to employees and customers.

Managers have less control over accountability than they do over control systems, organizational design, professional integration, or organizational adaptation because they lack influence over external groups, which have their own expectations regarding organizational and managerial performance. Health services is a particularly challenging field for managers because of the difficulties involved in specifying organizational performance and the contribution of a delivery system to health status in a community or for a population. These difficulties make agreement difficult to reach between those who provide services and external groups who seek to influence each other's expectations and behavior.

The Readings

Why not leave the management of health services organizations to those medical care professionals, including professional managers, who have been trained to direct them? If the organization does not produce quality services at reasonable cost, then consumers will choose to purchase services from competing organizations. Organizations better able to meet consumer demand will attract customers, while those not able to do so will lose customers.

MacStravic describes the benefits of involving patients in their own care, including lower costs, greater quality, and increased satisfaction for both patients and providers. By listening carefully to patients, one discovers ways to improve care. A satisfied patient can be a good will ambassador to the community.

Murphy and Pawasarat describe the development of a major medical center as a conflict over community objectives. Is the creation of a state-of-the-art, high-technology medical center worth the costs? Is the suburb's gain the center city's loss? The authors reveal conflict on many different levels.

Hanlon and Gladstein suggest that implementing programs to improve the quality of work life in health care settings is difficult because of the unique administrative structure and inherent complexities of modern hospitals. We wonder, however, whether different managerial behavior would have altered the unsuccessful outcome.

Vladeck suggests that, if hospitals are merely businesses, they will alienate those constituencies in society that founded and support them. If hospitals wish to compete effectively, Vladeck suggests, they must continue to provide services to those who need them, including patients who cannot pay.

Performance Requirements

The chapters in Section VI are discussed below in terms of the four performance requirements. In addition, Table VI.1 summarizes the authors' perspectives.

TABLE VI.1

Perspectives on Performance Requirements and Accountability

Readings	Goal Attainment	System Maintenance	Adaptive Capability	Values Integration
MacStravic	Quality care and costs	Patient & provider satisfaction	Marketing competition	
Murphy and Pawasarat	Whose goals?		Fit between organization & community	Community values in conflict
Hanlon and Gladstein	Quality of work life program did not improve performance		Significant change requires significant commitment	Lack of integration between union and managers
Vladeck		Full hospitals rarely close		Hospitals that do "good" will do well

GOAL ATTAINMENT

Murphy and Pawasarat ask whose goals are being attained in the development of a medical center. MacStravic argues that patient participation can promote goal attainment. Hanlon and Gladstein point out that the goals of the demonstration they describe were not attained for three reasons: lack of identification and involvement with the project by the union and by management, lack of department chief support and commitment of resources, and a poorly executed feedback process.

SYSTEM MAINTENANCE

MacStravic proposes a way of maintaining an organization with improved patient and provider satisfaction. Vladeck suggests that the problem of providing medical care to the poor is most severe in certain communities and among certain providers. He says that it is unlikely that society will allow that population to be ignored indefinitely. Providers serving the poor will eventually receive support. Their lack of financial stability in the short run may prove to be a successful competitive strategy in the long run (that is, of course, if they do not go out of business first).

ADAPTIVE CAPABILITY

Marketing intelligence can be a means to improving and creating a more satisfying fit between the organization and the patients it serves. Murphy and Pawasarat describe a misfit (or perhaps a partial fit) between organization and community. Perhaps the conflicts they describe are impossible to resolve.

Hanlon and Gladstein's article illustrates the faddishness of management innovations such as quality of work life. Managers sometimes attempt to replicate successful innovations in organizations that lack conditions conducive to success.

VALUES INTEGRATION

Murphy and Pawasarat describe how conflicting community values affect the creation of a medical center. Vladeck sees the manager as someone who effectively intervenes on behalf of patients and consumers in ways that can also benefit the organization. Hanlon and Gladstein point out the pitfalls in organizational performance when values of unions and management are not sufficiently integrated.

No one can argue that health services organizations should not be accountable to stockholders who are affected by their decisions. However, reasonable people might not agree on appropriate structures for and degrees of accountability in such organizations. Views will vary among stakeholders concerning the present effectiveness of the health services organization and whether patients and potential patients feel and will continue to feel satisfied.

What constituents and participants see as the obligations of health services organizations is changing. As of 1986, we see this as a move away from professional and social welfare models in the direction of market, self-determination, and performance accountability models. Vladeck argues that, sooner or later, the pendulum will swing back.

ADDITIONAL TOPICS OF INTEREST

There are a number of other interesting topics that are related to accountability. Accountability in HMOs, for example, is unique in that consumer bargaining power can be increased to the extent that consumers are effectively represented by employers or others in contractual negotiations with providers. Grievance procedures are also related to accountability and can be extremely important for patients and managers in improving services and avoiding malpractice. Patient participation in organizational decision making is a topic of interest in chronic-care institutions. The issue of marketing in health care is addressed in the readings in Section V, Adaptation. The selected bibliography below offers suggestions for further reading on topics related to accountability. Readers should also refer to the annotated bibliography at the end of the book.

SELECTED BIBLIOGRAPHY

Aaron, Henry J., and William B. Schwartz. *The Painful Prescription: Rationing Hospital Care*. Washington, DC: Brookings Institution, 1984.

American Hospital Association. "Patient's Bill of Rights." *New York Times*, 9 January 1973.

Bellin, Lowell E., Florence Kavaler, and Al Schwarz. "Phase One of Consumer Participation in Policies of 22 Voluntary Hospitals in New York City." *American Journal of Public Health* 62 (October 1972): 1370–78.

Blendon, Robert J. "Three Systems: A Comparative Survey." *Health Management Quarterly* 11, no. 1 (1989): 2–10.

Covell, Ruth. "Discussion of Kindig-Sïdel Paper." In *National Health Insurance*, edited by Robert D. Eilers and Sue S. Mayerman, 62–67. Homewood, IL: Irwin, 1971.

Denenberg, Herbert H. *A Shopper's Guide to Surgery: Fourteen Rules on How to Avoid Unnecessary Surgery*. The Pennsylvania Insurance Department, 18 July 1972.

Etizioni, Amitai. "Accountability in Health Administration." In *Selected Papers of the Commission on Education for Health Administration* 3–24. Education for Health Administration Series, vol. 2. Ann Arbor, MI: Health Administration Press, 1975.

Fleming, Gretchen V. "Hospital Structure and Consumer Satisfaction." *Health Services Research* 16 (Spring 1981): 43–67.

Gronbach, Robert C. "Hospital Employee Council." *Hospitals* 45, no. 9 (1971): 68–71.

Hacker, Richard L. "What Executive Managers Should Know about the Grievance Procedure." *Hospital & Health Services Administration* 25 (Spring 1980): 7–30.

Hofmann, Paul B. "Assessing Medical Efficacy: A Neglected Administrative Necessity." *Hospital Progress* 60 (October 1979): 45–47.

Knowles, John H. "The Responsibility of the Individual." In *Doing Better and Feeling Worse: Health in the United States*, edited by J. Knowles. New York: Horton, 1977.

Kovner, Anthony R., and Helen L. Smits. "Point of View: Consumer Expectations of Ambulatory Care." *Health Care Management Review* 3 (Winter 1978): 69–75.

Light, Harold L., and Howard J. Brown. "The Gouverneur Health Services Program—A Historical Overview." *Milbank Memorial Fund Quarterly* 45 (October 1967): 375-90.

Lloyd, Donald J. "The Medical Administrator's Role in the Physician/Patient Relationship." *Medical Group Management* 25 (September-October 1978): 24-32.

Luke, Roice D., and Robert E. Modrow. "Marketing and Accountability in Health Care." *Hospital & Health Services Administration* 26 (Summer 1981): 51-65.

McClure, Walter. "The Competition Strategy for Medical Care." In *Health Care Policy in America*, edited by S. E. Berki. *Annals of the American Academy of Political and Social Science* 468 (July 1983): 30-47.

Metsch, Jonathan M., and James E. Veney. "Consumer Participation and Social Accountability." *Medical Care* 14 (April 1976): 283-93.

Neuhauser, Duncan. "The Really Effective Health Delivery System." *Health Care Management Review* 1 (Winter 1976): 33-39.

Relman, Arnold S. "Dealing with Conflicts of Interest." *New England Journal of Medicine* 313, no. 12 (1985): 749-51.

Sheps, Cecil. "The Influence of Consumer Sponsorship on Medical Services." *Milbank Memorial Fund Quarterly* 50 (October 1972): 41-72.

Sigmond, Robert M. "A Community Perspective on Hospital Ownership." *Frontiers of Health Services Management* 1 (September 1984): 33-39.

Smith, David B. *Long-Term Care in Transition: The Regulation of Nursing Homes*. Ann Arbor, MI: AUPHA Press, 1981.

Speedling, Edward J., and Gary Rosenberg. "Patient Well-Being: A Responsibility for Hospital Managers." *Health Care Management Review* 11 (Summer 1986): 9-19.

Steckler, Allan, Leonard Dawson, Nancy Dellinger, and Anita Williams. "Consumer Participation and Influence in a Health Systems Agency." *Journal of Community Health* 6 (Spring 1981): 181-93.

Straus, Robert. "Hospital Organization from the Viewpoint of Patient-Centered Goals." In *Organizational Research on Health Institutions*, edited by Basil Georgopoulos, 203-22. Ann Arbor, MI: Institute for Social Research, The University of Michigan, 1972.

Summers, James. "Take Patient Rights Seriously to Improve Patient Care and to Lower Costs." *Health Care Management Review* 10 (Fall 1985): 55-62.

U.S. Department of Health, Education and Welfare. *Medical Malpractice*. Washington, DC: U.S. Government Printing Office, 1973.

Vladeck, Bruce C. *Unloving Care*. New York: Basic Books, 1980.

Williams, K. J. "Beyond Responsibility: Toward Accountability." *Hospital Progress* 44 (January 1972): 44-50.

24 | The Patient as Partner: A Competitive Strategy in Health Care Marketing

Scott MacStravic

This article title paraphrases the title of Joyce Riffer's article that appeared in the 16 June 1984 issue of *Hospitals* (Riffer 1984). Riffer discussed the patient as guest, noting the popularity of guest relations programs and describing how they function. The patient as partner idea incorporates a different perspective, based on involving the patient in the care experience for explicit and important purposes.

The idea of patients as participant contributors has parallels in other types of service. Lovelock and Young (1979) describe how customers could increase productivity of service industries, and Bowen (1986) discusses how customers should be managed as human resources of the organization, essentially as are its employees. While patients may have more physical limitations than the typical service customer, their potential for contribution is still great, especially when family members and significant others are included.

PATIENT CONTRIBUTIONS

There are a number of ways in which the actions of patients can aid the health care organization. Cooperative patients can:

Reprinted from *Hospital & Health Services Administration* 33 (Spring 1988): 15–24, with permission, Health Administration Press.

- Promote quality of care
- Reduce cost of care
- Add to provider profits
- Promote their own satisfaction
- Contribute useful marketing intelligence
- Use additional services
- Promote use of services by others.

QUALITY OF CARE

While the traditional view of the doctor-patient relationship has placed the patient in a dependent, passive role (Lorber 1975), current emphasis is on involving patients in their care. Stimulating intensive care unit (ICU) patients to engage in light exercise or to practice relaxation techniques has been shown to improve their status, as measured by levels of the stress-related hormone norepinephrine (Lindquist 1987). Giving patients control over pain-relieving drug infusions has, in addition to lowering costs, reduced the use of drugs and improved their effect (American Hospital Association 1985a). Patients who are active in their own treatment have been shown to recover faster (American Hospital Association 1985b). Encouraging and stimulating patients to be active, to make their own way to the bathroom, and to move about the unit promotes recovery and reduces dependence.

How patients and family members interact can have significant impact on both. Family members who participate in care of nursing home residents can reinforce family ties and reduce the sense of institutionalization among residents. Patients and residents who take care of their appearance can boost their own morale and that of their visitors. Patients who are frequently visited by family members are generally happier and feel better following the visits; they even do better after discharge (Van Dyke 1980).

How patients interact with providers has enormous impact on the quality of care they receive. Patients who are reluctant to communicate the full scope of their symptoms are placing the physician at a great disadvantage and those who fail to divulge the full scope of their concerns, often omitting the main reason for seeking a physician's services, are depriving the physician of the opportunity to address the entire problem (Stiles et al. 1979).

Patient compliance, both during a treatment episode and post-discharge, has great bearing on the effectiveness of treatment (Greene 1982). When patients and providers reach agreement on diagnosis and treatment, the results of treatment tend to be better (Starfield et al.

1979). Patients who seek health services in a timely manner promote the outcome quality of care; patients who are reasonable in demanding specific tests or treatments promote process quality and efficiency of care (Pratt 1976).

There are limits to what patients can do for themselves. Patients who expect to be waited on but are left to fend for themselves are likely to be dissatisfied. Providing service less than essential for quality patient care may result in a lawsuit (Ephraim McDowell Hospital v. Minks 1975). Just as patient consent is necessary to permit treatment, so is patient understanding and acceptance essential to patients' contributions to their own care.

REDUCING COSTS

Formal programs of patient participation in care giving, such as the Planetree Program in San Francisco, have been shown to reduce operating costs (Jenna 1986). Norman Cousins advocates providing hospital patients with special comedy programming on TV so as to keep them occupied and to make them feel better and less likely to demand nursing attention (American Hospital Association 1986). In areas where self-care is feasible, patients can substitute for staff, thereby reducing expense.

Those close to the patient can also reduce the cost of the patient's care. Good Samaritan Hospital of Portland, Oregon, for example, offers a 40 percent discount to patients who bring their own partner to help in care. This program has been shown to reduce staffing levels and, significantly, to increase the hospital's market share (Friedman 1985).

ADDED PROFITS

Reducing costs has significant potential for increasing profitability of services, programs, and organizations. In addition, patients' involvement in their own care has been shown to reduce length of stay, thus promoting profitability under diagnosis-related group (DRG) reimbursement (American Hospital Association 1985b). While speedy recovery is a valuable clinical quality measure, it has significant profit impact as well.

INCREASED PATIENT SATISFACTION

Probably the most frequently cited benefit of patient participation is its contribution to patient satisfaction. Participation in making treatment decisions restores to patients a sense of control and significantly affects their satisfaction (Speedling and Rosenberg 1986). Patient satisfaction is promoted when health care encounters can be tailored to individual wants and needs (Albrecht and Zemke 1985). This requires both that their needs be expressed and be fulfillable (Nyquist et al. 1985).

Other service industries have demonstrated how customer behavior promotes satisfaction. Having something to do while waiting for service both makes the wait seem shorter and promotes the sense that service has already begun (Maister 1985). Customers who are overly demanding and tell servers how to do their jobs are promoting their own dissatisfaction. By contrast, customers who make supportive comments to servers end up more satisfied (Bowen and Schneider 1985).

Customers who examine the layout, see how services are produced, and make choices based on available options and costs have been shown to be more satisfied (Upah and Fulton 1985). Customers who voice any complaints they have and give providers a chance to respond may end up more satisfied than those who had no complaints, and far more satisfied than dissatisfied customers who fail to mention their complaints (Fornell and Westbrook 1984).

In health care, patients who express their expectations and wishes to their physicians have been shown to be more satisfied as a result (Uhlmann et al. 1984). Patients who negotiate the problems to be addressed are more satisfied than those who are passively diagnosed and treated (Good and Good 1982). Patients who participate in addressing their own needs report higher satisfaction (Wallace 1986).

PROVIDER SATISFACTION

Patient behavior also makes a good deal of difference to provider satisfaction. In service industries, customers who are overly demanding and dictatorial promote server dissatisfaction while those who are supportive and thankful promote satisfaction (Bowen and Schneider 1985). Patients who fail to comply with physician advice are a major source of work stress and professional dissatisfaction (Linn et al. 1985). By contrast, patients who are informed and cooperative partners in care promote physician satisfaction (Douma 1980).

MARKETING INTELLIGENCE

Patients are perhaps the greatest potential contributors of marketing intelligence, that is, of usable market information. Customers can be one of the best sources of ideas on new products and services, if they are encouraged to focus on their actual experiences and perceived problems (Fornell and Menko 1981). Customers can be of substantial assistance in designing service experiences so as to meet their needs, expectations, and wishes. By reporting the specific causes of their satisfaction or dissatisfaction, they enable service organizations to respond appropriately (Czepiel 1980).

Patient and family feedback is a vital source of information, not only on how satisfied they are, but on what most affected their satisfaction. Where patients contribute specific, focused feedback on tangible, manageable events and experiences that made a difference to them, they become effective partners in health care marketing. By telling providers what specific actions demonstrate high quality in their eyes, patients become a part of the design and management process.

USING ADDITIONAL SERVICES

Established customers have always been the logical target for additional services. Patients who are satisfied with a particular program are prime prospects for related services. Expectant parents may well be interested in nutritional and financial planning assistance and classes on baby care, parenting, day care, and well-baby services, for example (Cassak 1986). Elderly patients may be interested in home care, respite care, Medicare gap insurance, nursing home care, and exercise programs tailored to their needs and capabilities.

If patients can be encouraged to think of themselves as permanent partners rather than one-time visitors, their potential use of services becomes almost unlimited. During a lifetime, patient contributions to the mission and prosperity of health care providers can amount to tens, even hundreds of times the value of any one episode. With experience, patient capabilities and contributions as partners are sure to increase.

PROMOTING USE BY OTHERS

Finally, patients may be encouraged to function as goodwill ambassadors in the community. Where they engage in positive word-of-mouth advertising, they will automatically contribute to attracting new patients (Stafford 1966). As a "reputational good," health care depends far more on recommendations by trusted acquaintances than do goods that can be carefully examined before purchase (search goods) or even tried before a commitment is made (experience goods) (Booth and Babchuk 1972).

While patients' comments to friends are a natural result of their satisfaction or dissatisfaction with care, there is great potential in managing, or at least influencing, their word-of-mouth activity (MacStravic 1985). Communications efforts can stimulate word-of-mouth rather than relying on nature (Healthcare Marketing Report 1986). For example, a California hospital has engaged all 75 members of a seniors' walking club as visiting goodwill ambassadors to make the rounds of local senior centers, service clubs, and their own neighborhoods (Bowen 1986).

The following is a list of potential contributions that patients as partners can make:

- Engaging in health-promoting activities while patients
- Controlling their own use of painkillers
- Interacting well with family members and significant others
- Interacting well with physicians and other care givers
- Complying with medical advice
- Seeking care as appropriate
- Giving informed consent
- Caring for themselves when appropriate
- Encouraging family or others to care for them
- Recovering quickly
- Expressing needs, expectations, concerns, and wishes
- Making informed decisions
- Providing practical feedback
- Using additional services
- Sharing good things about their experiences with providers with others

ELICITING DESIRED PATIENT BEHAVIOR

Given the substantial contribution potential represented by patient behavior, the challenge is to realize that potential by eliciting positive patient activities. While it is not possible within the scope of this article to describe all the ways in which each of the listed behaviors might be promoted, a few general suggestions are in order. The essence of these suggestions is to think of each patient as a human resource, just as we do our employees (Bowen 1986).

SELECTION

The critical first step in employee management is to select the right employees in the first place. Hiring those with the right skills, attitudes, and values may be the most important factor in an effective operation. This is at least partly true with respect to patients. Selecting the patients we intend to serve should include consideration of for whom can we do the best job; equally important is determining which patients can engage in what forms of participation. Special units, such as the Planetree Program, may be set aside for selected patients who have the greatest likelihood of effective participation, thereby promoting higher quality, lower cost, and greater satisfaction (Jenna 1986). Patients should be interviewed regarding the sort of relationship they desire with providers, so as to offer partnership only to those interested in and capable of such a role (Lazare et al. 1975).

TRAINING

Patients need to be educated in the roles they are to play. Knowing what is expected of them and how they can carry out their role is essential in promoting willingness as well as ability to contribute. Orientation of patients in person, by videotape, and in writing can supply motivation as well as the necessary information. The focus of training should be on helping patients to get the most out of their experience, while simultaneously contributing the most to the organization. Such training can have additional advantages in promoting satisfaction. Patients who understand what will happen to them and how they fit into the care routine are likely to enjoy their experiences more, as well as gain more from them.

FACILITATING AND SUPPORTING

Management has an obligation to facilitate and support any patient contribution it expects. Spatial layout, signage, and similar environmental factors should be used to promote desired patient behavior. Professional care givers should encourage and assist patients to do their part. Other patients can be especially helpful as peer role models for patients who are unsure of their capabilities or simply of how to go about specific tasks.

Managers, physicians, and employees also are role models; in treating each other well, they provide an example of proper interpersonal relations. Leadership examples are likely to be as effective in patient relations as they are in employee relations.

EVALUATION AND REWARD

Like any human resource, patients need to be evaluated and rewarded if their contributions are to be maximized and maintained. Financial rewards may suffice in cases where patient activities reduce costs and out-of-pocket costs can be reduced. Feedback and recognition by care givers, other patients, and volunteers may prove equally effective.

Maximizing choices available to patients is likely to prove an effective reward for their participation and contributions. Enabling patients to retain as much of the status they enjoy outside of the health care setting is likely to be valued. Promoting interactions among patients can provide interpersonal rewards and recognition as well as support. A simple "thank you" can work wonders.

Most of the rewards that patients experience are likely to be internal. Their sense of belonging, security, esteem, and even accomplishment can be enhanced far more through participation than through a conventional patient or even a pampered guest role. The comments of patients who have enjoyed such a partnership bear this out. Patients cite increased confidence and sense of self worth; family members and significant others find similar rewards (Jenna 1986).

GUEST VS. CUSTOMER VS. PARTNER

Thinking of the patient as a customer continues to elicit objections to the commercialization of an essential human service (Piper 1986). Treating patients as guests risks focusing on amenities and ignoring the reality that hospitals and nursing homes are not hotels; physicians are not the same as other service professionals. Patients as partners elevates their status above that of customers or guests—they become active participants rather than passive recipients.

Enabling providers to deal with patients as partners requires a good deal of effort. It requires special selection and education of physicians and employees (Haug 1979). All the human resources management effort needed for patients is equally essential for providers in order to develop and maintain a patient as partner program or policy.

The literature and patient feedback have informed us that patients wish to be treated as human beings with appropriate status and rights (Elliot 1984). Aside from the partnership benefits already cited, those who are able to develop and maintain successful partnerships with patients are also rewarded with self-satisfaction.

REFERENCES

Albrecht, K., and R. Zemke. *Service America: Doing business in the New Economy.* Homewood, IL: Dow Jones Irwin, 1985.

American Hospital Association. "Patients Support Greater Control Over IV Pain Drug Administration." *Hospitals* 59 (16 November 1985a): 52.

American Hospital Association. "Cooperative Care Tied to Quicker Recovery." *Hospitals* 59 (1 December 1985b): 59.

American Hospital Association. "Cousins: Hospital-Patient Teamwork Lowers Costs." *Hospitals* 60 (5 December 1986): 68.

Booth, A., and N. Babchuk. "Seeking Health Care From New Resources." *Journal of Health & Social Behavior* 13 (1972): 90.

Bowen, D. "Managing Customers as Human Resources in Service Organizations." *Human Resources Management* 25 (Fall 1986): 371.

Bowen, D., and B. Schneider. "Boundary-Spanning Role Employees and the Service Encounter." In *The Service Encounter*, edited by J. Czepiel et al. Lexington, MA: Lexington Books, 1985.

Cassak, D. "Extended Product Line." *Health Industry Today* 49 (June 1986): 12.

Czepiel, J. *Managing Customer Satisfaction in Consumer Service Businesses*, Report #10–109. Cambridge: Marketing Science Institute, 1980.

Douma, A. "Informed Patients and Physician Satisfaction." *Journal of the American Medical Association* 243 (6 June 1980): 2168.

Elliot, E. "My Name Is Mrs. Simon." *Ladies Home Journal* (August 1984): 18.

Ephraim McDowell Hospital, Inc. v. Minks. 529 S.W. 2nd 360 Kentucky (April 1975).

Fornell, C., and R. Menko. "Problem Analysis: A Consumer Based Methodology for the Discovery of New Product Ideas." *European Journal of Marketing* 15 (1981): 61.

Fornell, C., and R. Westbrook. "The Vicious Cycle of Consumer Complaints." *Journal of Marketing* 48 (Summer 1984): 68.

Friedman, J. "Good Sam Pushes Program to Bring 'Partner' to Hospital." *The Business Journal* (7 October 1985): 6.

Good, M., and B. Good. "Patient Requests in Primary Care Clinics." In *Clinically Applied Anthropology*, edited by N. Chrisman and T. Maretzhi. Dierdrecht, Holland: D. Riedel, 1982.

Greene, J. "Compliance with Medical Regimes Among Chronically Ill, Inner City Patients." *Journal of Community Health* 7 (Spring 1982): 183.

Haug, M., and B. Lavin. "Public Challenge to Physician Authority." *Medical Care* 17 (1979): 844.

Healthcare Marketing Report. "Videotapes Help Market OB Services." 4 (November 1986): 24.

Jenna, J. "Toward the Patient-Driven Hospital." *Healthcare Forum* 29 (May/June 1986): 8.

Lazare, A., et al. "The Customer Approach to Patienthood." *Archives of General Psychiatry* 32 (1975): 553.

Lindquist, R. "The Critical Difference in Critical Care." *University of Minnesota Public Health Magazine* (Winter 1987): 1.

Linn, L., et al. "Health Status, Job Satisfaction, Job Stress and Life Satisfaction among Academic and Clinical Faculty." *Journal of the American Medical Association* 254 (November 1985): 2775.

Lorber, J. "Good Patients and Problem Patients." *Journal of Health and Social Behavior* 16 (1975): 213.

Lovelock, C., and R. Young. "Look to Customers to Increase Productivity." *Harvard Business Review* 57 (May/June 1979): 168.

MacStravic, R.S. "Word of Mouth Communications in Health Care Marketing." *Health Progress* 66 (October 1985): 25.

Maister, D. "The Psychology of Waiting Lines." In *The Service Encounter*, edited by J. Czepiel et al. Lexington, MA: Lexington Books, 1985.

Nyquist, J., M. Bitner, and B. Booms. "Identifying Communications Difficulties in the Service Encounter." In *The Service Encounter*, edited by J. Czepiel et al. Lexington, MA: Lexington Books, 1985.

Piper, L. "Customer vs. Patient: A Sublime Difference in Hospitals." *Hospital & Health Services Administration* 31 (November/December 1986): 126.

Pratt, L. "Reshaping the Consumer's Posture in Health Care." In *The Doctor-Patient Relationship in the Changing Health Scene*, edited by E. Gallagher. Washington DC: U.S. Department of Health, Education and Welfare, 1976.

Riffer, J. "The Patient As Guest: A Competitive Strategy." *Hospitals* 58 (16 June 1984): 48.

Speedling, E., and G. Rosenberg. "Patient Wellbeing: A Responsibility for Hospital Managers." *Health Care Management Review* 11 (Summer 1986): 9.

Stafford, J. "Effects of Group Influence on Consumer Brand Preference." *Journal of Marketing Research* 3 (February 1966): 68.

Starfield, B., et al. "Patient-Doctor Agreement About Problems Needing Follow-Up Visit." *Journal of the American Medical Association* 242 (27 July 1979): 344.

Stiles, W., et al. "Interaction Exchange Structure and Patient Satisfaction with Medical Interviews." *Medical Care* 17 (June 1979): 66.

Uhlmann, R., T. Inui, and W. Carter. "Patient Requests and Expectations. *Medical Care* 22 (July 1984): 681.

Upah, G., and J. Fulton. "Situation Creation in Service Marketing." In *The Service Encounter*, edited by J. Czepiel et al. Lexington, MA: Lexington Books, 1985.

Van Dyke, C. "Family Centered Health Care Recognizes Needs of Patients, Families, Employees." *Hospital Progress* 61 (August 1980): 54.

Wallace, C. "Hospital's 'Personalized' Care Unit May Boost Share, Patient Satisfaction." *Modern Healthcare* 16 (3 January 1986): 36.

<table>
<tr><td>25</td><td># The Politics behind the Building of a High-Tech, High-Cost Medical Center</td></tr>
</table>

25 | # The Politics behind the Building of a High-Tech, High-Cost Medical Center

Bruce Murphy
John Pawasarat

Milwaukee County Executive John Doyne called it "the realization of a dream." The dream was to create a medical center that would put Milwaukee at the cutting edge of medical technology, train needed doctors, improve people's health and boost the local economy.

And the best part was that it would cost very little—at least that's what backers said.

To judge by publicity about the Milwaukee Regional Medical Center, the dream has been realized.

The center, located on county land in Wauwatosa, has touted itself as a magnet for out-of-town patients, as the most important institution in town for attracting skilled physicians and applying new medical knowledge, as one of Milwaukee's major economic assets.

In the public mind, the concept of the medical center may be less precise, but the glittering new buildings of member organizations such as Froedtert Memorial Lutheran Hospital and the Medical College of Wisconsin hold a certain allure. They have helped crystallize the widespread impression that the huge medical complex out on the county grounds is vital to our health and economy.

Behind that image, however, is a stark economic reality: the staggering

Reprinted from *The Milwaukee Journal Magazine*, 28 June 1987, 10–51, with permission, Bruce Murphy and John Pawasarat.

costs of these institutions. And those costs raise the most basic question: Was the medical center really necessary?

An in-depth examination of that question suggests the answer could be no. If decisions during the last 35 years creating the medical center had been made differently, southeastern Wisconsin might have had an equally effective medical system at much less cost. And construction of the center, however worthy the goals and intentions, has been a major factor in creating a situation marked by duplication of hospital programs and excess capacity.

The costs to the public of the medical center are enormous. The best estimate is that patients are charged about $35 million annually to support education connected to a medical college that many experts say is unnecessary.

The public also pays as much as hundreds of millions of dollars per year because of an excess of doctors and hospitals in southeastern Wisconsin.

Rather than getting an inexpensive ride to the medical forefront, county taxpayers have paid well over one-half billion dollars to help underwrite a regional medical center that, as one expert says, is more dependent on property taxes than most such institutions in the United States.

However, the true public cost of the medical center only can be estimated: No full accounting of tax money spent to support it is available from county officials. Nor have local business leaders ever demanded a cost-benefit analysis of an institution that required one of the largest investments of any project in state history.

That lack of accountability is no accident. It springs from the fact that crucial political and business figures have been convinced of the need for the medical center. Milwaukee's civic heavyweights created the center largely by operating behind the scenes, and today, the operation of that complex remains misunderstood by the public.

This is the story of the creation of that medical center, an inside account of how political power is wielded in Milwaukee. It is the story of long-running turf battles that pitted hospital against hospital, business leaders against county politicians and health planners, Milwaukee against Madison and, in the end, narrow private interest against the welfare of the community.

THE BEGINNING: A TROUBLED MEDICAL SCHOOL

There was a time when a high-priced item like the regional medical center never could have been financed publicly in Milwaukee. For much of this century, the city was dominated by the so-called "Sewer Social-ists." While they championed progressive causes such as child labor laws, they maintained a fiscally conservative, pay-as-you-go approach to city services, refusing to borrow money to pay for public works.

The situation left some key business leaders feeling that Milwaukee was suffering from civic paralysis. In 1948, they formed the Greater Milwaukee Committee—a group that would do much to change things. The GMC leaders argued that public money of all kinds, often raised through deficit financing, was necessary for progress. They pushed for government funding of projects such as the airport terminal, the War Memorial Center, expressways and the county zoo.

Frank Zeidler, Milwaukee's last Socialist mayor, suspected their motives. He believed the GMC agenda promoted "glamour projects," favored by suburbanites at the expense of the city.

Thus, the GMC avoided Zeidler and pushed its agenda through county government. And its leaders favored a behind-the-scenes approach: They could influence politicians more easily in an atmosphere free from public scrutiny.

As the county became the conduit for the GMC agenda, the county came to dominate local government, while the city became more of a maintenance organization handling services such as police and fire protection.

John Doyne, who in 1960 became the first county executive, became known for his ability to whip the County Board into line on GMC projects. To GMC members, he was "Johnnie," an easy companion, a politician they could count on. Doyne, however, argues that the associa-tion worked both ways: "The Greater Milwaukee Committee asked for my support of the Performing Arts Center and I asked for their support of the medical center."

In fact, the idea for the medical complex first came from John Hirsch-boeck, longtime dean of the old Marquette University Medical School.

For decades, his school had used Milwaukee County General Hospital as a makeshift teaching facility, relying on volunteer community doctors to train interns. Hirschboeck first proposed a university medical center— a teaching hospital affiliated with MU—as early as 1952.

Marquette's problem appeared to be solved after millionaire Kurtis Froedtert died in 1951, leaving more than $5 million in his will to create a hospital "as soon as practicable." The four trustees of the will—led by attorneys Joe Rapkin and Leon Foley of the Foley & Lardner law firm— publicly announced their intention to build a teaching hospital for MU's medical school.

Instead, under Rapkin's direction, the money was invested in the Mayfair and Southgate shopping centers. Rapkin said later that there wasn't enough money at the time to build the hospital, although others say that it could have been done, especially if the trustees had taken advantage of federal matching money available then for hospital construction.

The delay turned out to be profitable both for the trust and for the law firm, which handled the investment. Probate court records show that the firm charged the estate as much as $71,000 a year for this work. In addition, the trustees collected more than $500,000 in trustee fees by 1968, with each trustee earning as much as $14,000 per year.

The delay in construction had enormous consequences. Had a university medical center been built in the early 1950s, it could have become the prime facility in town for the provision of specialized care.

Instead, the city's obvious need for such care was filled in a piecemeal fashion, as various hospitals competed to become medical centers. An inefficient and wasteful system arose. By the early 1970s, the duplication of specialized care had gotten to the point where, according to one study, Milwaukee had twice as many surgery units as necessary.

In addition, the delay all but destroyed the MU Medical School. Partly at the urging of the Froedtert trustees, Hirschboeck began replacing volunteer physician supervisors with full-time faculty. The idea was to gear up for the university medical center, which could not cut corners as a county hospital for the poor did, and these new staff costs would be paid for by patient fees at the new hospital.

But as Froedtert Hospital was delayed, the medical school's deficit skyrocketed. In 1952, the school broke even. In 1962, its yearly loss approached $400,000. By 1965, the accumulated 13-year deficit — money borrowed from Marquette University — topped $4 million.

As the debt mounted, MU administrators began to flirt with the idea of closing the school. Hirschboeck knew he had to come up with some way to save it. He also knew that the GMC's support was crucial.

As early as 1959, he tried to win GMC favor and broaden the appeal of the medical center proposal by including in the planned complex not just MU and Froedtert Hospital, but Milwaukee Children's Hospital, Curative Workshop and the Blood Center as well.

Initially, the idea generated little enthusiasm, including among GMC leaders. The outlook was discouraging. But Hirschboeck had gained an important new ally: Father John Raynor. Raynor took over as MU president in 1965, but he began working on the medical school problem as early as 1962 as academic vice president.

Hundreds of pages of Marquette internal documents, some of them labeled confidential, found on public shelves in the MU library, offer a revealing look at Raynor's style: his phone conversations with government officials transcribed word for word or his contacts with the right politician to get a county position paper leaked to him. To beef up Marquette's political clout, Raynor hired staff members with good political connections and added civic heavyweights as university board members.

Raynor and Hirschboeck came up with an ingenious carrot-and-stick approach to sell the medical-center idea. The stick was a direct threat made in December 1964: Without a medical center, Marquette would close the city's only medical school. The carrot was a proposed new source of federal funding for regional medical complexes, which was touted in the press as a sure thing.

County Executive Doyne faced a critical choice. The creation of Medicare and Medicaid meant Inner City patients could get care from hospitals nearer to where they lived than the county grounds in Wauwatosa. If Doyne closed County Hospital, he would default on the county's investment in the facility. But to keep it open, he needed MU's participation in creating a high-grade medical center that would attract private patients.

The project was expensive. As then-supervisor William O'Donnell explained to the press, Milwaukee County could not afford the medical center without federal financing.

But it appeared the federal money would be there. "That's really when we started talking about a medical center," Doyne says, "when the federal government started the talk about regional medical centers."

Meanwhile, MU officials began meeting privately with GMC members. A key convert was Edmund Fitzgerald, then recently retired chief executive officer of Northwestern Mutual Life Insurance Co. [NML]. (He died last year.) One of the GMC's top power brokers, Fitzgerald was a master of the soft sell.

Fitzgerald all but took over medical-center planning. He asked Doyne to call a meeting of community leaders to discuss the idea and appoint a fact-finding commission. Before the meeting, he wrote Doyne to inform him who should be invited; at the meeting, he made the motion to create the fact-finding commission. The commission was chaired by Joseph Heil, then president of the Heil Co., and Fitzgerald was a member.

A confidential MU memo quotes Fitzgerald as saying that things were set up in such a way that he could control the contents of the Heil Report. In the end, Fitzgerald also made one key addition to the report. Fearing that some GMC members preferred a medical school affiliated with the University of Wisconsin, he wrote, "The financial burden of a medical school is beyond the capacity of an institution without an endowment such as Marquette."

In fact, the medical school's endowment had no value and already was surpassed by its debts. But Fitzgerald's claim assured Marquette's participation.

In January 1967, the Heil Report was released, supporting the creation of a medical center modeled on Hirschboeck's proposal. It emphasized the need for tertiary, or specialty, care, noting that Milwaukee was one of only three major metropolitan areas without a medical center to provide it.

The report was marred by a huge oversight: It never did a survey of Milwaukee's many community hospitals (with the exception of Children's) to determine what tertiary care was offered there.

But support for the medical center was a foregone conclusion by the time the Heil Report came out. It seemed to be the only way to save the medical school and assure that Milwaukee got its fair share of federal funds. It offered an incentive for the construction of Froedtert Hospital, which still was being delayed. And it was the kind of glamour project the GMC and Milwaukee County always had supported.

In a private memo, Raynor noted what that support meant. He paraphrased O'Donnell's private declaration to civic leaders that "our people in this community are willing to be taxed for these services."

Ironically, now that public support of his financially troubled medical school was assured, Raynor intended to get rid of the school.

MILWAUKEE COUNTY TO THE RESCUE

To this day, only a handful of people fully understand Marquette's strategy to solve its financial plight in the 1960s. Publicly, Raynor sought government funding to save the medical school. But Marquette records shows that privately he had decided, months before the Heil Report was issued, to let the GMC take the school off MU's hands.

Former MU academic vice president John Cowee says Raynor thus hoped to devote all of MU's financial and administrative resources to upgrade the university. Raynor wanted to launch a $30 million fund drive for the university, and he didn't want the medical school to eat up any of the money.

By the same token, he couldn't afford any negative publicity that might arise if the medical school were scrapped. According to Cowee, Raynor was partly concerned about the feelings of medical school alumni, who were potential donors. But Raynor also was worried about alienating the entire community.

As he put it in one of his confidential memos, "I did not want Marquette University to be accused of being a traitor to metropolitan Milwaukee."

As a result, Raynor and Cowee never divulged their strategy, even to top aides. Only certain members of the GMC knew the truth.

University of Wisconsin President Fred Harrington unwittingly provided the perfect excuse for MU to give away its medical school. Letters written by his key assistant, Wally Lemon, showed that UW feared that if the MU Medical School got state funding, it might get some of the money UW wanted for its proposed $130 million hospital in Madison. Harrington began arguing that it would be unconstitutional for the state to fund a Catholic medical school.

In response, MU and Fitzgerald arranged for Fitzgerald to recommend that Marquette and the medical school separate legally, and for Raynor to announce that he agreed. That was what happened in 1967.

The new school bore the Marquette name, but the board included no Jesuits and was dominated by GMC leaders. In essence, a group of businessmen had taken over a medical school.

Ultimately, Raynor won all that he had hoped to win. He unloaded the medical school without alienating the community; the $30 million fund drive, with strong support from the GMC, was a tremendous success. And he was able to collect on the entire debt the medical school owed the university.

But the medical school was left with no endowment, no property or facilities of its own and no connection to a university. It was renting space in an MU building. Had it been a business, the owner would have closed the doors. Instead, the business leaders who now ran the college turned to private donors and state government to bail it out.

There was little success with private donors. One major factor was that in 1970, the medical school changed its name to the Medical College of Wisconsin. That alienated many alumni who might otherwise have been donors.

Beginning in 1969, the state had answered the Milwaukee demand for funding of medical education with an annual allocation of $1.5 million. To override UW opposition, Milwaukee's political leaders had found a new source for funds for the payments: an unprecedented tax on state breweries. As Raynor explains, opposition to the tax never arose because executives from all three breweries sat on the MU board.

But after a private fund-raising campaign by the medical college stalled in 1972, Milwaukee's business leaders once again began to flex their political muscle in Madison.

"I was feeling pressure," former Gov. Patrick Lucey recalls. "I knew that if the medical school collapsed, I'd be under pressure from the civic leaders of Milwaukee to create one at UWM."

The cheaper route would be to increase the state's subsidy of the school.

Lucey appointed a state task force headed by David Carley, a prominent Democrat and high-powered Madison businessman with close ties to Lucey. Carley took up the medical college cause with a vengeance. His task force supported increased funding for the school and recommended that the college create a new position: president.

As it turned out Carley had created a job for himself, and after he was appointed president in 1974, the college made a dramatic turnaround, winning both federal and state grants.

With the help of the GMC, Carley also rekindled the private sector's excitement about the medical center. The medical college raised $17.6 million, the largest private fund drive in Wisconsin history. When added to $8 million from the state and $2 million in Milwaukee County money, there was enough to build a very impressive medical sciences building by 1978.

But Milwaukee's medical school was never able to garner the amount of state support that went to the UW Medical School. So the GMC leaders who took over the medical school turned to their old ally, Milwaukee County. Ultimately, it was John Doyne, not David Carley, who was the real savior of the medical college.

Throughout the 1950s, Milwaukee County had provided little support of the medical college faculty at County Hospital. Then, in the early 1960s, the federal government began providing National Institutes of Health funding for medical personnel. The grants usually were awarded on a matching basis, with the local portion provided by the county.

Based on that experience, Doyne had high hopes for federal support of a medical center. President Lyndon B. Johnson initially had proposed paying 90% of the operating costs – salaries and equipment – of regional medical centers. But the money never came.

Both Doyne and O'Donnell occasionally have complained about the trap into which they fell.

In 1977, for instance, Doyne declared that "Milwaukee County cannot afford to subsidize the medical school so that they can survive." But as the years went by, the county had spent so much on the medical center that it could not default on its investment.

As a result, the county's payments for medical education steadily have increased. by 1973, the county was paying $2.75 million for more than 100 faculty positions – compared with $600,000 for 55 positions in 1963.

In addition, County Hospital was paying millions of dollars more for the training of residents and provision of education and research facilities.

By 1986, according to the best measure available (accounting figures used by Medicare), the county was paying some $27 million for medical education.

Where did this money come from? Much of it was passed on to patient fees and third-party payers like Blue Cross and Medicare. the rest was underwritten by the property tax, which covered the yearly deficit of County Hospital and medical care for the indigent. In the mid-1970s, that deficit reached a high of $15 million one year. Since 1967, some $150 million of property taxes have gone to cover the deficit.

These figures are only estimates, compiled by analyzing proposed budgets of Milwaukee County. The exact amounts of the county's yearly deficits — and its payments for medical education — are unknown because county officials did not provide actual costs for any of the past 25 years.

Several hospitals affiliated with the medical college, including Froedtert and Children's, also pass medical education costs on to patients. The exact amount of these payments also is unknown. One recent study by Lewin and Associates, using a conservative computation method, estimated that other Milwaukee hospitals pay an extra $24 million annually to support the medical college.

The one thing that can be said with certainty is that the medical college budget has skyrocketed since the Carley Task Force examined it. By 1985–'86, it was $112.4 million — a 540% increase over the 1972–'73 budget of $17.5 million.

County residents were doubtless unaware of it, but they had become key benefactors of a vastly expanded medical school — indeed, of the entire Milwaukee Regional Medical Center.

DOWNTOWN LOSES, WAUWATOSA WINS

The Greater Milwaukee Committee letterhead said it all: "It Can Be done." Once the GMC decided on the appropriate policy, its objective was to cut through public discussion that might slow down action.

In the case of the regional medical center, the first major policy question was where to locate it.

On the face of it, a Downtown Milwaukee location had overwhelming advantages. Downtown's key asset was the number of hospitals located there. In the 1960s, there were nine medical facilities within a mile of MU's medical college. They could have been used in creating a Harvard-style medical center, in which a medical school links up with nearby community hospitals.

"That would have been a cheap way to have a medical center," says Ralph Andreano, former administrator of the State Division of Health. "Instead of putting your money into bricks and mortar, you could put it into training and educational infrastructure."

Recognizing these advantages, some argued in favor of a Downtown medical center. Doyne and the GMC however, preferred Wauwatosa. The decision may have made no sense economically, but there was political logic to it.

By 1974, the medical college had become dependent on its ever-increasing county subsidy. But, as one Greater Milwaukee Committee insider puts it, "It was a little bit of a hot potato to acknowledge how much it was costing." The solution, critics say, was to hide the subsidy within County Hospital's budget.

In a paper delivered to the GMC in 1976, NML executive Donald Mundt said the true reasons for choosing the county site "were largely unspoken [at least in public] in the community." From the medical college's perspective, Mundt explained, the site was chosen "simply because of the substantial financial support given the medical school directly and indirectly by Milwaukee County."

Milwaukee County needed the medical center, Mundt explained, because County Hospital had become a "white elephant" largely because Medicare and Medicaid had made it easy for poor patients to go elsewhere for treatment.

The county site, Mundt charged, "was not the best location from a health care delivery standpoint" or "an education standpoint, and it was certainly not the best location for controlling costs."

But by the time of Mundt's paper, the location issue long since had been settled, with consequences some consider devastating for the city.

The City of Milwaukee had demolished hundreds of housing units for hospital expansion. For Children's Hospital alone, it cleared 100 housing units. Now that a medical center was to be built in Wauwatosa, these expansion plans never would be realized and some institutions that had been clustered Downtown left. Curative Workshop moved to the medical center, and Children's Hospital is now following. Some believe the Blood Center will eventually move, also.

Downtown also lost a source of employment. A recent report said the medical center now provides 7,654 jobs.

But the biggest cost associated with the Wauwatosa location was the price of keeping County Hospital going after Medicare and Medicaid were created. At the time, Milwaukee had too many hospital beds; community hospitals easily could have absorbed the patients left at County. As then-County Board Chairman William O'Donnell put it, without the medical school, "there would be no sense of operating County General Hospital—we could just buy care for those who need it and get out of the hospital business."

Instead, the county upgraded its outmoded hospital. Today, the budget for the Milwaukee County Medical Complex (the new name for County Hospital) is $112 million. It is impossible to estimate how much money the county has spent over the years to duplicate medical care provided by other local hospitals. Conservatively speaking, it probably has cost the community many millions of dollars.

In retrospect, state Sen. John Norquist (D-Milwaukee) argues, "This is an example of what happens when you "get things done.' Instead of closing County Hospital when Medicaid came in, they made everything move out to it. So the biggest losers were the poor. They lost jobs, they lost access to medical care. And the impact on the West Side was to have more empty lots and less economic development."

THE BATTLE OVER CONTROL AND COSTS

Once the question of location was settled, members of the medical center became embroiled in a dispute over the issue of cost and control: Who would control the medical center and who would pay for running it?

The key player in negotiations over the issue and the man who pushed through the private-sector agenda was longtime Greater Milwaukee Committee executive secretary Rudy Schoenecker.

In 1968, County Executive Doyne told business leaders in a private memo that he expected the county to retain 100% control of the medical center "because this is going to involve a considerable amount of public funds."

But Doyne felt he needed the private sector's support to create the complex, and he was used to working closely with the Greater Milwaukee Committee. He set up a medical center steering committee with membership that largely had been recommended by Schoenecker and GMC leader Edmund Fitzgerald.

Doyne had stacked the deck against himself. Supervisor William O'Donnell, his right-hand man, pushed for county control of the medical center. But he was badly outnumbered by private-sector members. The steering committee voted to create a private, non-profit corporation as the governing body and voted to put only three county representatives on this 18-member council. The compromise assured that the county would not control the medical center council. In fact, it allowed each member so much autonomy that the council became a kind of debating society.

Even today, the council lacks the power needed to direct the development of the medical center or eliminate duplication of facilities.

The county fared just as poorly on the cost issue as it did on the control question. Doyne and the County Board passed a "cost-sharing ordinance" that charged private-sector members a pro-rated amount for the expense of developing and maintaining the medical center grounds.

Well before the ordinance was passed, Schoenecker began meeting privately with County Supervisor Charles Mulcahy and attorney T. Michael Bolger, who represented the medical school, to work out a strategy to whittle down the costs for private members.

"We had more breakfasts at the University Club than I had with my wife," Bolger recalls.

Schoenecker says, "A lot of it was done without a lot of blabbing."

The private members created an alternative cost-sharing ordinance, and Schoenecker and Mulcahy began lobbying Doyne and the County Board. As the negotiations went on, tempers flared on both sides.

Finally, an exasperated Doyne declared publicly, "This is as good a deal as they're going to get, and if they don't agree, I've got news for them."

Three months later, Schoenecker arranged a private meeting at the Milwaukee club, where Doyne discussed the situation with business leaders, including members of the medical college board. Within days, Doyne announced his support of the revised cost-sharing ordinance.

The key reason for Doyne's capitulation is suggested by a letter he wrote to county supervisors, noting that the cost-sharing ordinance was a problem for the medical school.

"I am sure that the school cannot raise almost $500,000 annually and still stay in business," he wrote.

The private sector members got "90% of what we requested," in the estimate of Del Jacobus, chairman of the medical center council.

If anything, Jacobus understated the case. Under the old ordinance, the Medical College of Wisconsin was charged $776,000 for its share of yearly services and capital improvement costs. The new ordinance cut this figure by 93%, to $50,000 annually. Other private-sector members enjoyed a similar reduction in costs—which was welcome news for supporters of the proposed Froedtert Hospital, the next addition to the medical center.

THE PRICE OF FROEDTERT

By the early 1970s, several Milwaukee hospitals had introduced programs for state-of-the-art specialty care in specific fields. But some of these services were duplicated, and complaints were growing about the high costs and the excessive numbers of hospital beds and programs.

Despite this, creation of the hospital called for in the will of industrialist Kurtis Froedtert, who died in 1951, remained an issue.

Many medical experts felt a Froedtert Hospital was unnecessary and that any medical program or facility bearing Froedtert's name would be approved by the courts. But ever since 1967, the Greater Milwaukee Committee had favored making Froedtert Hospital part of the regional medical center.

Sy Gottlieb, then the director of the Hospital Area Planning Committee, felt there was no need to build Froedtert Hospital. "I got slapped down a couple of times by GMC members for suggesting it be built as part of a wing on some other hospital," he says.

In 1976 some surprising opposition to Froedtert developed within the GMC leadership. Even more surprising was the company leading the way: Northwestern Mutual Life. It was an ironic turnabout.

Back in the mid-'60s, the two business leaders most responsible for creating the medical center were NML executives Edmund Fitzgerald and Donald Slichter. Now Francis Ferguson, the company's chief executive officer, and Donald Mundt, the executive vice president, had some serious reservations.

Ferguson reportedly had heard complaints about the Froedtert project from fellow members of the Columbia Hospital board. Ferguson asked Mundt to prepare a report on Froedtert for the GMC.

Mundt, then president of the Lutheran Hospital board, had spent countless hours as a volunteer in the health care field. He had a superb grasp of the issues, and he wrote a devastating critique of the new hospital project.

Mundt argued that the Froedtert facility would add to the city's surplus of 1,600 hospital beds, which cost the community an estimated $32 million per year. Milwaukee hospitals, he noted, already provided most of the specialty care Froedtert was supposed to offer.

Mundt argued that the new hospital was unneeded and that County Hospital probably should be closed. by duplicating specialty care, Mundt predicted, the new hospital "will likely have the most substantial effect on costs of any action ever taken in the Milwaukee area."

In the 10 years since the medical center planning began, Mundt wrote, "there have been fantastic changes in the community hospitals, with over $325 million spent on them since 1967, and with $97 million additional in the works."

The real reason for building Froedtert, Mundt suggested, was that the medical school preferred to maintain its own hospitals where it could continue to add staff and facilities without regard to cost.

"The Froedtert Hospital will be largely for private patients of the medical school staff for increasing the school's income," Mundt wrote. "The community would be far better off to raise the legitimate financial needs of the medical school in a more direct manner."

Mundt's conclusions were resisted by those who sat on the boards of Froedtert and the medical school. Among other GMC leaders, "There were a lot of people who agreed," according to one observer. "But they felt it was so far down the line it would produce less trauma to go ahead than to derail it."

Once the GMC leadership made its decision, the city's business leaders, including Ferguson and Mundt, closed ranks to support it. As in the past, the County Board approved the project. But after that, there was some unexpected opposition.

Under state law, the new hospital had to be approved by the Southeastern Wisconsin Health Services Administration. As Eleanor Vogt, a former member of that agency, recalls, the Froedtert supporters "hadn't done their homework. They ran into a brick wall."

Ironically, it was a key Froedtert supporter, medical college president David Carley, who had helped build that wall. As chairman of a 1971 state health policy task force, Carley had helped produce a voluminous study intended to rationalize health planning. The state adopted his recommendation that all plans to construct or expand hospitals must receive state approval.

Now, Carley wanted Froedtert built, and he didn't care whether it was the rational thing to do.

Questions raised by the Southeastern Wisconsin Health Services Administration added fuel to a growing controversy. the agency estimated that Milwaukee residents would pay a $14 million annual surcharge for medical care if Froedtert were built. After a tie vote by the board, the issue was kicked upstairs to the man who had the final say on the application: Ralph Andreano, head of the State Division of Health.

Given the growing excess of hospital beds and care in Milwaukee, Andreano was astounded by the suggestion that Froedtert be built.

"When I discovered there was something called the Greater Milwaukee Committee," he recalls, "I couldn't believe this group of businessmen were so naive about hospitals."

According to Andreano, he was lobbied by many top business leaders, including former Allen-Bradley Co. chief I. Andrew (Tiny) Rader, former Marine Bank chief John Geilfuss and former Universal Foods Corp. chief Robert Foote.

Andreano, however, wouldn't budge.

"Andreano turned us down a couple of times," Carley recalls, "so I had to go back to the man who had put me there [at the medical school] and remind him of that." Carley took his case to Gov. Patrick Lucey.

"Lucey was Andreano's boss," Carley notes. "He was helpful."

After Carley met with Lucey, Andreano suddenly changed course. He began to demand a merger, preferably between Deaconess and Lutheran hospitals in Downtown Milwaukee, to reduce the city's surplus of beds. Without the merger, he declared, he wouldn't approve Froedtert's application. In essence, Andreano was justifying the addition of an unnecessary facility by reducing hospital beds Downtown.

The tactical shift did not fool Deaconess President Ken Jamron. "Deaconess became the one you kick," he charges, "because none of the moguls of industry were on its board."

Deaconess eventually yielded to the pressure and announced its intention to seek a merger. Andreano then approved the Froedtert application.

With barely concealed glee, Carley declared that, "For those few critics of the way the medical school participated in the negotiations, I can only say some people can't stand success."

The construction of Froedtert added 285 hospital beds to a community which, according to Froedtert's application, already had 2,000 surplus beds. It added more teaching beds for a medical school which, according to the Carley task force of 1973, already had more than enough by national standards.

As for its contribution to specialty care, for the most part Froedtert simply began handling specialties already existing at County Hospital. Froedtert and medical college officials reportedly met with County Hospital's chief of medicine and dictated an agreement to "share" clinical programs. County agreed to give Froedtert 15 of its clinical specialties, which handled an average of 127 patients. The number of beds at County was reduced by 143 when Froedtert opened.

In 1981, its first full year of operation, Froedtert Hospital had a daily average of 141 patients. Without the programs given it by County Hospital, it would have served 14 patients per day, filling 5% of its beds. As of 1986, Froedtert's daily average had increased to 156 patients. In essence, Milwaukee had constructed a $43 million hospital with a $60 million annual budget to serve, on a daily basis, a handful of new patients.

If anything, these figures understate the amount of unnecessary spending. In 1986, Froedtert and County hospitals together actually served fewer patients than did County Hospital alone in 1979. Yet the combined budget for the two hospitals was $172 million in 1986, a 125%

increase since 1979, when County Hospital alone had a budget of $76 million.

This rate of inflation—double that of other Milwaukee hospitals during this period—provides dramatic proof that an excess of beds and a duplication of hospital programs simply increase the cost of medical care.

As Mundt predicted, there was a benefit for the Medical College of Wisconsin. Today, Froedtert's patients are charged anywhere from $6 million to $15 million annually for medical education, depending on whose figures you believe.

In addition, with the construction of Froedtert Hospital, the maintenance and development costs associated with the medical center continued to escalate: by 1980, the total topped $160 million. As County Supervisor Richard Bussler put it, Froedtert Hospital had become "an abysmal disaster." It was Children's Hospital that ultimately felt the fallout from that disaster, as business leaders finally began to have second thoughts about medical care costs.

THE BATTLE OVER CHILDREN'S HOSPITAL

Both the board and medical staff of Children's Hospital often were divided on whether the hospital belonged Downtown or at the medical center. But all agreed that the No. 1 goal was to remain a free-standing hospital with as little connection as possible to other institutions.

"We need a free-standing hospital so we're not competing with any other department for our equipment and resources," explains Jon Vice, current president of Children's. "I don't pay attention to other hospitals in town. I don't care if St. Francis and St. Luke's merge. I'm only concerned about Children's."

Going back to 1959, Children's Hospital had been included in the proposed plan for a regional medical center. In the mid-'60s, Children's president Ed Logan, a key supporter of the medical center, delayed building a new facility for Children's to await the creation of the medical center. In the 1970s, the city's business leaders again asked Children's to put off construction because all charitable dollars were needed to support the medical college's new facility, built in 1978.

By 1976, according to Bob Lawrence, who replaced Logan as Children's president, "our board was frustrated. We needed a new hospital in 1967. We felt we couldn't wait forever for the medical center to take form." As a result, in July 1976, Children's announced plans to build Downtown.

Given the private sector's preference for relocating Children's on the county grounds, the Downtown project faced an uphill battle.

The situation grew worse as the merger talks between Deaconess and Lutheran hospitals fell apart. Andreano had approved Froedtert Hospital based on the promised merger, and his successor, Robert Durkin, was adamant about enforcing that policy. Durkin made it clear that no new hospital construction would be approved until a merger occurred.

For three confused years, Children's flipflopped between various locations for a new hospital, waiting for the state and the city's business leaders to resolve the disputed merger. Children's appeared to be leaning toward building Downtown, but shortly after the Deaconess-Lutheran merger was completed, it announced its intention to move to the county grounds.

Despite a public storm of protest over this decision, only two county supervisors opposed a rent-free lease for Children's. The old coalition of the GMC and the county was once again at work, further expanding the medical center.

In the past, money seemingly had been no object in pursuing this goal. Now the business community had gotten the religion of cost control, and along with many county and state officials, believed that a medical center location provided the best chance for Children's to share resources with other hospitals.

County officials were the key players in carrying out this strategy. Initially, they lured Children's to the medical center by offering it a surprising amount of autonomy.

"But once we went public with our decision to move out to the medical center," says Paul Donnelly, Children's president from 1978 to 1984, "then the county started to try to whittle us down."

The county's main ally was Linda Reivitz, secretary of the State Department of Health and Social Services, who had the power to reject the hospital's application.

Reivitz ultimately forced Children's to cut its proposal back by 48 beds, to a 142-bed hospital. But Children's hired lobbyist and former legislator Bill Broyderick and the law firm of Foley & Lardner, and together they pushed the proposal through without any other reductions.

In the end, the inexorable logic of the medical center took over. Because each private-sector member has full autonomy, even the combined opposition of business leaders and Milwaukee County is hard put to force these institutions to share facilities.

Because the county is so committed to the medical center, it continues to give in to private-sector demands. The county had to agree to build a new, $17 million emergency and trauma center to encourage some sharing of facilities between the Milwaukee County Medical Complex and Children's Hospital (which will rent space in the facility).

Ald. Paul Henningsen, who was a critic of the medical center when he served on the County Board, predicts that if Children's has any difficulties making it economically, the county will be asked to provide further subsidies.

That seems a safe prediction, given the history of the medical center. For 20 years, Milwaukee County has invested heavily in the complex, without ever stopping to ask the obvious question: Is it worth it?

HOW WE'VE PAID THE PRICE

Since the mid-1960s, the Milwaukee Regional Medical Center has been a kind of sacred cow in Milwaukee. In writing about one of its proposed components in 1976, Donald Mundt of Northwestern Mutual Life said, "The community has not had the information it needs to make an informed decision on the Froedtert proposal" because of "the failure of the press to properly report it, the reluctance of the health-care community to speak frankly because of possible retaliation by the medical school," and "because it appears that the 'power structure' of the community is either supporting the project or at least not opposing it."

Today, all of those factors continue to prevent a realistic appraisal of the entire medical center from being made. In addition, the medical center is by now a fait accompli: Even its one-time critics have decided it must be supported, now that it has been completed.

Medical center supporters once hoped federal regional medical program funds would pay for as much as 90% of operating costs. Other than a few million dollars for initial planning of regional programs, no such money arrived because the program was killed.

Some argued that the medical center was needed to save the medical school and thus to keep up the supply of doctors.

In fact, statistics provided by the medical college show that only 34% of graduates since 1970 have stayed to practice medicine in Wisconsin. That relationship is even more tenuous for Milwaukee County.

Even if more medical college graduates did stay in Wisconsin, that would only add to the oversupply of doctors. A recent study by the State Department of Health and Social Services estimates that Wisconsin has 23% to 26% more doctors than it needs, and that Milwaukee County has 60% more doctors than needed.

This oversupply, the study suggests, may encourage duplication of sophisticated medical technology, such that Milwaukee County could pay a $1.3 billion surcharge for unnecessary medical care by the year 2000.

The study concluded that there was no justification for continued financial support of the Medical College of Wisconsin by the Legislature.

To James Kuperberg of the Wisconsin Hospital Rate Setting Commission, "The basic policy question that has not been addressed is: Do we want to be an exporter of physicians? We certainly don't need the number of doctors we're producing in this state."

Some argued that a medical center would draw more out-of-state patients to Milwaukee. It's true that patient referrals to Milwaukee have significantly increased in the last 20 years. About 27% of Froedtert's patients and 21% of patients at the county's hospital come from outside the metropolitan area.

But it seems likely these out-of-town patients would have been drawn to upgraded specialty programs at other Milwaukee hospitals. Today, even with the competition from the medical center, there are more out-of-state referrals to community hospitals, with about 18% of St. Luke's patients and 12% of St. Mary's patients coming from outside the metropolitan area.

Some argued that a medical center would centralize medical care, reducing inefficient duplication. In fact, as Mundt argued, it "led to empire building and duplication."

Medical center doctors have duplicated programs already existing at community hospitals, including open-heart surgery and neonatology. Now there is talk of creating a new Heart Institute and moving the Blood Center to the medical center, which could add to the duplication and increase Milwaukee County's costs.

By constructing Froedtert Hospital and keeping the county hospital's doors open, the medical center contributed hundreds of unnecessary beds to the city's surplus, at a cost of millions of dollars a year.

The medical center, in fact, hasn't even centralized care on its home court. Kuperberg notes that between Froedtert and the county's hospital, "There is a duplication of management, of patient services and infrastructure."

Given what knowledgeable observers refer to as the medical center's "Balkan kingdoms" and "Byzantine politics," future prospects for consolidation seem dim. Everyone seems to agree that some form of central governance is needed. No one seems to know how to get medical center members to accept it.

Proponents of the medical center believed it would upgrade Milwaukee's specialty medical care. Today, the medical college claims to have developed some 15 specialty treatments at the medical center, while community hospitals argue that only about five are unique to the medical center.

Most agree the center has become known for kidney and liver transplants, limb replantation and laser retinal surgery. But some medical experts suggest that the medical college could have developed these treatments at community hospitals.

In response to this suggestion, medical college president Ed Lennon says: "A doctor that has to go 10 miles away is not the same as someone who's just down the hall."

Lennon also argues that community hospitals are less focused on specialty care. "You need an academic health center because there's got to be a place where inquiry is the order of the day."

Some people supported the medical center as an economic development measure. A study commissioned by the medical center showed that it has a $459 million positive impact on the local economy. Others suggest that this impact just as easily could have occurred had the medical college worked through community hospitals.

Supporters of the medical center argued that its benefits would far outweigh its costs. Back in 1967, the Greater Milwaukee Committee's Heil report concluded that it "would require comparatively little to finance the development of . . . a first-rate medical center."

Of all the claims made to support the medical center, that one ranks as the most monumental mistake.

Since the initial creation of the medical center in 1967, Milwaukee County has spent about $325 million in property taxes for health-related costs at Milwaukee County's institutions. In addition, the county spent more than a quarter of a billion dollars in capital and interest payments for projects at the medical center, with most of the spending occurring in the past 12 years.

The sting of these costs is heightened by the fact that they are financed by Milwaukee's property tax.

Comparing the Medical College of Wisconsin with the UW Medical School in Madison is illuminating: While about 60% of the Madison school's budget comes from federal and state funding, only 15% of the medical college's budget does. The difference is largely made up by Milwaukee County residents through hospital fees, health insurance and property-tax payments. Although the vast majority of medical college students do not come from Milwaukee and will not practice in the county, their training is heavily subsidized by county residents.

That local tax burden is all the more significant when support of the medical center is added.

"Nationally, it's not common to have a medical center underwritten by local government," says Gottleib. "Usually, the local government funding has been the weak portion, and the private hospital and university funding has been the strong portion."

Richard Cooper, dean of the Medical College of Wisconsin, says the spending has not been without benefit for Milwaukee County.

"They paid a lot. They get a lot. The county is investing in state-of-the-art medical systems. They serve the goals of medical education, but they also serve the needs of county residents."

But truly the most unusual aspect of all these costs is that they can be only estimated. County officials cannot provide exact figures for the medical center for any of the past 25 years.

"There isn't any ongoing tally of county costs for the medical center," says Emil Stanislawski, director of Milwaukee County's Department of Administration. "Pieces of it come from different budgetary units. It's a real difficult task to sit down and try and identify every project related to the medical center over two decades."

Chuck Brotz, budget administrator of the county Department of Health and Social Services, said, "It's definitely true that you don't find the county costs for the medical center in any one neat place. That's a commentary on the county's accounting system, but I'm not sure I'd want to lay a blast on it for that."

If it seems incredible that a major governmental agency has never totalled the amount it is spending publicly, it is one small measure of how the push to create a medical center has affected community priorities in the last 20 years.

Back in the early 1960s, Milwaukee County paid very little to support its hospital because most care was provided free by faculty associated with the medical college. Today, spending on the medical college has gotten so out of hand that officials either cannot or will not reveal what it is costing taxpayers.

In the early '60s, the Greater Milwaukee Committee's prime concern was the need to prevent hospital duplication and promote medical efficiency. Today, as a result of its push to build up the medical college and the medical center, Milwaukee has a much more costly health-care system with an excess of hospital beds and doctors.

The situation has led the Metropolitan Milwaukee Association of Commerce to suggest that the state be given the power to close hospitals. given the private sector's previous success at undermining the state's power over hospitals, the recommendation is more than a little ironic.

The way decisions were made on the medical center has defenders.

"With anything of this kind, there's a hell of a lot done behind the scenes," says Francis Ferguson, formerly head of Northwestern Mutual Life and a major GMC leader. "But I don't see anything sinister about that. That's really the only way things can get done."

That belief, with its lack of faith in an open and democratic system of policy-making, consistently has characterized the actions of the power brokers who dictated the nature of Milwaukee's medical center.

Whether the leadership came from the city's political, business or academic sectors, the secret agenda and the back-room deals have been the preferred tools to determine medical policy.

For more than two decades, the city's power brokers presumed that the public good could best be determined without involving most of the public. In the case of the Regional Medical Center, that presumption would appear to be wrong.

<table>
<tr><td>26</td><td>Improving the
Quality of Work
Life in Hospitals:
A Case Study</td></tr>
</table>

26 | Improving the
Quality of Work
Life in Hospitals:
A Case Study

Martin D. Hanlon
Deborah L. Gladstein

Over the past decade, managers and organizational change specialists have devoted considerable attention to the quality of work life within complex organizations. Many have come to accept that an organization should be responsive to the social and psychological needs of its employees—a position supported by a growing body of empirical data showing that improvements in quality of work life, or QWL, are often linked to improvements in organizational effectiveness.[1] Previous efforts to improve QWL were limited to non-unionized, private sector firms. More recently, however, several major unions have become co-sponsors of QWL projects, and the joint labor-management project has become an innovation in U.S. labor relations.[2] Currently, there are hundreds of QWL projects in different types of work organizations throughout the United States.

Hospitals have not been a major setting for QWL projects, despite the urgent demands on healthcare executives to increase operating efficiency and raise employee morale. In part, the newness of QWL and other forms of organizational development change strategies may explain their limited impact in medical care organizations.

However, several organizational change specialists have identified a more fundamental set of problems.[3] Basically, they argue that behavioral science knowledge produced in private, profit-making (usually indus-

Reprinted from *Hospital & Health Services Administration* 29 (September-October 1984): 94–107, with permission, Health Administration Press.

trial) organizations may have little practical value within the radically different environment of the hospital. The conceptual framework used to determine the success or failure of a project in a goods-producing organization may be ill-suited to an organization devoted to saving human lives. In manufacturing firms, work redesign, employee problem-solving groups, and other quality of work life strategies are justified by documented increases in productivity—generally expressed as greater output of goods produced per unit of labor time.

As healthcare executives know, it is often difficult to apply standard productivity measures in a medical care context. Hospital performance goals, such as improving the quality of routine patient care or enhancing clinical research capabilities, may entail different or conflicting change strategies. Moreover, the dual hierarchy of medical and administrative authority characteristic of modern hospitals complicates the process of organizational change. Weisbord and Stoelwinder note that physicians generally have limited interest in the improvement of administrative functioning and often fear that better management, however defined, may result in limits to their professional autonomy.[4] The complexity of the hospital, lack of goal clarity, and the conflicting interests of different employee groups are formidable barriers to improving operating effectiveness and the nature of work life within the organization.

Whether or not quality of work life programs *can* be effectively carried out in hospitals is still an open question; data on the subject are very limited. Healthcare executives must learn more about the specific structural constraints that impede QWL efforts in hospitals as well as the actual benefits to be gained. These empirical issues provide the focus of this paper.

A quality of life project was carried out in a well-known teaching hospital in a large city in the eastern United States. The project spanned a three-and-a-half-year period from 1974 to 1978. In terms of duration, scope of activities, and budget, the quality of work life project at Parkside Hospital (not the actual name) was perhaps the largest such project ever attempted in this country.[5] Our evaluation data indicate that it was largely a failure. There were some improvements in affected areas of the hospital as well as less tangible gains in employee morale and communications, but the results hardly justify the financial and human resource costs incurred.

The significance of the Parkside project lies in its careful attempt to document the entire course of project activities and to measure the various outcomes. These findings provide insight into why the objectives of improving organizational effectiveness and quality of work life are so difficult to realize within the context of the hospital, but they also point to means of improving the likelihood of success in future QWL projects.

PROJECT DESCRIPTION

The Parkside quality of work life project was conceived as a joint labor-management experiment sponsored by the hospital administration and the two major unions representing Parkside employees. The latter include the local of a national healthcare employees union — referred to here as the Hospital Workers' Union — which represented most of the nonprofessional employees at the hospital, and the local affiliate of the statewide nursing association, which represented RNs. The Parkside chapter of the city-wide association of interns and residents was included in the original agreement; however, the group lost NLRB union certification shortly after the beginning of the project and had no subsequent involvement. Of the two remaining employee groups, only the Hospital Workers' Union had a major policy presence during the course of the project.

The Parkside project was one of several quality of work life projects initiated by the Institute for Social Research of the University of Michigan and the American Center for the Quality of Working Life in Washington, D.C.[6] Funding for research and consulting activities were provided by the National Center for Health Services Research. The authors of this article, who at the time were associated with the Columbia University Graduate School of Business, directed the project evaluation. The research strategy was based on a comprehensive multiple measurement approach and included survey questionnaires, interviews, archival data gathering, and several hundred hours per year of on-site participant observation.

The project had two principal objectives common to most QWL projects: (1) to increase the hospital's performance effectiveness and thereby improve the standards of patient care; and (2) to improve the quality of work life of hospital employees. A hospital-level steering committee composed of union and management representatives was the project's official policy-making body. The steering committee was responsible for technical and resource support for all intervention activities and for diffusing useful innovations from the target or "experimental" areas to the institution at large. The steering committee was the principal client of an outside team of organizational development consultants responsible for facilitating change.

As in most QWL projects, there was an attempt to encourage employee participation at all levels, with particular attention to low status nonprofessional employees. The project was intended to have a leveling influence within the hospital. Traditional means of exercising authority would give way to a more participative, democratic style of interaction among employees. Theoretically, at least, the physician, the nurse, and the housekeeper would have an equal say in suggesting new ways to improve patient care and the quality of work life.

The project operated in several different parts of the hospital and encompassed a variety of activities, including improving communications within the nursing division, setting up a training program in interpersonal skills for nursing and housekeeping personnel, modifying work procedures on selected nursing floors, and improving the functioning of the hospital's clinical services. The latter project, the largest component of the overall Parkside project, is the focus of this article. The clinical services project offers the best illustration of the problems and potential of this type of organizational change.

THE CLINICAL SERVICES PROJECT

In the spring of 1977, the administrative director of the clinical services division met with a member of the consulting team to discuss ways of improving the functioning of the 20 departments within the division. The departments included radiology, nuclear medicine, respiratory therapy, the hospital library, and the blood bank. There was a consensus within the division and among the hospital's 30-odd nursing units that major improvements in administrative procedures were needed. Coordination problems seriously affected the relationships between several of the clinical departments and the nursing units. This compromised the quality of patient care. There were serious morale problems as indicated by high rates of employee turnover and absenteeism.

A common perception was that service department chiefs, many of whom were physicians with international reputations, were, at best, mediocre administrators with little sensitivity for the human side of management. The clinical services director, a Ph.D. in hospital administration, came to Parkside the previous year from a similar position in a smaller hospital. He was competent, energetic, and committed to the QWL project as a framework for transforming the widespread sentiment that "something must be done to turn things around" into a coherent program of change.

Two specific sets of activities emerged—a large-scale survey feedback project and a smaller "organizational mirroring" project.

SURVEY FEEDBACK

The survey feedback project at Parkside was based on the action research model of organizational change.[7] Questionnaire survey data are collected on employee attitudes — data that are subsequently used as a resource for identifying and solving problems among employee groups. In most applications of the model, Parkside included, the questionnaire is readministered at a later time point. The two or more waves of survey data provide the basis for evaluating project outcomes. The survey instrument used in the Parkside project was adapted from the Michigan Organizational Assessment Package.[8] It contained 26 item clusters that measured employee perceptions of different aspects of organizational functioning and quality of work life, including the level of trust among work groups, job satisfaction, supervision, and standards of patient care.

The questionnaire was administered to employees in the 14 clinical services departments that had substantial daily contact with nursing units. The plan called for feedback of data to employees in the form of summary statistics on departmental performance and comparative division-level statistics. To minimize threats to trust, employees did not receive data on departments other than their own; department chiefs and administrators did, however, and this created some antipathy toward the project.

Following the identification of problems from the survey data, the consultant's role shifted to providing technical and interpersonal assistance to intra-departmental working groups. These groups were responsible for generating ideas for changing work procedures to improve the functioning of the department. The consultant team anticipated that some changes would impact several departments and require the assistance and approval of the hospital-wide labor-management steering committee. However, other minor changes could be implemented with the blessing of middle management within a particular department.

The survey feedback literature indicated that data feedback is most effective at the work group level; department-wide problem solving is too unwieldy to produce useful results.[9] However, the consultant team did not have the resources to assist all work groups within the division. To deal with the problem, the consultants and the clinical services director chose five administrators from within the clinical services hierarchy as project facilitators. Each was trained to run feedback meetings, elicit and refine suggestions for change, and follow these suggestions through to implementation.

Consistent with the overall research design, the evaluation research team used a multiple measurement approach to assess the outcomes of the clinical services project. In addition to the two waves of questionnaire data—the second round of administration was carried out shortly after the end of the year-long project—the team attended most of the survey feedback meetings, conducted extensive participant observation using the Structured Naturalistic Observation method,[10] and interviewed all key personnel following project termination. Each facilitator was instructed to write a capsule summary of each meeting, fill out a standardized meeting rating form, and provide data on the process and content of feedback.

The initial survey administration yielded 350 completed questionnaires. The return rate varied considerably among the departments and appeared to be related to the degree of involvement of the department chief. The instrument's internal structure was verified and scale reliabilities for each of the 26 performance and QWL measures were computed by means of varimax factor analysis. Overall, scale reliabilities were quite adequate; coefficients ranged from .62 to .93 and most were between .80 and .85. T-tests were used to identify significant changes in departmental scores over the course of the survey feedback project.

The feedback literature indicated that how the data are used (if at all) is predictive of the direction and magnitude of change.[11] There were substantial differences in data utilization within the initial group of 14 departments. Some department chiefs, reacting to implicit negative criticism of their performance from the first round of survey data, refused to participate in feedback activities. The time commitment required for feedback drained the initial enthusiasm of some chiefs and administrators. "We didn't know what we were getting ourselves in for" was a frequent complaint.

Interview and observational data enabled the research team to make predictions about change outcomes for each of the clinical departments. Predicted outcomes for the final group of 10 departments that participated in both questionnaire administrations and the rationale for the predictions are presented in Figure 26.1. As indicated, these process data led the research team to expect performance improvements in four departments—the blood bank, the library, chemistry, and radiology—and no change in the others.

The actual performance data are reported in Table 26.1 (pages 472–73) and are generally consistent with the predicted outcomes.

In departments where little or no feedback activity was observed, such as pathology and respiratory therapy, there were no significant performance changes over the course of the project. Positive changes occurred in radiology, blood bank and, to a lesser extent, in the library and micro-

FIGURE 26.1

Predicted Directions and Sources of Change
in the Clinical Services Departments

Predicted Change	Source
Blood Bank positive	Project — Talked over issues; feedback resulted in regular meetings Nonproject — Reorganization of department Organizational mirroring project New office arrangements New work structure New telephone system New administration
Chemistry positive or none	Project — In-service education program started After initial meetings, meetings were stopped because not seen as beneficial Nonproject — New chairman
Library none or negative	Project — Meetings held, but people became cynical when a lot of time was spent with little results
Microbiology none	Project — Feedback given, but no need was seen for more meetings since employees saw problems as institutionwide and insoluble
Pathology none	Project — Results reported, but meetings stopped because people thought they were a waste of time
Radiology positive change	Project — Feedback in May 1978 Nonproject — New chairman New departmental structure Four supervisors replaced
Radiotherapy none	Project — No feedback
Rehabilitation medicine none	No one could say; had lost track after limited exposure
Respiratory therapy none	Project — Discussions about managers who were gone by the time of the survey

biology. For example, blood bank employees reported increased job satisfaction, greater work group effectiveness, and more willingness to work with employees in other departments. The chemistry department was the exception to the predicted pattern. There were significant declines in freedom and variety on the job, support from co-workers and personal sense of achievement.

The second wave instrument included a number of questions about the operation and outcomes of the survey feedback project. The results were not encouraging. Fewer than half (47.7%) of the surveyed employees indicated receiving feedback from the first questionnaire. Within this group, 37.7% felt that the results were presented "clearly," 38.6% indicated "somewhat clearly," and 23.7% responded "not clearly at all." In response to a question about the use of survey results, 39.1% felt they were not used, 34.4% said that data were limited to airing feelings and criticisms, 15.6% said data were used to solve problems, and 10.9% responded that results were used to set goals. Overall, 69.6% of the employees felt that the survey results were not at all useful, 26.1% rated them somewhat useful, and only 4.3% gave a rating of extremely useful.

ORGANIZATIONAL MIRRORING

Unlike the survey feedback project, the organizational mirroring project was modest in scope. The consultant team collaborated with employees from the blood bank, radiology, and selected nursing units in the design of a mirroring card—essentially a problem-reporting form distributed to all employees in these areas of the hospital. A nurse, for example, would use the card to list all problems she or he encountered in routine contacts with blood bank or radiology.

The card also allowed employees to cite examples of superior performance and offer words of praise. Employees in the two target clinical departments completed a comparable form rating the performance of nursing unit staff. Data were summarized and fed back to enable employees to see how they were perceived by their counterparts in the other division—hence, the "mirroring" aspect of the exercise. Integrated problem-solving groups involving employees from nursing and one or the other of the clinical departments would follow. Each of the groups included no more than a dozen employees from both divisions and represented a wide range of job titles.

Most of the data from the survey feedback project involved general evaluations of departmental functioning. In contrast, the mirroring data were limited to immediate and specific concerns, such as setting deadlines for next-day blood requisitions. While most employees were recep-

TABLE 26.1

t-Tests for Each Department—Time 1 vs. Time 2†

Scale	Department									
	Blood Bank	Chem-istry	Library	Micro-biology	Nuclear Medicine	Patho-logy	Radio-logy	Radio-therapy	Rehabili-tation Medicine	Respira-tory Therapy
1. Importance of co-workers			.060–*							
2. Importance of extrinsic rewards										
3. Importance of achievement				.053*						
4. Satisfaction with co-workers			.025	.046–			.002			
5. Satisfaction with extrinsic rewards				.008–						
6. Satisfaction with achievement										
7. If do job well, greater extrinsic rewards										
8. If do job poorly, someone will get angry		.023–								
9. If do job poorly, co-workers help		.054–*								
10. If do job well, greater sense of achievement		.000–	.067*–					.032–	.068–	
11. Freedom on the job		.008–								
12. Variety on the job		.100–*					.01			

13. Not enough time to get work done				
14. Work group listens and trusts				.001
15. Work group is competent	.094*			.003
16. No matter what, others criticize	.061*	.067*-		
17. Conflict between groups				
18. Discuss problems with other groups	.011		.083-*	
19. Different groups work well with each other	.097*			
20. Supervisor listens, encourages, sets example				.001
21. Director listens, encourages, sets example				.002-
22. Director is informed of department activities				.017-
23. Have a say in how to do work				.044
24. Have a say in policies	.024			
25. Hospital is improving	.005			
26. Satisfaction with working at Parkside				

†Empty cells indicate no significant differences
*significant if 1-tailed test used
–becomes more negative over time

tive to the goals of the mirroring project, the card device did not work. Few nursing unit personnel filled them out, and completed cards were often lost.

Sensing the need for some type of interdepartmental forum, the consultant team set up the integrated problem-solving groups despite the lack of a working data base. Two groups were formed. One involved radiology and nursing personnel; the other, employees from nursing and the blood bank. Within a short period of time, the groups devised their own performance measures and proceeded to gather data. Unfortunately, lack of research competence rendered the data almost worthless. Still, the idea of joint problem-solving groups had caught on and employees continued to meet on a regular basis (usually weekly).

In the end, both interdepartmental groups proposed innovations that promised to improve the coordination between nursing units and the clinical department. The radiology-nursing group established new procedures for filing and retrieving X-rays, and devised a new, improved method for queuing patients who were being transferred to and from radiology. After meeting for several months, the joint group felt that its original mission had been accomplished. Its report noted that the project "has proved successful as measured by the wide ranging problem solving in both departments." The group intended to reconstitute itself from a temporary working group into a permanent, interservice committee.

By this time, however, the clinical services director had abandoned his earlier support for the project. Opposition from department chiefs, the slow pace of change, and the difficulty in managing a diffuse, multidepartment project had taken a toll. The project's overall failure obscured the gains being made by the mirroring working group. Neither the clinical services director nor the director of nursing responded to the group's report. Without further institutional sanction, the radiology-nursing working group failed to meet again.

The blood bank mirroring committee followed a similar course. The group proposed several innovations, which included delegating sole responsibility for ordering and tracking blood to the unit clerk (this led to a decrease in the number of multiple phone calls required to complete blood orders), and integrating blood bank personnel into the orientation program for new nurses. Despite these successes, the group stopped meeting after the consultants left the hospital, as no support from senior management was forthcoming.

DISCUSSION

From the perspective of the Columbia evaluation research team and in the minds of most participants, the Parkside QWL project failed to meet its dual objectives of improving organizational functioning and employee quality of work life. The meager results of the survey feedback project hardly justified the tremendous expenditure of staff time and resources. The mirroring projects led to a number of innovations and demonstrated the benefits of maximizing employee participation in the change process. But the experiments failed to engage the support of key decision makers, and this effectively foreclosed the institutionalization of change and the diffusion of innovation within the larger hospital system.

The Anatomy of Failure

The failure of the clinical services project at Parkside supports the pessimistic observations of organizational change experts cited earlier. By and large, the project's demise is consistent with previous research on factors that predict the outcomes of QWL projects.[12] There were at least three major factors contributing to failure.

LACK OF UNION AND MANAGEMENT OWNERSHIP

A comparative study of 16 quality of work life projects found that ownership—how much constituent groups identify with and are involved in a project—is a major factor in predicting success or failure.[13] At Parkside, the lack of union leadership involvement was clear from the start. For both the Hospital Workers' Union and the Nurses' Association, project sponsorship was largely a matter of political expediency—to demonstrate to the public that unions were committed to the goal of better patient care. Management committment was equally weak. The hospital director, who assumed the post after the project was established, was pledged to stabilize the financial status of the hospital and implement a management control system.

A collaborative union-management relationship and employee participation are central to the QWL model. These were at odds with the authoritarian management style that the director felt was necessary to meet his goals. The threat of layoffs which existed throughout the project's operating period precluded all but a hostile and distant relationship between union and management. The directors of clinical services and nursing accurately saw few political gains in visibly supporting the QWL project, and gradually withdrew their support. This doomed the project in their respective divisions.

LACK OF PHYSICIAN SUPPORT

Project involvement was a liability for physician department chiefs. First, the initial survey data were viewed, with some justification, as a negative performance evaluation. Second, the diffuse nature of the project and the complex structure of committees and working groups precluded immediate solutions to any problems. Moreover, the lack of "hard data" limited the willingness of department chiefs to commit resources to project objectives. The abstract goals of improving organizational functioning and quality of work life were not sufficient to overcome the political and philosophical misgivings of department chiefs.

POORLY EXECUTED FEEDBACK PROCESS

Soon after the survey feedback project was underway, it became clear that its scope was much too large. Initially, 14 departments and over 1400 employees were included within the boundaries of the project. The consultant team, the clinical services director, and his cadre of facilitators did not have time to supervise project activities and provide support to the numerous employee working groups. They assumed that the survey data would reveal specific and well-defined organizational problems that could be approached in a rational, deliberate manner by interdepartmental problem-solving teams. Instead, the data were too detailed to be clearly interpretable and employees found support for conflicting positions. Departmental leadership underestimated the difficulties inherent in a data-based change effort. The implicit message to staff was: "Take the data and run with it"—a strategy that proved to be unworkable.

LESSONS FOR FUTURE PRACTICE

For several months, the two interdepartmental working groups that were the core of the mirroring project provided a vibrant example of QWL in action. Supervisors and subordinates met together, if not as equals, then as partners in a common task. Employees were committed to improving their departments—a commitment that sometimes meant coming in for a meeting on one's day off or taking project work home to prepare for the next meeting.

Consistent with QWL philosophy, employees believed that improving how their department functioned and improving the quality of their jobs were closely intertwined. The failure of the Parkside project is sharpened by the possibilities for constructive change that might have occurred if the working groups had received support from management. In hindsight, the Parkside experience suggests a number of guidelines for attempting quality of work life/organizational improvement projects in hospitals.

1. *Keep It Small.* The survey feedback component of the clinical services project received most of the available consulting time and the atten-

tion of the clinical services director and his staff. It was largely a failure. The organizational mirroring component—a low-cost, makeshift effort—produced innovations in operating procedures and quality of work life. As noted, the feedback project fell under its own weight. The clinical services director and the consultants were spread too thin to provide sufficient attention. A project of this type demands a lot of energy; it is not self-starting. As the feedback process began to flounder within the various departments, management began to withdraw support, which in turn reduced employee commitment. The project was caught in a vicious circle; each sign of failure provided the impetus for further withdrawal which insured the project's eventual demise.

The evidence presented here suggests that survey feedback or other modes of QWL/organizational improvement projects should involve no more than one or two departments. Moreover, participative problem solving works best in day-to-day operations, with specific problems. In the mirroring project, problem solving involved a half-dozen employees from each of two divisions at most, representing a diversity of occupational roles, from first-level supervisors to housekeeping staff. Initially, several participants did not know each other, but knowledge of one another's generic work duties enabled them to get specific problems "on the table" quickly.

In contrast, the survey feedback project focused on abstract, department-wide data that required a lot of consultant time to be meaningfully interpreted. Data seldom "speak for themselves." When the information consists of complex, attitudinal data, problems of interpretation become difficult. It is more useful to rely upon performance problems (lost X-rays, late blood requisitions, incomplete lab reports) as the focus of change efforts rather than attitudinal data (level of satisfaction with supervisor, opportunities for using skills). This is because the face validity of performance data is likely to be greater, and employees are more willing to participate in QWL activities when there are specific and measurable outcomes in organization performance. Attitude change measures should be included in any systematic evaluation of a QWL project; enhanced job satisfaction is just as important and real as, for example, reducing the number of recorded complaints between two linked departments. But attitude change may not be a strategically useful primary objective.

2. *Provide Support.* Once employees were given a legitimate forum for discussing means of improving QWL and department effectiveness, there was no shortage of excellent ideas. Tapping this latent reserve of ideas for creative organizational change is a challenge for healthcare executives. The Parkside case suggests that the critical factor is not whether employees working in problem-solving groups are able to diag-

nose organizational shortcomings and offer solutions—the answer in this case is strongly affirmative. The critical factor is whether or not management is willing to provide the support necessary to implement proposals for change. This is the "ownership" issue discussed above—an issue that is especially critical in hospitals because the complex management structure means that the backing of a single upper-level manager is not enough to assure implementation.

Any non-trivial change project is likely to involve more than one hierarchy of authority. At Parkside, the directors of clinical services and nursing, as well as the physician department chief, had effective veto power over the project. All three represented "management" in an abstract sense, but each maintained a semi-autonomous power base. Implementing an employee's idea for changing a specific working procedure must, by necessity, involve managers in all affected hierarchies.

The Parkside project shows the promise of QWL interventions in hospitals and the formidable problems of implementation. While there is an obvious need for improving quality of work life and the effectiveness of hospitals, successful change efforts must first address the critical issues of project scope and management ownership.

The healthcare executive who is planning a QWL project must be aware that employees responsible for improving their work environment who are denied access to management-controlled resources for implementing change are likely to become disillusioned. The manager must be committed to the goals of the project and be willing to engage the support of his or her counterparts in other lines of management. This commitment and the ability to focus upon small-scale problem solving at the workforce level are probably the most crucial factors in a project's outcome.

REFERENCES

1.   Davis, Louis E., and Albert B. Cherns (Editors), *The Quality of Working Life. Volume One: Problems, Prospects and the State of the Art; Volume Two: Cases and Commentary.* New York: The Free Press, 1975; Cummings, Thomas G., and Edmond S. Molloy, *Improving Productivity and the Quality of Work Life.* New York: Praeger, 1977.

2.   Drexler, John A., Jr., and Edward E. Lawler III, "A Union-Management Cooperative Project to Improve the Quality of Work Life." *Journal of Applied Behavioral Science*, Vol. 13, No. 2, 1977; Nadler, David A., Martin D. Hanlon, and Edward E. Lawler III, "Factors Influencing the Success of Labour-Management Quality of Working Life Projects." *Journal of Occupational Behaviour*, Vol. 1, No. 1, 1980.

3.   Weisbord, Marvin R. "Why Organization Development Hasn't Worked (So Far) in Medical Centers," *Health Care Management Review*, Vol. 1, No. 1,

1976; Stoelwinder, Johannes U., and Peter S. Clayton, "Hospital Organizational Development: Changing the Focus From 'Better Management' to 'Better Patient Care,'" *Journal of Applied Behavioral Science*, Vol. 14, No. 3, 1978; Nadler, David A., and Noel M. Tichy. "The Limitations of Traditional Intervention Techniques in Health Care Organizations." In Margulies, Newton, and John D. Adams (Editors), *Organizational Development in Health Care Organizations*. Reading, MA: Addison-Wesley, 1982.

4. Weisbord, Marvin R., and Johannes U. Stoelwinder, "Linking Physicians, Hospital Management, Cost Containment and Better Patient Care." *Health Care Management Review*, Vol. 4, No. 2, 1979.

5. For a description of the theoretical model underlying the Parkside Project, see: Nadler, David A., "Hospitals, Organized Labor and the Quality of Work: An Intervention Case Study," *Journal of Applied Behavioral Science*, Vol. 14, No. 3, 1978. A summary overview of the entire project including the research methodology is presented in: Nadler, David A., and Deborah Gladstein, "A Case Study of Abortive Collaboration: The Labor/Management Quality-of-Working-Life Project at Parkside Hospital." In Margulies and Adams, op. cit., Chapter 9.

6. Lawler, Edward E. III, and John A. Drexler, Jr., "Dynamics of Establishing Cooperative Quality-of-Worklife Projects." *Monthly Labor Review*, 1977.

7. Nadler, David A. *Feedback and Organizational Development: Using Data Based Methods*. Reading, MA: Addison-Wesley, 1977.

8. Nadler, David A. *Michigan Organizational Assessment Package*. Ann Arbor: Institute for Social Research, 1975.

9. Nadler, 1977, op. cit.; Klein, Stuart M., Allen I. Kraut, and Alan Wolfson, "Employee Reactions to Attitude Survey Feedback: A Study of the Impact of Structure and Process." *Administrative Science Quarterly*, Vol. 16, No. 4, 1971.

10. Nadler, David A., Dennis N. T. Perkins, and Martin D. Hanlon, "Structured Naturalistic Observation." In Stanley Seashore, et al. (Editors), *Observing and Measuring Organizational Change: A Guide to Field Practice*. New York: Wiley-Interscience, 1982.

11. Nadler, David A. "The Use of Feedback for Organizational Change: Promises and Pitfalls." *Group and Organization Studies*, Vol. 1, No. 2, 1976; Harris, Reuben T. "Improving Patient Satisfaction Through Action Research," *Journal of Applied Behavioral Science*, Vol. 14, No. 3, 1978.

12. Nadler, Hanlon, and Lawler, op. cit.

13. Ibid.

<table>
27 | The Dilemma between Competition and Community Service
</table>

27 | The Dilemma between Competition and Community Service

Bruce C. Vladeck

The growth of competitive behaviors—and, perhaps more importantly, competitive ideologies—in the nation's hospitals is widely perceived to create a conflict between competition and traditional patterns of community service. But in fact, there is no dilemma, at least not in the sense of having to choose between two relatively unpalatable alternatives. A rededication to community service is going to be the most effective competitive strategy hospitals can adopt. Community service is not a luxury hospitals can afford to abandon in the pursuit of a competitive strategy. It is, rather, the core of an effective competitive strategy.

To make this point, I want to address four different subjects: competition as a theoretical economic principle, competition from a historical perspective, the nature of the poor and the financing of care for this segment of the population, and the competition between hospitals and doctors. These topics may seem unconnected, and in some ways they are, but they can be drawn together to crystallize the central argument.

THE ECONOMICS OF COMPETITION

First, I think we're really quite naive in the health care sector, or perhaps we're self-delusional in our concept of what competition is and how competitive markets are likely to work. In most real markets, with the exception of those for bulk commodities like grain or chemicals or

Reprinted from *Inquiry* 22 (Summer 1985): 115-21, with permission, Blue Cross and Blue Shield Association.

oil, most competition is not about price. Most competition in a real economy is some variant of what for 40 years economists have called "monopolistic competition," in which competitors seek to distinguish themselves from one another on the basis of nonprice characteristics. It could be product differentiation; it could be location; it could be image; it could be marketing. But the capacity to differentiate the product by something other than price is seen by most real firms as the most effective strategy. Kodak is not the low-price producer or supplier of photographic film or equipment; Budweiser is not the low-price beer. But both of them have been concerned that their market shares would grow too great and that they would run into antitrust problems. Their successful long-term strategies have not been price competitive.

Second, much of what we are now describing as competition in the health care environment, be it PPOs or HMOs or related relationships, would probably in most other sectors of the economy be defined as illegal "tying" arrangements under the Robinson-Patman Act and antitrust law. Not that there's anything wrong with them from a legal point of view, or even from a health services point of view. It's just that it's a funny kind of competition.

What we're moving toward in many of the more so-called competitive sectors of the health system is a form of "bilateral monopoly," with a cartel of large purchasers on one side and some number of suppliers on the other. A lot of things can be said for that kind of relationship, but it certainly doesn't look like competition in the Economics 101 sense of pure markets under perfect market conditions. It's awfully hard to have a competitive market when one buyer has a 40% market share and insists on behaving like a very aggressive and largely indifferent monopolist.

The notion that the Medicare Prospective Payment System is procompetitive shows how confused we've become about what competition really is, and how willing we are to accept political rhetoric from an administration needing to justify a 180 degree turn in policy. The underlying reality in financing hospital care is that the single biggest guy on the block — the only one whose market share is growing — has decided that he's going to make his own rules and not really listen to anybody else. That's what's going to determine the shape of health care financing and service arrangements in coming years.

It's also hard to pursue classical competitive strategies when you start with an industry that's functioning at 65% capacity on the one hand, but is characterized by a lot of local monopolies on the other. Again, that leads to competitive strategies that look a lot different than price competition in the classical economics sense.

All this is not to say health care is not becoming more competitive — it clearly is—and not to say that institutions won't need to compete effectively to survive—certainly they will. But the narrow notion of competition as having something to do with price per se is highly misleading. A competitive market dominated by two very large, very noncompetitive payers implies certain things about what the effective strategies are likely to be. And while the biggest payer is not very susceptible to traditional economic inducements, it is very susceptible to short-term political forces, and that says something else about the strategies for hospitals in the years to come.

One last thing on this general point of competition and theory, in relation to care of the indigent: The problems of caring for both the "covered" and the "uncovered" indigent have been with us a long time. It's true that in the short run a lot of the forces that are creating this so-called competitive climate are going to shrink the margins that have been available in the past from other payers and make it more difficult to subsidize care for the nonpaying. But if one looks at where the margins customarily have been and at who's been providing care to nonpaying customers, it's hard to make the argument that that should have a direct effect either. It's something of a cop-out to attribute problems of meeting the needs of the medically indigent to a competitive environment. The problems take on a different character under current circumstances, but they're not new problems.

SOME HISTORICAL PERSPECTIVE

Hospitals, it's important to remember, were initially created to serve the poor. You don't have to go back many years to see that in most hospitals, most of the patients weren't paying. There was a very simple reason for that: Before roughly the time of the First World War, if you could afford to get medical care outside a hospital, you'd be crazy to go into one. There was very little the institution could do for you, and most of what it could do could be done in your own home just as well. Most of the older hospitals in this country were originally created as facilities for poor people who had nowhere else to go, whether they were very sick or not.

It's also only since the Second World War that we've come to expect that hospitals would be able to meet their costs from patient service revenues. Before the Second World War, more than half of hospital revenues came from charity and from direct public subsidies. The only exception to that pattern was in the 10% to 20% of the hospital market that involved physician-owned proprietary hospitals, which were supported largely by patient fees. But most nonprofit hospitals, like most public hospitals, until very recently did not count on patient revenue providing anything like all of their financial requirements.

They certainly didn't count on any surplus or debt capacity arising from patient service revenue to generate capital. Through the mid-1950s, the great bulk of all capital for hospital construction and modernization came either from charity or from public subsidies. The use of equity and debt, and the use of patient service revenue to finance hospital capital, is really only a phenomenon of the last 20 years or so.

What we've seen in this country is a substantial change in what might be called the social contract between government and other major forces in society, on the one hand, and hospitals, on the other. Before the Second World War, voluntary hospitals were granted a tax exemption and a variety of other subsidies as well as a number of other forms of favored legal treatment, including, for instance, until very recently, exemption from coverages of employers under labor laws or minimum wage laws.

Most voluntary hospitals in this country grew up with the mission of taking care of their own, whether their own constituted a religious community or an ethnic community or all of a smaller rural or suburban community. The expectation was that they would figure out how to take care of their own, and that they would provide services whenever they could within the limits of the revenue they could raise.

This social contract changed somewhat during the Second World War, as the population learned about the advances of modern medicine and the benefits available from it. The new social contract was embodied in the Hill-Burton program. Communities built hospitals with Hill-Burton grants and loans and, in exchange, made certain assurances to the federal government. One of the assurances was that they would continue service to the poor according to historic levels. It was only then that we really began to talk about hospitals as a community resource.

What happened next was an explosion of private insurance, an explosion in medical technology, the increasing recognition of hospitals as "houses of hope," in the language then used, and an increasing improvement in the kinds of health care services available to an increasingly insured middle class.

This process culminated in the enactment of Medicare and Medicaid, yet another new form of the social contract. What Medicare and Medicaid said to the hospital community was: "Take care of our clients exactly the same way as you take care of your private customers; let them have semiprivate rooms, don't discriminate on the basis of payment source, and we will pay the cost associated with that care."

What happened as a result hardly needs repeating, but it's fair to say that hospitals didn't entirely keep their end of the bargain. In retrospect, the post-Medicare and Medicaid growth in expense looks a lot greater than anyone can justify. The proliferation of capacity also looks a lot greater than anyone can justify. Competition among institutions was a primary source of both of these phenomena, and has a lot to do with the fix we're currently in. At least twice in the post-Medicare period, when public policy makers got particularly upset about increases in hospital costs, the hospital industry committed itself to voluntary efforts to reduce the rate of cost increase as a way of precluding other forms of public intervention. Neither was successful.

Hospitals' margins grew throughout that period as well, to the point where you really could question the extent to which the hospital community had played fair under the social contract established in 1965. The industry could not discipline itself because of competition within its ranks. Despite a 20-year dialogue between public and private sectors about the cost implications of the entitlements and the payment mechanisms created under Medicare and Medicaid, each time the industry recommitted itself to doing something without direct public intervention, cost growth accelerated still further. That led by the beginning of this decade to unacceptable budgetary problems. Everyone knows about the problems with the Medicare Trust Fund. And throughout the 1970s and into the early 1980s, Medicaid costs for state governments rose 30% faster than state revenues in general.

What really created PPS in its present form was the increasing irritation and anger with the hospital community on the part of policy makers. A lot of what has happened over the last couple of years – the Medicaid programs and PPS and PROs and a variety of other things – is really a conscious effort on the part of policy makers to mount a punitive initiative toward hospitals. William Guy has talked about how hospitals missed their chance in 1972 and 1975 and 1978 to come to some better accommodation with Medi-Cal, which culminated in the selective contracting scramble in California. You hear much the same kind of rhetoric among a lot of the congressional staff: "It's time these guys got theirs" is basically the message they are giving us.

Part of that message is the newest social contract, reflected in the Tax Equity and Fiscal Responsibility Act of 1982, the 1983 revisions to the Social Security Act, and the various Medicaid programs. The big payers – the public payers and increasingly the private payers – are saying to hospitals collectively, "Here's how many dollars we're prepared to spend. We can call it a budget neutral amount; we can call it a total Medicaid budget amount; we can call it a capitation rate under a private plan. But this is the limit, the ceiling, the cap. This is all you have in the coming year, and do the best you can."

There's been substantial reaction from hospitals that this new attitude represents a withdrawal, a reneging, a going back on commitments made in the past, and to some extent it is. But it's important to recognize the extent to which the collapse of the preexisting understanding was really arrived at mutually by both sides to the deal.

It is particularly important that, rather than beating their breasts about it, hospitals recognize their obligation to respond as energetically and creatively as they can under this new set of rules — not to cop out by dumping community services, by dumping patients, by dumping populations, but to acknowledge that these are the rules of the game whether they like it or not for the foreseeable future, and to accept that their continuing obligation is to do the best they can under those rules.

HOSPITALS AND THE POOR

The most obvious observation about the problems of providing care to the medically indigent is that the poor are not distributed at random throughout the population. The poor are concentrated — perhaps increasingly concentrated — in a relatively small number of areas. What this means is that the problem of providing medical care to the poor is not equally everybody's problem. It's a particular problem — and a particularly serious problem — for some communities and for some providers. Much of the anxiety about the impact of competition on the health care system has arisen from the recognition that some institutions are in a substantially better position to ignore this population.

It seems unlikely, however, that society will accept permanently ignoring that population. As we've seen in at least four Northeastern states and in Florida, if the hospital community itself does not collectively undertake some sort of redistributive response in terms of the haves subsidizing the have-nots, those redistributions will be imposed externally. If they are imposed externally, they will be a lot less comfortable for the hospitals involved than those that hospitals impose on themselves. Whether such nonregulatory, nonexternally imposed redistribution is possible in a competitive environment, I don't know. But it is the crux of what people are worried about in terms of the impact of competition on the poor.

It is useful, although terribly oversimple, to distinguish between those who have Medicaid and those who have no coverage at all for health care services — two groups that might be called the old poor and the new poor.

Most of the old poor — children, the elderly, the disabled — are covered by Medicaid; they are, in our current notion, the deserving poor.

Much of the concern about the impact of Medi-Cal and other Medicaid payment cutbacks arises from the confusion we have created in hospital financial offices over the last few years in the distinction between average and marginal costs. In fact, hospitals are very high fixed-cost operations; marginal costs for most hospitals most of the time are only a small fraction of average costs. Many hospitals have learned from experience with Medi-Cal that, depending on other sources of revenue, a payer that has 10% or 15% of the market in an industry with a substantial excess of capacity over demand, and which meets marginal costs, is worth having. It is important to recognize the need — once you're up and going — to cover those marginal costs.

Another group of people, some 25 million of them, have no health care coverage at all. But that population, which includes many people who have lost health insurance benefits as a result of losing employment and a substantial number of unregistered aliens, is not always going to remain poor. The uninsured tend to go on and off insurance coverage. I wonder whether institutions that are unwilling to treat them when they're having problems are going to be looked at very favorably when they are back to being paying customers.

There's no question that in the current political environment, public and policy attitudes toward services to the poor are substantially less generous than they've been in the recent past. If you take a long enough historical perspective, however, this is not the inevitable course of history. This is the swing of a pendulum, and sooner or later it is going to swing back. The question is, how will hospitals be positioned when the pendulum starts to swing back? How will the institution be perceived by the public as the public becomes increasingly sympathetic to putting back in the necessary dollars to serve indigent populations?

HOSPITALS AND DOCTORS

The real competition that hospitals face in the balance of this decade and the decades to come is not among one another, but from physicians. Between 1960 and 2000, the ratio of physicians to population will roughly double. This is happening in an environment where many parts of the country already have a relatively abundant supply of physicians.

What we are facing in the hospital industry, in health care in general, is a very serious shortage of patients. I don't know where that patient shortage is coming from. Maybe patients are responding to economic incentives as insurance benefits change, or maybe the population is getting healthier and using health services less. But it's going to be competition over those patients and who gets to do the expensive procedures that will be driving the system.

Again a bit of historical perspective is useful. It's only since the Second World War that doctors have become so dependent on hospitals. Young physicians perceive admitting privileges as an absolute necessity to the practice of medicine. One can associate this with the technologies that developed after the Second World War, but there were other social and political forces as well.

But the technologies are starting to shift, and the social and political forces are shifting as well. It's increasingly clear that ophthalmologists, plastic surgeons, and, increasingly, urologists and other types of surgeons are less and less dependent on hospitals for most of the work they do.

In the short run, as the physician supply continues to grow and as hospital utilization continues to fall, and as physicians and hospitals become more competitive with one another, the competition between physicians and hospitals will be oriented toward the most lucrative markets. But there aren't enough of those markets to go around. As the physician supply continues to grow, and as the major payers move away from fee for service to some form of either capitated or fee schedule payment, physicians, like hospitals, will get less and less picky about whether the patient is paying the average price and instead will become more and more concerned about whether they're paying anything at all.

Again, it's not so long ago that most physicians in private practice — and this is not just American Medical Association mythology — did treat some patients for free and did provide de facto sliding scales tied to patients' ability to pay. That all went out the window with the development of "uniform, customary, and reasonable" charges and Medicare and Medicaid. But the economic pressures for physicians to keep markets, even if it means discounting prices, remain, and will be reinforced both by physician supply phenomena and by the movement away from fee for service. While competition between hospitals and physicians now tends to be over the best-paying patients, it's only a matter of time before any patient will begin to be attractive.

At this point, I want to propound what I call "Vladeck's theorem": Full hospitals rarely close. I state this cognizant that a hospital is a political and social, as well as an economic, institution. Someone from New York can speak with a significant degree of expertise on the closing of hospitals. A lot of hospitals there that lost a lot of money in recent years have been quite busy and have remained open, and a lot of hospitals that have not lost much money have closed.

The key to survival is having a justification for survival, and that justification is not the bottom line. It's having patients who perceive you as a provider of a needed service. I think once we get by the first generation of anxiety about competitive forces, we will all come to recognize that a poorly paying patient or even a nonpaying patient may be better in a competitive environment than no patient at all. Certainly the revenue that the nonpaying patient generates is no less than that of the absent patient. But as we get more sophisticated in our cost accounting, we will realize that the cost to the institution of serving that nonpaying patient isn't a whole lot greater than that for the nonexistent patient either.

SUMMING UP

Where does this lead, particularly in the short to medium run? First, the pivot to the whole system has got to be Medicare, the one buyer that has 40% of the market on the hospital side and that's pushing a third of the physician market and a lot bigger share of the market for certain kinds of specialists and for general practitioners, family doctors, and general internists in particular communities.

The Medicare population is going to be the only source of increasing demand for services in the years ahead. There are only three cohorts in the population that are likely to grow substantially over the next decade. These are children, as a result of the little bubble on the population curve, who are going to be healthier than they've ever been and who have never used a lot of inpatient services to begin with. We baby boomers are beginning to age into an era in which we will use slightly more health care services, but that's running against the trend of the decline in utilization in the 35–64 population. There is going to be explosive growth in the over-75 population, people who use a lot of institutional services and are going to continue to do so. So that 40% market share we're looking at for Medicare as a floor is going to continue to grow. All the net growth in demand, certainly for inpatient services, and probably for outpatient services as well, is going to come from that sector.

This means two things. One is we've got to fix the Prospective Payment System. There's a lot to be said for PPS, but I have yet to hear any rational justification whatsoever for uniform national rates. I've never seen a federal policy that is so extraordinarily redistributive in terms of dollars from one part of the country to another be enacted into law and implemented — all without the kind of screaming that I expect we'll begin to hear next year.

The second thing we have to do is to relegitimate the hospital in the eyes of the public and of policy makers. It is critical to recognize the extent to which public perceptions of hospitals, which have historically been quite favorable, have changed in recent years, and the extent to which those changes in perceptions have colored public policy developments. I don't think we can do that solely by advertising. It's very difficult to convince the public of a proposition that fundamentally isn't true.

The way to legitimate the hospital in the eyes of the public is to go back, in a sense, to the era in which hospitals were valued and were looked up to and were protected by public policy because they were perceived as providing an essential community service that no one else would — because they existed for the purpose of providing community service, rather than because the vice-president for marketing and strategic planning told them that was a good thing to do. To the extent that hospitals are perceived as necessary community resources, they will be supported and maintained as necessary community resources. To the extent that they are not, the kind of risk hospitals are facing now will only get worse.

You can't compete effectively under any set of rules in any sort of game if you don't know who you are and what you are and why you're there. The hospital industry has become particularly susceptible to a substantial degree of faddism. As it passed the $100-billion-a-year level several years ago, a whole new army of consultants and vendors and newsletter peddlers sprung up, whose stock in trade is to scare the hell out of potential customers so they will buy what they are selling. A little fear is probably good for the soul, but it has created a climate in which it's all too easy to lose sight of why hospitals are in business in the first place.

We've all been saving for a rainy day. I would suggest that in some communities the rainy day might be here already. What surpluses are for in the first place are to meet a basic institutional mission, not to worry entirely about the next generation. We also need to rediscover the most effective competitive strategies — ways of generating revenue from other than patient care.

I think it's critical that we rediscover the role of philanthropy in support of hospitals. There are a lot of philanthropic dollars out there. Americans are very generous; they give a lot of money to health care. But they give increasingly smaller shares of it to hospitals. The reason they do, as I've found over the last year or so, is that people won't give you money unless you can effectively make a case why they should. The dollars are out there if you can convince people that you have a case for them. To do that you have to have a case.

We are talking about a phenomenon that is not purely a phenomenon of economics, that is at root a social and very political phenomenon. We live in a political economy, not a textbook economy, and the most effective strategies for survival in a political economy involve the attitudes of the public and of important decision makers and policy makers about the legitimacy of the institutions involved. That's really the basic message.

The worst mistake hospitals can make is to confuse a swing of the social policy pendulum with the path of history. If hospitals don't do everything they can, as hospitals always have, to serve their communities in the tough times, when times get a little less tough the community may not care as much about them as it did in the past.

NOTE

This paper is a slightly revised version of a speech on "The Dilemma Between Competition and Community Service" presented at the annual meeting of the California Hospital Association on Oct. 18, 1984. I am extremely grateful to CHA for having invited this unreconstructed Easterner to make such a presentation and for having permitted, even encouraged, its republication in this form. Special thanks are due to Michael Nolen, director of education and conference planning at CHA, and to Allen Toon, publications editor. An earlier version of this paper appeared in CHA Insight, Nov. 28, 1984.

Annotated
Bibliography

The following is a representative list of books and journals relevant to health services management and delivery. The books marked with an asterisk are particularly insightful and useful.

Aaron, Henry J., and William B. Schwartz. *The Painful Prescription: National Hospital Care.* Washington, DC: Brookings Institution, 1984.

Analyzes the British system's response to tight budget limits and draws inferences about how Americans would respond should they undertake to reduce the growth of medical spending.

Aiken, Linda H., and David Mechanic, eds. *Applications of Social Science to Clinical Medicine and Health Policy.* New Brunswick, NJ: Rutgers University Press, 1986.

Twenty-five chapters on sociology. See, in particular, Freidson's article on the medical profession in transition.

American College of Healthcare Executives. *The Evolving Role of the Hospital Chief Executive Officer.* Chicago: American College of Healthcare Executives, 1984.

Suggestions for the role of the hospital CEO, based on a 1983 survey. (Note: ACHA is now the American College of Healthcare Executives.)

American Hospital Association. *Vision, Values, Viability, Environmental Assessment 1989-1990.* Chicago: American Hospital Publishing, 1988.

Assessment of the hospital environment in 1989-90.

Austin, Charles J. *Information Systems for Hospital Administration.* 3d ed. Ann Arbor, MI: Health Administration Press, 1988.

Information systems and how they can become effective management tools.

Bellin, Lowell E., and Lewis E. Weeks. *The Challenge of Administering Health Services: Career Pathways.* Washington, DC: AUPHA Press, 1981.

A collection of 17 articles on a variety of careers within health services management.

Blum, Henrik. *Planning for Health*. 2d ed. New York: Human Sciences Press, 1981.

Development and application of social change theory. A systems approach.

*Brown, Lawrence D. *Politics and Health Care Organizations: HMOs as Federal Policy*. Washington, DC: Brookings Institution, 1983.

The interplay between politics and policy on the federal HMO development effort. Part one on HMO management is excellent.

*Cochrane, A.L. *Efficiency and Effectiveness*. London: Oxford University Press, 1972.

Propounds the use of randomized clinical trials to evaluate clinical procedures and the delivery of health services.

Coddington, Dean C., and Keith D. Moore. *Market-Driven Strategies in Health Care*. San Francisco: Jossey-Bass, 1987.

Strategies for gaining and sustaining competitive advantage in health care marketing.

Commission on Education for Health Administration. Series on *Education for Health Administration*. Vol. 1, *The Report of the Commission on Education for Health Administration*, 1975. Vol. 2, *Selected Papers of the Commission on Education for Health Administration*, 1975. Vol. 3, *A Future Agenda*, 1977. Ann Arbor, MI: Health Administration Press.

Report of the commission and related projects and papers.

Cowen, Dale H. *Preferred Provider Organizations: Planning, Structure and Operation*. Rockville, MD: Aspen, 1984.

Background on PPOs and how to start and operate a PPO.

Davis, Fred, ed. *The Nursing Profession: Five Sociological Essays*. New York: Wiley, 1966.

Original essays by William Glaser (nursing leadership), Anselm Strauss (structure and ideology), Hans Mauksch (organizational context), Fred Davis (collegiate nursing), and Esther Brown (nursing and patient care).

*Donabedian, Avedis. *Aspects of Medical Care Administration*. Cambridge: Harvard University Press, 1973.

Sections on basic values, distinctive characteristics of medical care, program objectives, and assessment of need and supply. Extensive references.

Donabedian, Avedis, Solomon J. Axelrod, Leon Wyszewianski, and Richard L. Lichtenstein. *Medical Care Chartbook*. 8th ed. Ann Arbor, MI: Health Administration Press, 1986.

Basic data tables taken from published sources on population characteristics, disease prevalence, organization of health care manpower, costs, and quality of care.

*Enthoven, Alain C. *Health Plan: The Only Practical Solution to the Soaring Cost of Medical Care*. Reading, MA: Addison-Wesley, 1980.
Proposed competition among health care providers.

Flood, A. B., and Scott, W. R. *Hospital Structure and Performance*. Baltimore, MD: Johns Hopkins University Press, 1987.
Describes program of research examining the relation between the structural characteristics of hospitals and the quality and cost of care experienced by patients.

Freidson, Eliot. *The Hospital in Modern Society*. Glencoe, IL: Free Press, 1963.
Original articles by George Rosen (history), W. A. Glaser (international comparisons), Charles Perrow (goals and power structure), Mary Goss (patterns of bureaucracy), Patricia Kendall (learning environment), Rose Coser (alienation and structure), and others. Excellent book on hospitals from a sociological perspective.

*____. *Profession of Medicine: A Study of the Sociology of Applied Knowledge*. New York: Dodd, Mead, 1970.
An insightful study of the social organization of the medical profession.

Fuchs, Victor. *How We Live*. Cambridge: Harvard University Press, 1983.
Choices concerning how we live. The book is organized in terms of life cycle categories such as birth, childhood, and old age.

Georgopoulos, Basil S., ed. *Organization Research on Health Institutions*. Ann Arbor, MI: Institute for Social Research, The University of Michigan, 1972.
Original articles summarizing the then current state of organizational research primarily within hospitals.

Georgopoulos, Basil S., and Floyd Mann. *The Community General Hospital*. New York: Macmillan, 1962.
A quantitative study of ten community hospitals; based on extensive employee interviews.

Glaser, William A. *Social Settings and Medical Organization: A Cross-National Study of the Hospital*. New York: Atherton Press, 1970.
Sections on religious input into hospitals, the status of women and nursing, economics, urbanism, and social changes.

*Griffith, John R. *The Well-Managed Community Hospital*. Ann Arbor, MI: Health Administration Press, 1987.
Classic systems approach to hospital management.

*Joint Commission on Accreditation of Hospitals. *AMH/88*. Chicago: JCAH, 1987.
Accreditation manual for hospitals.

Kaluzny, Arnold D., D. Michael Warner, David G. Warren, and William N. Zelman. *Management of Health Services*. Englewood Cliffs, NJ: Prentice-Hall, 1982.
Health services management text. A survey of applicable concepts and methodologies basic to behavior, operations research, financial management, and the law.

Kane, R. A., and R. L. Kane. *Long-Term Care Principles, Programs and Policies.* New York: Springer, 1987.

Overview and analysis of problems, issues, and programs in long-term care.

Kotler, Philip, and Roberta N. Clarke. *Marketing for Health Care Organizations.* Englewood Cliffs, NJ: Prentice-Hall, 1987.

Application of business techniques to health care organizations.

*Kovner, Anthony R. *Really Managing: The Work of Effective CEOs in Large Health Organizations.* Ann Arbor, MI: Health Administration Press, 1988.

Focus on what makes four CEOs effective in large health care organizations.

*____. *Really Trying: A Career Guide for the Health Services Manager.* Ann Arbor, MI: Health Administration Press, 1984.

A collection of personal observations and recommendations focusing on the art and politics of management. Uses case studies, interviews, maxims, and a manager's correspondence to convey the context of health services management.

Kovner, Anthony R., and Duncan Neuhauser. *Health Services Management: A Book of Cases.* 3d ed. Ann Arbor, MI: Health Administration Press, 1989.

Companion book of cases to this edition of *Readings and Commentary.* Uses the same organizing approach in categorizing problems and issues of management.

Lewis, Irving J., and Cecil G. Sheps. *The Sick Citadel: The American Academic Medical Center and the Public Interest.* Cambridge, MA: Oelgeschlager, Gunn and Hain, 1983.

Issues and problems facing the academic medical center from both historical and public interest perspectives.

Longest, Beaufort B., Jr. *Management Practices for the Health Professional.* 3d ed. Reston, VA: Reston Publishing, 1984.

Text for clinicians with management responsibilities who want to improve management skills.

*Luft, Harold S. *Health Maintenance Organizations: Dimensions of Performance.* New York: Wiley, 1981.

Research findings on HMO performance. Detailed empirical analysis of issues that have significant policy implications.

MacEachern, Malcolm. *Hospital Organization and Management.* 2d ed. Chicago: Chicago Physicians' Record Company, 1946.

For perhaps 20 years, this was the standard textbook for hospital managers. Over 1,000 pages long. Now largely out of date.

McMillan, Norman H. *Marketing Your Hospital*. Chicago: American Hospital Association, 1981.
Brief application of business techniques in marketing hospital services.

____. *Planning for Survival: A Handbook for Hospital Trustees*. Chicago: American Hospital Association, 1978.
Brief application of business techniques in hospital long-range planning.

Mechanic, David, ed. *Handbook of Health, Health Care, and the Health Professions*. New York: Free Press, 1983.
Thirty-four chapters on macro and clinical issues, epidemiology, delivery and management, occupations, and research perspectives.

____. *Readings in Medical Sociology*. New York: Free Press, 1980.
Twenty-nine readings on people, health, and the environment; identification of disease in populations and in clinical settings; reactions to health and illness; and the macro and micro systems of health care and social policy.

Neuhauser, Duncan. *Coming of Age: A 50-Year History of the American College of Hospital Administrators and the Profession It Serves, 1933–1983*. Chicago: Pluribus Press, 1984.
The only history of hospital administration as a profession.

The Organization and Development of a Medical Group Practice. Cambridge, MA: Ballinger, 1976.
Consolidated reference source of steps and decisions necessary for group practice formation.

Pascarelli, Emil F. *Hospital-Based Ambulatory Care*. Norwalk, CT: Appleton-Century-Crofts, 1982.
Collection of 36 articles on hospital-based ambulatory care.

Peterson, John, David Manchester, and Arthur Toan. *Enhancing Hospital Efficiency: A Guide to Expanding Beds without Bricks*. Washington, DC: AUPHA Press, 1980.
How hospitals can provide more services to physicians and patients without expanding present bed supply.

Rakich, Jonathan, and Kurt Darr, eds. *Hospital Organizations and Management*. 2d ed. New York: SP Medical and Scientific Books, 1978.
Collection of 41 reprinted articles.

Rakich, Jonathan, Beaufort B. Longest, and Kurt Darr. *Managing Health Services Organizations*. 2d ed. Philadelphia: W. B. Saunders, 1985.
Standard text and case studies in health services management.

*Redman, Eric. *The Dance of Legislation*. New York: Simon & Schuster, Touchstone, 1973.
A marvelously written tale by a staff member for Senator Warren Magnuson who recorded the drafting and passage of the National Health Service Bill (P.L. 91-623). A superb description of the political and legislative process.

*Rosenberg, Charles E. *The Care of Strangers.* New York: Basic Books, 1987.

Historical view of hospitals in the United States.

*Seay, J. David, and Bruce C. Vladeck, eds. *In Sickness and in Health: The Mission of Voluntary Health Care Institutions.* New York: McGraw-Hill, 1988.

What distinguishes voluntary hospitals in an increasingly commercial health care environment.

Sheldon, Alan. *Managing Change and Collaboration in the Health System.* Cambridge, MA: Oelgeschlager, Gunn and Hain, 1979.

Case studies and analyses on hospital collaboration.

Shortell, Stephen M. *A Model of Physician Referral Behavior: A Test of Exchange Theory in Medical Practice.* Chicago: Center for Health Administration Studies, University of Chicago, Research Series No. 31, 1973.

A research study of referral patterns in private medical practice.

*Shortell, Stephen M., and Arnold D. Kaluzny. *Health Care Management: A Text in Organizational Theory and Behavior.* 2d ed. New York: Wiley, 1983.

Defines and outlines effective and successful management of health organizations. Focuses on theoretical approaches and research results.

Shortell, Stephen M., and William C. Richardson. *Health Program Evaluation.* St. Louis: Mosby, 1978.

Text on health program design, analysis, and evaluation.

Smith, David B., and Arnold D. Kaluzny. *The White Labyrinth: A Guide to the Health Care System.* 2d ed. Ann Arbor, MI: Health Administration Press, 1986.

Text on how organizations in the health sector work and on approaches to changing these organizations.

Snook, I. Donald, Jr. *Hospitals: What They Are and How They Work.* Rockville, MD: Aspen, 1981.

Introductory approach to organization, internal operations, and functions of the hospital.

Somers, Anne R., ed. *The Kaiser-Permanente Medical Care Program: One Valid Solution to the Problem of Health Care Delivery in the United States.* New York: Commonwealth Fund, 1971.

Southwick, Arthur F. *The Law of Hospital and Health Care Administration.* 2d ed. Ann Arbor, MI: Health Administration Press, 1988.

Basic graduate text on health law.

Starkweather, David B. *Hospital Mergers in the Making.* Ann Arbor, MI: Health Administration Press, 1981.

Six case studies of hospital mergers with an organization theory perspective.

Starr, Paul. *The Social Transformation of American Medicine.* New York: Basic Books, 1982.

Classic history of the development of American medicine.

Stevens, Rosemary. *In Sickness and in Wealth: American Hospitals in the Twentieth Century.* New York: Basic Books, 1989.

Together with Rosenberg's *The Care of Strangers,* this book provide a fine history of American hospitals.

Strauss, Anselm, Shizuku Fagerhaugh, Barbara Suczek, and Carolyn Wiener. *Social Organization of Medical Work.* Chicago: University of Chicago Press, 1985.

The management of chronic care in acute hospitals from a clinician's perspective.

U.S. Department of Labor, Manpower Administration. *Job Descriptions and Organizational Analysis for Hospitals and Related Health Services.* Rev. ed. Washington, DC: U.S. Government Printing Office, 1971.

Produced in cooperation with the American Hospital Association. This lengthy book describes what over 200 different hospital employees do. A good reference book.

*Vladeck, Bruce C. *Unloving Care.* New York: Basic Books, 1980.

A thorough critique of nursing homes and their problems.

Williams, Stephen J., and Paul R. Torrens. *Introduction to Health Services.* 3d ed. New York: Wiley, 1988.

The title says it.

Wilson, Florence, and Duncan Neuhauser. *Health Services in the United States.* Rev. 2d ed. Cambridge, MA: Ballinger, 1987.

A basic description of laws, personnel, institutions, and financing of health services.

Witt, John A. *Building a Better Hospital Board.* Ann Arbor, MI: Health Administration Press, 1987.

Practical approach to hospital governance.

Young, David W., and Richard B. Saltman. *The Hospital Power Equilibrium: Physician Behavior and Cost Control.* Baltimore, MD: Johns Hopkins University Press, 1985.

The influence of physicians and cost control. Uses two hospitals as case examples.

Relevant Journals

In addition to their other merits, many of the journals listed below feature book reviews and announcements of new books.

Administrative Science Quarterly
    Editorial Office ASQ
    Malott Hall, Cornell University
    Ithaca, NY 14853

American Journal of Public Health
    American Public Health Association
    1015 Eighteenth Street, N.W.
    Washington, DC 20005

College Review
    American College of Medical Group Administrators
    1355 South Colorado Boulevard, Suite 900
    Denver, CO 80222

Frontiers of Health Services Management
    Health Administration Press
    1021 East Huron Street
    Ann Arbor, MI 48104–9990

Group Health Journal
    Group Health Association of America, Inc.
    624 Ninth Street, N.W., Suite 700
    Washington, DC 20001

Health Affairs
    Project Hope
    Millwood, VA 22646

Health Care Management Review
    Aspen Publishing, Inc.
    7201 McKinney Circle
    Frederick, MD 21701

Health Matrix
    National Health Publishing
    99 Painter's Mill Road
    Owings Mills, MD 21117

Health Services Management Research
    Longman Group
    Fourth Avenue
    Harlow Essex
    CM195AA
    United Kingdom

Health Services Research
Health Administration Press
1021 East Huron Street
Ann Arbor, MI 48104–9990

Hospital & Health Services Administration
Health Administration Press
1021 East Huron Street
Ann Arbor, MI 48104–9990

Hospitals
American Hospital Association
840 North Lake Shore Drive
Chicago, IL 60611

Inquiry
Blue Cross and Blue Shield Association
840 North Lake Shore Drive
Chicago, IL 60611

Journal of Ambulatory Care Management
Aspen Publishing, Inc.
7201 McKinney Circle
Frederick, MD 21701

Journal of Health Administration Education
Association of University Programs in Health Administration
1911 North Fort Myer Drive, Suite 503
Arlington, VA 22205

Journal of Health and Social Behavior
American Sociological Association
1722 N Street, N.W.
Washington, DC 20036

Journal of Health Politics, Policy and Law
Duke University Press
6697 College Station
Durham, NC 27708

Journal of Long-Term Care Administration
American College of Health Care Administrators
8120 Woodmont Avenue, Suite 200
Bethesda, MD 20814

Journal of Mental Health Administration
Association of Mental Health Administrators
840 North Lake Shore Drive
Chicago, IL 60611

Journal of Nursing Administration
J.B. Lippincott Company
East Washington Square
Philadelphia, PA 19105

Journal of Public Health Policy
   Journal of Public Health Policy, Inc.
   23 Pheasant Way
   South Burlington, VT 05401

Medical Care
   J.B. Lippincott Company
   East Washington Square
   Philadelphia, PA 19105

Medical Care Review
   Health Administration Press
   1021 East Huron Street
   Ann Arbor, MI 48104–9990

Medical Economics
   Medical Economics Company
   680 Kinderkamack Road
   Oradell, NJ 07649

Medical Group Management
   Medical Group Management Association
   1355 South Colorado Boulevard, Suite 900
   Denver, CO 80222

The Milbank Quarterly
   Cambridge University Press
   1 East 75th Street
   New York, NY 10021

Modern Healthcare
   740 Rush Street
   Chicago, IL 60611

New England Journal of Medicine
   Massachusets Medical Society
   10 Shattuck Street
   Boston, MA 02115–6094

Nursing Administration Quarterly
   Aspen Publishing, Inc.
   7201 McKinney Circle
   Frederick, MD 21701

Public Health Reports
   Government Printing Office
   Superintendent of Documents
   Washington, DC 20402

Social Security Bulletin
   Social Security Administration
   5401 Security Boulevard
   Baltimore, MD 21235

Topics in Health Care Financing
    Aspen Publishing, Inc.
    7201 McKinney Circle
    Frederick, MD 21701

Trustee
    840 North Lake Shore Drive
    Chicago, IL 60611

REFERENCE SOURCES AND SERIALS

Code of Federal Regulations
    Government Printing Office
    Washington, DC 20402

Current Literature in Health Services
    Cumulative Guide to Hospital Literature
    American Hospital Association
    840 North Lake Shore Drive
    Chicago, IL 60611

Excerpta Medica: Health Economics and Hospital Management
    E.M.
    Box 211
    1000 AE Amsterdam
    Netherlands

Federal Register
    Office of the Federal Register
    National Archives and Record Service
    Washington, DC 20402

GAO Reports
    General Accounting Office
    441 G St., N.W.
    Washington, DC 20548

Harvard Business School (Case Studies)
    Publishing Division
    Operations Department
    Boston, MA 02163

Health Care Financing Review
    Health Care Financing Administration
    Department of Health and Human Services
    Government Printing Office
    Washington, DC 20402

Hospital Abstracts
    H.M.S.O.
    P.O. Box 569
    London SE1 9NH
    England

Hospital Literature Index
American Hospital Association
840 North Lake Shore Drive
Chicago, IL 60611

NTIS Newsline
National Technical Information Service
5285 Port Royal Road
Springfield, VA 22161

NTIS Weekly Abstract: Health Planning and Health Services Research
National Technical Information Service
5285 Port Royal Road
Springfield, VA 22161

Vital and Health Statistics
National Center for Health Statistics
Public Health Service
Government Printing Office
Washington, DC 20402

Index

absenteeism, 162, 298, 426, 467
academic health center, 16, 359–85
access to care, 38–43, 52, 197, 358, 372, 375, 384, 415
accountability, xiv-xxiii, 2, 22, 67, 93, 99, 127, 191, 206–8, 211, 214, 237, 284, 361, 365, 416; hierarchy of, 206–9, 212, 214, 292; medical staff and, 217–18, 292
accounting, xiv, 110, 198; department, 162–64, 190, 329–31; general ledger, 144, 146, 147; payroll, 198–99, 210; system, 110, 165
accounts payable (A/P), 138, 147, 198
accounts receivable (A/R), 109–10, 138, 146–47
accreditation, 6, 66, 121, 122, 323, 325, 426
acuity. *See* variance analysis, health care specific
adaptation strategy, 10, 43, 44–49
adaptive capability, 97, 98, 191, 192, 265–66, 351, 353–54, 428, 429
administrative communication center (ACC), 249–50
admissions, 30, 171, 173, 289, 376, 379, 402
AGIL schema, xxii
Allison, Robert, 71
Alta Bates Hospital, 128–29
alternatives, generation of, 319, 321, 326, 328, 338
ambulance service, 82, 424
ambulatory care, xiii, 16, 20, 92, 148, 188, 226, 263, 317–19; facilities,

285; surgery center, 188, 318, 327, 371, 378–80, 382, 383, 387
American Academy of Medical Directors (AAMD), 271
American College of Healthcare Executives (ACHE), 9–11, 56–59; board of governance, 59, 60, 65; Code of Ethics (1941), 56–58; Code of Ethics, 59–70; Committee on Ethics, 58–59; history, 56–58
American College of Hospital Administrators (ACHA), 56
American College of Surgeons (ACS), 57
American Federation of State, County, and Municipal Employees, 203
American Healthcare System (AHS), 318
American Hospital Association (AHA), xix, 56, 58, 65–69, 256, 357, 433, 434; board of trustees, 69
American Medical Association (AMA), 357, 487
ancillary services, 201, 212, 227, 228, 239, 403, 442
Andreano, Ralph, 455, 456, 458
Androscoggin Valley Hospital (NH), 424
Anthony, Robert, 149
Arrow, Kenneth, 38–39, 40
Association of American Medical Colleges (AAMC), 361
audits, 61, 117, 169, 170; financial, 198; medical, 178, 336

authority, 22, 93, 308–10, 428; structure, 40, 72, 93, 123–24, 206
autonomy: organizational, 94–95, 127, 407; professional, 43, 309–13

Batalden, P., 182
Becker and Gordon's schema, xxii, xxiii
Bedford, Norton, 149
Billings, John Shaw, 345
Blue Cross, 164, 243, 378, 417–18, 450
boards: conflict and, 124–25; performance, 99, 121–31; recruitment, 128; role of, 98. *See also* governance; trustees
Bolger, Michael, 453
Bolman and Deal's typology, xxiii
Boston Consulting Group (BCG), 379–82
Boulding, Kenneth, 38–41
Bowen, D., 432
break-even ratio, 138, 139, 144
Brotz, Chuck, 462
Brown, Ray, 75
budgets, xv, 74, 95, 97, 103, 110, 134, 147, 149–55, 199, 202, 213, 222, 237, 240, 243, 244, 245, 361, 366, 465, 484; flexible, 158–59
Bureau Common Reporting Requirements (BCRR), 137

California Hospital Association (CHA), 168, 490
California Medical Association (CMA), 168, 169
California Medical Insurance Feasibility Study (CMIFS), 168–70
capital sources management, 199
Caplow, Theodore, xxi, xxii
Capra, Fritjoh, 398
Cargill, V., 183
Cavafy, 423
centralization, 203, 248–49, 257, 262, 385
certificate of need, 19, 285
Chandler, A., 370
change: managing, 127, 128, 359–67; strategies for, 253–54
Chi Systems study, 254, 256–57

chief executive officer (CEO), 25, 66, 95, 103, 122, 125, 127, 129, 184, 222
chief operating officer (COO), 24, 28, 31, 32
clinical support services, 201–2, 244
closed system performance: measurement alternatives, 113–16; measures selection, 116–19
Codman, E. A., 91
collateral organization, 104, 207
collective bargaining, 203
communication, 71, 103, 153, 204, 207, 212, 249, 262, 265, 275, 280, 283, 284, 290, 300, 322, 323, 326, 328, 334, 338, 339, 435, 467; effective, 18, 319; skills, 74–76; systems, 109, 247–50, 255–58
community service, xvii, 2, 20, 48, 65, 66, 82, 83, 107, 370, 400, 416, 418, 427
CompCare, 417, 418
competition, xvii, 5–7, 17, 22, 44–45, 61, 67, 107, 124, 282, 293–96, 316, 318, 323, 334, 342, 348, 369, 381–83, 386, 406, 409, 428, 480–90
competitive strategy, 433–42, 480, 481
Comprehensive Health Center, 132
conflict, 102, 122–25, 130, 211, 271, 300, 355, 427, 428, 429, 472; of interest, 62–63, 68; resolution, 99, 103–5
control, xiv–xxiii, 14, 37, 40, 49, 262, 271, 275, 284, 285, 332, 353, 354, 361, 411; systems, 93, 426
Cooper, Richard, 462
cooperative model, 409–10
Coronary Care Unit (CCU), 233, 330, 380
corporate culture, xix, xx, xxi, xxiii, 49, 182, 185, 415; restructuring, 385, 387
corporate structure, future, for voluntary hospital, 188
cost accounting, 95, 110, 116, 119, 488
cost analysis, 107, 443
cost containment, 27, 42, 316, 317,

324, 334, 342, 375, 382, 384, 390–91
cost control, 6, 45, 104, 191, 197–99, 202, 237, 451–53, 498
costs, measurement system, 117
Cousins, Norman, 434
Cowee, John, 447, 448
Curative Workshop, 451
cybernetic model, 102–13, 119

Daniels, N., 41
data systems: accounts payable, 138, 147, 198; accounts receivable, 109, 146–47; departmental, 109; materials management, 110; medical records, 4, 28, 57, 59, 95, 109, 176, 181, 322, 336, 357; order entry, 109; payroll, 110; physical plant management, 110
Dayton, K. N., 124
Deal, Terrence, xxiii
Dearden, John, 149
debt to equity ratio, 123
decentralization, 19, 193, 334, 373, 385, 391; medical staff, 284; system, 248–50, 255–57
decision making: process, 277–79; strategic, 130, 282–98
Deming, Edwards, 101, 180–86
DeRusso, John, 75
diagnosis-related groups (DRGs), 19, 92, 153, 160–61, 236, 243, 244, 317, 332, 334, 434
diagnostic center services, 20, 188
dietetics, 4, 92, 151, 169, 221, 228, 233, 234, 239, 250, 321, 404, 413
diversification, 191, 193, 385, 388, 390; acute care hospitals and, 233; management perspective on, 234; mental health services and, 233; product, 46, 224–35; vertical integration and, 231–35
division model (medical staff), 266, 322, 327–34, 338, 341
Donnelly, Paul, 458
Donovan, L., 298
Doyne, John, 442–53
Durkin, Robert, 458

education, xix, 2, 57, 65, 122, 163, 183, 200, 215, 228, 233, 234, 243, 349, 354, 361, 362, 365, 366, 385, 388, 398, 424; educators, obligations of, 85–88; health administration, 9, 50–53, 69–70, 89; medical, 27, 262–63, 360, 443, 450, 451; patient, 361–62
Eichna, L. W., 362
Einstein, Albert, 398
Ellwood, P., 335
emergency medical services (EMS), 416
emergency room (ER) service, 107, 156, 157, 174, 183, 188, 190–91, 211, 228, 231, 262, 348, 424, 456; emergicenters, 354
environment, competitive, 67, 224, 285–86, 291, 293, 351, 356, 370, 384, 391; complexity, 4, 5, 45, 183, 347, 350
environmental assessment, 213, 288, 373
environmental change, 43, 45, 50, 288, 353, 354, 376
ethics, xiv, 10, 11, 85, 217. *See also* American College of Healthcare Executives
Etzioni, Amitai, xxi–xxiii
Evashwick, C., 283
expectation setting, 102–8; conflict resolution, 104–5; cooperation and, 103–4; as incentive, 110–13

Fairfax Hospital (VA), 335
family practice (FP), 262, 324, 352, 402
FARMCARE, 420
Federal Health Planning Act (1966), 57
Federal Trade Commission (FTC), 57
fee-for-service payment, 198, 201
Ferguson, Francis, 454, 463
finance: cost accounting department, 7, 190, 199, 216, 329; internal and external audits, 198; patient accounting, 198; payroll and accounts payable, 198
financial analysis, 199–200; variance, 149–65

financial planning, 5, 199, 436
Fitzgerald, Edmund, 446, 447, 448, 452, 454
flexible budget, 158–59
Foley, Leon, 444
Foote, Robert, 455
Frankena, W. K., 85
Freidson, Eliot, 40, 42, 261
Friesen, Gordon, 248–49, 256–57
Froedtert, Kurtis, 444, 454
Froedtert Memorial Lutheran Hospital (WI), 442, 445, 447, 453–57, 458, 460
Fuchs, Victor, 361
full-time equivalent (FTE), 135, 138, 143, 148
functional organization, 220–21
functional units, 237, 238, 242, 321; management of, 240, 243, 244
Fundamental Interpersonal Relations Orientation–Behavior (FIRO-B), 271

Gardner, John, 365
Geilfuss, John, 455
General Electric Multiple Factor Matrix, 379–82
General Motors, 232
goal attainment, xviii–xxiii, xxvii, 9–12, 97, 191, 192, 265, 266, 351, 353, 354, 428
Goldsmith, S., 124, 372
Good Samaritan Hospital (OR), 435
Gottlieb, Sy, 454, 462
governance, xix, 20, 83, 93–95, 99, 177, 193, 196–97, 202, 208, 221–22, 262, 263–66, 284, 322, 356, 357, 361, 452; boards, performance of, 121–30; effectiveness of, 9, 121–31. *See also* boards; trustees
Greater Milwaukee Committee (GMC), 444–52, 454, 455, 458–60
grievance procedure, 58, 63–65, 430
group practice, xiii, 5, 7–8, 17, 21, 71, 76, 192, 194, 264, 391, 402
Guest, Robert, 353

Harrigan, K. R., 225, 227, 229
Harrington, Fred, 448

health administration education. *See* education
health care: equal access and, 40–41, 42, 43, 52; delivery, 43–50; future of, 41–43, 317–19; government policies and, 49–50; market failure and, 38–40, 42; pre-1980s, 37–41; professional dominance in, 40, 42
Health Care Financing Administration (HCFA), 181, 182
health maintenance organizations (HMOs), 4, 17–18, 21, 22, 28, 35, 36, 44, 47, 48, 51, 57–58, 71, 200, 201, 212, 228, 239, 262, 283, 285, 323, 335, 354, 377, 382–84, 390, 399, 407, 411–14, 416, 430, 481; group model, 323; rural, 407, 417, 418–20; of Wisconsin, 411
Heil, Joseph, 446, 447
Henningsen, Paul, 459
Heyssel, R., 284–85
hierarchy, xv, 191–93, 206–7, 209, 212–13, 215, 217, 267, 277, 279, 308; duel, 465; formal, 275–76
Hill-Burton Act (1946), 57, 67, 483
Hirschboeck, John, 444, 446, 447
Hitt, D., 340
home care, 92, 188, 226–28, 233, 317, 318, 327, 378, 379, 380, 381, 388, 437
horizontal growth, 36, 49
horizontal integration, 222, 224
hospice, 233, 264, 318, 378, 379, 382, 387
Hospital Corporation of America (HCA), 122–23, 182
hospitals: administration, 74, 80–89, 408, 415; community and, 10, 66–67, 82, 189, 295, 424, 461; competition, 130, 287, 288; cooperative, 351, 407–21; cost of, 84–85; diversification and, 233; for-profit, 222, 283, 284; investor-owned, 94, 122, 192, 318, 372, 376, 378, 384; medical staff, 66, 205, 262, 319–22; operation of, 83; paradigm shifting, 400–401; physicians and, 264; purpose of, 82–83; traditional paradigm and, 398–400
hospitals, nonprofit, 94, 283, 284,

291, 296, 350, 357, 397, 398, 482;
manager and, 5–6; organization,
102–19; physician-owned, 503;
quality of care, 167–81; rural, 407,
421; size, 196, 237, 283, 284, 286,
415; teaching, 5, 7, 123, 191,
236–45, 341, 349, 352, 356, 363,
366; voluntary, 188, 376, 384,
397–407
housekeeping department, 72, 119,
193, 203, 204, 211, 216, 218, 221,
239, 321–22, 404

incentive systems, xvii, xix, 93,
95–96, 97, 99–100, 110–13, 154–58,
192, 332, 379
incident reports, 95, 175–78
independent corporate model, 266,
322, 323–27, 328, 332, 341, 342
independent practice association
(IPA), 8, 47, 335
industrial medicine, 380
Infantile Paralysis Society, 352
information management systems, xv,
xvii-xix, 6, 8, 95, 97, 98, 127, 192,
198, 214, 222, 243, 388–89, 391–92,
426
insurance, health, 203, 413, 419;
companies, 11, 42, 45–46, 50, 168,
198, 199, 224, 379, 413–14, 417,
419; competition among, 44–45;
national, 49, 190; private, 198; *See
also* Blue Cross
integration, xix, xxi, xxii, 74, 126,
127, 270, 376; backward
(upstream), 225, 228, 318; forward
(downstream), 225, 228; integrated
systems, 44; vertical, 46
intensive care unit (ICU), 107, 171,
218, 220, 330, 380, 434
internal management report (IMR),
132–48; samples, 138, 139. *See also*
management indicators
International Classification of Disease, 114

Jacobus, Del, 453
Jamron, Ken, 456
Johns Hopkins Hospital, 193, 221,

237–45, 332, 333, 345; organizational design, 238
Johnson, Robert Wood, Foundation,
271, 275
Joint Commission on the Accreditation of Healthcare Organizations
(JCAHO), 57, 83, 92, 197, 323,
405

Kahn, R., xx
Kaiser Permanente Medical Group,
323
Katz, D., xx
Kellogg, W. K., Foundation, 36
Klion, Stanley, 75
Kropf, R., 124, 372
Kuperberg, James, 460

labor relation negotiations, 72, 73,
112, 464
Lao Tzu, 1
laundry department, 119, 157, 201,
203, 222, 223, 233, 234, 247, 404
Lawrence, Bob, 457
Lawrence and Lorsch's schema, xxi,
xxii
Lemon, Wally, 448
length of stay (LOS), 105, 173, 177
Lennon, Ed, 461
Lewin and Associates, 450
Lewis, Irving J., 360
licensure laws, 215–16, 323, 325
Life Orientation Survey (LIFO), 271
Locke, E., 298, 299
Logan, Ed, 457
Longest, B., 372, 373
Lorsch, J., xxi, xxii
Lovelock, C., 432
Lucey, Gov. Patrick, 448–49, 456

maintenance department, 74, 110,
216, 219, 404
malpractice, 47, 99, 106, 217, 325,
350; medication errors, 178, 179,
180
management, xiv, 20, 216, 219,
475–76; activities, 8, 23, 24, 25,
137; beliefs, 10, 76–77; clinical,
132–48; control, 96, 149–65, 425;
decentralized, 236–45, 310; effec-

tiveness of, 6, 7, 18–22, 27, 33, 74,
76, 78, 103, 191; financial, 151,
154; materials, 101, 204, 321; middle, 214–21; senior, 74–76, 309,
326; style, xix, 10, 76, 77–78
management, hospital: indicators,
13–48; information systems, 72, 99,
244; leaders, 51, 66, 86–89, 243,
282–86, 309, 311–12, 326, 335, 337;
middle, 211, 212–23, 397, 414
management indicators: characteristics of, 133–34; financial management, 143–148; health center services, 141–43; organization and
display, 136–41; personnel management, 148; reception, 143; summary statistics, 137–41; total
encounters, 137–38; use of,
134–37
managerial effectiveness, 18–22;
evaluating, 22–25; expectations for,
25; sample episodes, 29–32; skills
for, 74–76, 81–82; style, 76–79;
transferability of, 26; visible results
and, 27–28
managers, health service: business
vs., 3–5, 36; opportunities for,
263–64
market: competitive, 404; conditions,
288, 332; development, 377, 385;
failure, 38–40, 42; growth potential, 379; health care, 433–40;
share, xx, xxi, 6, 16, 95, 114, 126,
181, 189, 191, 372, 376, 476
marketing, 6, 21, 22, 119, 124, 153,
197, 222, 273, 327, 329, 330, 331,
347, 369–71, 378, 380, 385, 387,
404–6, 425, 428, 435–37
Marquette University Medical School,
444–48
Maryland Health Services Cost
Review Commission, 240
Massachusetts General Hospital, 107
matrix organization, 218–21; functional organization of, 220–21
Mayo Clinic Medical School, 183
Medicaid, 4, 138, 146, 243, 349, 355,
378, 384, 416, 446, 451, 452, 483,
484, 485, 487
Medi-Cal, 484, 486

medical care organization (MCO),
52–53
medical center, 270–81, 294, 351,
359–67, 415, 420, 427, 428, 442,
463; teamwork contexts and,
270–74
Medical College of Wisconsin, 442,
448, 453, 457, 460, 461, 462
Medical Management Analysis System, 167–80; data retrieval coordination, 177; implementation
model, 176
medical practice, history of, 45
medical records, 4, 28, 57, 61, 95,
109, 151, 176, 181, 216, 217, 322
medical school, 13–27, 221, 238, 242,
274, 349, 352, 356, 360, 372,
443–53, 455, 456, 459, 461; dean,
363–65; faculty, 362–64, 367
medical staff: accountability and,
217–18; conjoint, 201; organization
structure, 262; responsibility centers and, 211–12
Medicare, 4, 106, 138, 198, 199, 203,
214, 236, 243, 349, 355, 376, 378,
384, 401, 417, 420, 437, 446, 450,
451, 481, 483, 484, 487, 488
mental health services, diversification
and, 233
midlevel practitioner (MLP), 138,
141, 142
Miles, R. E., 370
Milwaukee Children's Hospital, 445,
451, 457–59
Milwaukee County Medical Complex,
444, 451, 452, 454, 456, 457
Milwaukee Regional Medical Center,
442–43; history, 443–47
Mintzberg, H., 187, 189–90, 206,
370, 371, 372, 373
mission statement, 103, 213
Mizrahi, T., 185
Mulcahy, Charles, 453
multihospital systems, 222–23
Multiple Employer Trust, 418
multi-unit systems, 5, 11, 36, 44, 45,
47, 51, 122, 189, 191, 194, 221–23,
283, 294, 295, 317, 328, 341, 354,
357, 371, 378, 382, 383, 384
Mundt, Donald, 451–59

National Center for Health Services Research, 466

national health insurance, 49, 190

National Health Service Corps, 132

National Labor Relations Act, 350

National Labor Relations Board (NLRB), 466

National Rural Health Care Association, 420

New England Journal of Medicine, 107, 183

New York Academy of Medicine, 360

New York University Medical Center, 2

Norquist, John, 452

Northwestern Mutual Life Insurance Co. (NML), 446, 451, 454, 459, 463

nurses/nursing: change strategies, 253–58; directors of, 30, 190, 216, 238, 242, 243, 333; hospitals and, 308–9; licensed practical (LPN), 247–50, 254, 257, 258; modular, 258; physicians and, 102, 193, 202, 214; practitioner, 402; primary, 193, 246, 247, 251–52, 253–58; problems of, 309–10; quality of care and, 177, 184, 202, 216; recruitment and, 243, 310, 311; registered (RN), 76, 246–52, 254, 255, 257–58, 298, 299, 302–13, 424, 466; shortage, 265, 298–99, 399; staff, 178, 240, 255, 310, 333, 335; supervisor, 220, 265; task autonomy and, 309–12; team, 250–51, 252, 254–70; utilization, 246–58; work satisfaction and, 298–314

nursing home, xii, 4, 5, 19, 35, 71, 188, 190, 194, 226–30, 233, 283, 378, 382, 383, 387, 436, 439; for-profit, 6–8; manager and, 6–7

obstetrics-gynecology (OB-GYN), 23, 31, 32, 118, 170, 220, 229, 238, 283, 322, 324, 329, 330, 336, 380

O'Donnell, William, 446, 447, 449, 451, 452

operating room (OR), 30, 115, 119, 172, 211, 217

organization: collateral, 104, 206, 207–9, 212, 214, 220, 223; decentralized, 10, 47, 193; efficiency vs. effectiveness, xx; flow of influence within, xvi; for-profit, 96, 194, 221, 222, 318, 342, 419, 464; formal, 47–48, 192, 206, 335; functional, 214–16, 202–22, 321, 322; goals of, xviii, xix, xxii, 3, 6, 8, 9, 263, 321, 355, 360, 386, 426; heliocentric view of, xiv–xvi; matrix, 190, 214, 215, 218–20, 332, 354, 398; mirroring, 473–74; not-for-profit, 15, 67, 194, 350, 407, 452; objectives, 24–29, 316; organization theory and, xviii–xxiv; performance requirements of, xviii–xxiv, 47, 354, 374, 425, 426; problems within levels of, xvii–xviii; strategic adaptation, 44–49; structure, xvii, xix, 28, 196–204, 262, 287, 326, 375, 386; theory, xiii, xiv, xvii, xxiv, 386; transformation process, 346

organizational activities, 71–74; motivating, 71–73; negotiating, 73; resource management, 74; scanning, 73

organizational design, 204–23; alternative, 319–22; collaboration, 209–10; components of, 206–8; criterion for, 205; decisions, 208–9

organizational design, hospital, 321–22; divisional model, 322–34; independent-corporate model, 322, 323–27; parallel model, 335–42; physician vs. administrator, 322

organizational skills, 74–76

outcome screening criteria for hospitals, 171–74

outpatient department (OPD), 171, 174, 189, 220, 226, 228, 229, 231–33, 262, 264, 371, 380, 401, 424

Papanicolaou test, 115

parallel model, 266, 322, 328, 335–42

Parsons, Talcott, xxii

pathology, 172, 193, 238, 262, 284, 362, 413, 414, 469, 470, 471

patients: care of, xxii, 2, 3, 65, 110, 158, 163, 179, 191, 193, 232, 240, 242, 244, 299, 300, 324, 334, 348, 353, 361, 362, 363, 365–67, 384, 398, 402, 465, 467; contributions of, 423–37; -doctor relationship, 433–34; education of, 359–61, 366; feedback, 437, 439; need, 42–43; satisfaction, 200, 202, 426–28, 433–35, 438; self-pay, 143, 144; training, 433–34
Patton, G., 270, 271
Pauly, M., 284
pediatrics, 220, 238, 262, 283, 322, 324, 329, 330, 379, 380
performance, classification measurements for, 114
performance, monitoring of, 108–10
performance requirements: adaptive capability, 10, 11, 98, 192, 265–66, 353–54, 428, 429; goal attainment, 9–10, 97, 192, 265, 352, 428; system maintenance, 10, 98, 192, 265, 352–53, 428; values integration, 1, 98, 192–93, 266–67, 355–56
Peters, J., 121, 128
Pfeffer, J., 124
pharmacy, 61, 109, 119, 150, 151, 177, 216–17, 247, 336, 402
physical medicine and rehabilitation, 61, 191, 330, 470, 471; physical therapy, 119, 217, 219, 411, 414, 420
physician assistants, 356, 400
physician leaders: administrators, 275–76; case study, 291–95; contractual relationship of, 287–88; defined, 283; strategic orientation of, 287, 306–11; training of, 319–20
Physician-in-Management Seminars (PIMS), 271, 272, 275
physicians: administrators and, 244, 275, 318, 320, 350, 397, 465; autonomy, 42, 318, 319, 377, 399; chiefs of service (clinical chiefs), 14, 18, 27, 28, 76, 126, 184, 190, 191, 216, 240, 243, 262, 267, 282, 291, 294–96, 321, 326, 333, 336; credentialing, 28, 61, 67, 177, 323,

324, 325, 336, 337; hospitals and, 48, 50, 167–80, 190, 223, 261, 264, 266, 273, 282–306, 316, 317, 342, 383, 384, 402, 404, 407, 413, 417, 419, 486–88; medical centers and, 273, 274; nurses and, 102, 202, 214, 266, 402, 405; organization of, 44, 47–48, 197, 200, 212, 214, 221, 265, 323, 327, 338, 340, 342; patients and, 49, 229, 317, 402; private practice and, 170, 231, 294, 361, 387, 389; quality of care and, 323, 325, 337, 399; recruiting, 8, 72, 201; responsibility centers, 211–13; rural, 105, 202, 399, 411; supply of, 130, 334, 354, 443, 459, 486, 487; time orientation of, 320; trustees and, 73, 123, 126, 127, 129, 208, 262, 284, 290, 322, 400, 412, 420
Planetree Program, 434
planning: financial, 5, 199, 436; long range, xix, 2, 72, 73, 105, 110, 213, 222, 337; strategic, 11, 124, 165, 188, 196, 197, 199, 283, 289–91, 334, 336, 337, 385, 397, 404, 406
plant maintenance, 119, 222
poor, care of the, 82, 189, 451, 482, 485–87
preferred provider organization (PPO), 36, 45, 51, 228, 230, 335, 382, 481
primary care, 45, 215, 318, 361, 366, 407
primary health center, 132, 378, 391
primary nursing. *See* nursing
problem solving, 264, 272, 275–78, 477, 478
professional review organization (PRO), 484
professional standards review organization (PSRO), 61
prospective payment system (PPS), 317, 332, 369, 390, 399, 410, 481, 484, 488. *See also* diagnosis-related groups
provider satisfaction, 435
psychiatric services, 82, 119, 175, 220, 238, 329, 380

purchasing department, 7, 157, 188, 216

quality assessment, 73, 95, 97, 118, 150
quality assurance (QA) programs, 27, 61, 97, 99, 167–69, 175–77, 182, 323–25, 336–37, 348, 350, 426
quality control, 72, 109, 112, 405
quality of work life (QWL), 427–29, 464–74; failures, 475–76; improvement of, case studies, 466–73

Rader, Andrew, 455
radiology, 61, 104, 105, 151, 152, 193, 228, 238–40, 262, 284, 333, 379, 467, 469–71
Rapkin, Joe, 444, 445
Rawls, J., 41
Raynor, Father John, 445–48
Regional Health Systems Agency, 416
regulatory agencies, 7, 383, 401
responsibility center (RC), 105, 193, 210–12, 214, 216, 218; conflicting criteria and, 210–12, 214, 216, 218, 219, 229
responsibility center managers (RCM), 210
return on equity (ROE), 399
Reivitz, Linda, 458
Riffer, Joyce, 432
Riverside Hospital (VA) study, 254, 255–56
Robinson-Patman Act, 481
rural hospitals, 407–21; advocacy, 416–17. *See also* Rural Wisconsin Hospital Cooperative
Rural Wisconsin Hospital Cooperative, 408, 420–21; basic model, 409–10; HMO development, 418–20; mission and goals, 408–9; multiple employer trust, 417–18; reactions to, 410–11; shared-service development, 411–15
Rush-Presbyterian-St. Luke's Hospital (Chicago, IL), 332

St. John's Hospital (CA), 335

St. Mary's Hospital (Milwaukee, WI), 254, 257, 419
Scarborough Centenary Hospital (Toronto), 256–57
Schein, Edgar, xxi, xxiii
Schoenecker, Rudy, 452, 453
shared services, 31, 188, 407, 411–15
signal detection/evaluation, 108, 109
SIVA schema, xxii
Slichter, Donald, 454
Sloan, F., 284
Snow, C. C., 370
Southeastern Wisconsin Health Services Administration, 455
Stanislawski, Emil, 462
State Insurance Commissioner, 416, 419–20
strategic content, 377–87
strategic decisions, 283; complexity of, 286–87; decentralization and, 391; strengths and limitations of, 295–96
strategic planning, 165, 404
strategy, 44, 52, 191, 346, 370, 371, 375; competitive, 432–39; corporate, 99, 122, 124, 130, 370, 371; defined, 370; deliberate, 372; emergent, 372; factors affecting, 383–87; formulation, 372–77; growth, 378; implementation, 370–72, 387–92; intended, 371; market penetration, 377; need for, 376–77; new market development, 377–78; product-service refinement, 378
strategy implementation, 387–92; complexity, 388, 390; degree of agreement, 389–90; diversity, 389; divisibility, 388; reversibility, 388–89
structural support system (SSS), 246–60; primary, 253–58
surgery/surgeons, 82, 112, 171, 172, 178, 181, 184, 190, 200, 208, 218, 229, 233, 238, 242, 263, 264, 322, 324, 330, 331, 333, 377, 379, 445, 460, 487; ambulatory, 318, 327; chief of, 329, 336

task rewards, 312–13

Tax Equity and Fiscal Responsibility
Act of 1982, 484
teamwork, 272; clear representative
structures and, 275–79; decision
processing, 277–79; hierarchy and,
275–77
teamwork context, medical centers
and, 270–74
technical support system (TSS),
246–71
tertiary care facilities, 226–29, 232,
360, 447
Theory Z management, 49
third party payment, 146, 228–33,
377–78, 381, 384, 390, 401, 404
trustees, 20, 25, 27, 29, 57, 83,
121–31, 176, 183, 185, 238, 240,
244, 289–93, 365, 367, 377, 385,
445; as governing body, xix,
196–98
Tseng, S., 121
turnover, staff, 95, 97, 128, 137, 138,
148, 265, 266, 298, 300, 310, 311

"uncompensated care," 49
Union of Hospital and Health Care
Workers #1199, 203
Urmy, Norman, 74

variables: competitive environment
and, 285–86; dependent models,
288–91; status, 30, 301
variance: causes of, 152–54; controllable, 152, 163; data quality,
164–65; detail, 158–64; direct,
161–64

variance analysis, 97, 99, 149–65;
data, 164–65; defined, 149; health
care specific, 161–64; incentives
and, 154–58; price (rate), 159–60;
quantity (use), 160–61; reports,
150–52; volume, 158–59
vertical integration, 222, 225–31;
consumer and, 226; distribution
and, 229–30; diversification and,
231–35; examples of, 225; four
stages of, 225–26; of hospital services, 228; management perspective, 230–31; output and, 226–27;
production and, 227
Vice, Jon, 457
Vogt, Eleanor, 455
Voluntary Hospitals of America
(VHA), 318

Wausau Hospital study, 254–55, 258
Wisconsin Blue Cross, 417
Wisconsin, HMO of, 411
Wisconsin Health Services Adminis-
tration, Southeastern, 455
Wisconsin Hospital Association, 416
Wisconsin, University of, 446, 448
Wisconsin. *See also* Rural Wisconsin
Hospital Cooperative
Wolf, G., 299, 311
work satisfaction, 265, 266, 299, 312,
473

Young, R., 432

Zeidler, Frank, 444

About the Editors

ANTHONY R. KOVNER, M.P.A., Ph.D., is currently Professor of Health Policy and Management at the Robert F. Wagner Graduate School of Public Service, New York University. He also serves as Senior Program Consultant to the Robert Wood Johnson Foundation and is Director of the Foundation's Hospital-Based Program to Improve Rural Health Care. Dr. Kovner is a member of the Board of Trustees of Lutheran Medical Center and Augustana Nursing Home in Brooklyn, New York. Before joining NYU, he was Chief Executive Officer of the Newcomb Hospital of Vineland, New Jersey, and Senior Health Consultant to the United Autoworkers Union in Detroit, Michigan. His most recent book, *Really Managing: The Work of Effective CEOs in Large Health Organizations*, was published by Health Administration Press in 1988.

DUNCAN NEUHAUSER, M.H.A., M.B.A., Ph.D., is Professor of Epidemiology and Biostatistics, Keck Foundation Senior Research Scholar, Professor of Medicine, Adjunct Professor of Organizational Behavior, and Codirector of the Health Systems Management Center (all at Case Western Reserve University). He is coauthor with Kovner of *Health Services Management: A Book of Cases*, second edition. Other works include *Health Services in the United States*, second edition, with Florence Wilson (Ballinger, 1974) and *Coming of Age, A History of the American College of Hospital Administrators and the Profession It Serves* (Plenum, 1984). He is Editor of *Medical Care* and of *Health Matrix*.